Update on Temporal Bone Imaging with Emphasis on Clinical and Surgical Perspectives

Editors

GUL MOONIS
AMY FAN-YEE JULIANO

NEUROIMAGING CLINICS OF NORTH AMERICA

www.neuroimaging.theclinics.com

Consulting Editor
SURESH K. MUKHERJI

February 2019 • Volume 29 • Number 1

ELSEVIER

1600 John F. Kennedy Boulevard • Suite 1800 • Philadelphia, Pennsylvania, 19103-2899

http://www.neuroimaging.theclinics.com

NEUROIMAGING CLINICS OF NORTH AMERICA Volume 29, Number 1
February 2019 ISSN 1052-5149, ISBN 13: 978-0-323-65477-7

Editor: John Vassallo (j.vassallo@elsevier.com)
Developmental Editor: Casey Potter

Neuroimaging Clinics of North America (ISSN 1052-5149) is published quarterly by Elsevier Inc., 360 Park Avenue South, New York, NY 10010-1710. Months of issue are February, May, August, and November. Business and editorial offices: 1600 John F. Kennedy Blvd., Suite 1800, Philadelphia, PA 19103-2899. Business and editorial offices: 6277 Sea Harbor Drive, Orlando, FL 32887-4800. Periodicals postage paid at New York, NY, and additional mailing offices. Subscription prices are USD 397 per year for US individuals, USD 653 per year for US institutions, USD 100 per year for US students and residents, USD 451 per year for Canadian individuals, USD 832 per year for Canadian institutions, USD 525 per year for international individuals, USD 832 per year for international institutions and USD 260 per year for Canadian and foreign students and residents. To receive student/resident rate, orders must be accompanied by name of affiliated institution, date of term, and the *signature* of program/residency coordinator on institution letterhead. Orders will be billed at individual rate until proof of status is received. Foreign air speed delivery is included in all *Clinics* subscription prices. All prices are subject to change without notice. POSTMASTER: Send address changes to *Neuroimaging Clinics of North America*, Elsevier Health Sciences Division, Subscription **Customer Service, 3251 Riverport Lane, Maryland Heights, MO 63043. Telephone: 1-800-654-2452 (U.S. and Canada); 314-447-8871 (outside U.S. and Canada). Fax: 314-447-8029. E-mail: journalscustomer service-usa@elsevier.com (for print support); journalsonlinesupport-usa@elsevier.com (for online support).**

Reprints. For copies of 100 or more of articles in this publication, please contact the Commercial Reprints Department, Elsevier Inc., 360 Park Avenue South, New York, NY 10010-1710. Tel.: 212-633-3874; Fax: 212-633-3820; E-mail: reprints@elsevier.com.

Neuroimaging Clinics of North America is covered by *Excerpta Medical/EMBASE,* the RSNA Index of Imaging Literature, *MEDLINE/PubMed (Index Medicus),* MEDLINE/MEDLARS, SciSearch, Research Alert, and Neuroscience Citation Index.

PROGRAM OBJECTIVE

The goal of *Neuroimaging Clinics of North America* is to keep practicing radiologists and radiology residents up to date with current clinical practice in radiology by providing timely articles reviewing the state of the art in patient care.

TARGET AUDIENCE

Practicing radiologists, radiology residents, and other healthcare professionals who utilize neuroimaging findings to provide patient care.

LEARNING OBJECTIVES

Upon completion of this activity, participants will be able to:
1. Review common imaging findings in pediatric hearing loss.
2. Discuss temporal bone imaging as part of treatment planning in patients with congenital syndromes and hearing loss.
3. Recognize decision-making pearls from a surgical perspective during a radiographic analysis of the ear and lateral skull base.

ACCREDITATION

The Elsevier Office of Continuing Medical Education (EOCME) is accredited by the Accreditation Council for Continuing Medical Education (ACCME) to provide continuing medical education for physicians.

The EOCME designates this enduring material for a maximum of 15 *AMA PRA Category 1 Credit*(s)™. Physicians should claim only the credit commensurate with the extent of their participation in the activity.

All other healthcare professionals requesting continuing education credit for this enduring material will be issued a certificate of participation.

DISCLOSURE OF CONFLICTS OF INTEREST

The EOCME assesses conflict of interest with its instructors, faculty, planners, and other individuals who are in a position to control the content of CME activities. All relevant conflicts of interest that are identified are thoroughly vetted by EOCME for fair balance, scientific objectivity, and patient care recommendations. EOCME is committed to providing its learners with CME activities that promote improvements or quality in healthcare and not a specific proprietary business or a commercial interest.

The planning committee, staff, authors and editors listed below have identified no financial relationships or relationships to products or devices they or their spouse/life partner have with commercial interest related to the content of this CME activity:
Vanesa Carlota Andreu-Arasa, MD, PhD; Anja Bernaerts, MD; Larissa T. Bilaniuk, MD; Mary Beth Cunnane, MD; Hugh D. Curtin, MD; Bert De Foer, MD, PhD; Kathryn E. Dean, MD; Akifumi Fujita, MD, PhD; Daniel Thomas Ginat, MD, MS; Justin S. Golub, MD, MS; Mai-Lan Ho, MD; Sachin Jambawalikar, PhD; Amy Fan-Yee Juliano, MD; Alison Kemp; Ana H. Kim, MD; Raekha Kumar, BSc, MBBS, MRCP, FRCR; Pradeep Kuttysankaran; Joshua E. Lantos, MD; Kristen Leeman, MD; Ravi Kumar Lingam, BSc(Hon), MB BCh, MRCP, FRCR, EBiHNR; Michael Z. Liu, MS; Gul Moonis, MD; Suresh K. Mukherji, MD, MBA, FACR; Aaron N. Pearlman, MD; Tiffany Peng, MD; Apoorva T. Ramaswamy, MD; Naoko Saito, MD, PhD; Karuna V. Shekdar, MD; Anne Marie Sullivan, MD; Edward K. Sung, MD; Philip Touska, MBBS, BMedSci (Hons), FRCR; Ram Vaidhyanath, DMRD, DNB, FRCR, EBiHNR; John Vassallo; Elizabeth K. Weidman, MD.

The planning committee, staff, authors and editors listed below have identified financial relationships or relationships to products or devices they or their spouse/life partner have with commercial interest related to the content of this CME activity:
Osamu Sakai, MD, PhD, FACR: is a consultant/advisor to Boston Imaging Core Lab and receives royalties/holds patents with Gakken Medical Shujunsha Co., Ltd. and Medical Sciences International, Ltd.

UNAPPROVED/OFF-LABEL USE DISCLOSURE

The EOCME requires CME faculty to disclose to the participants:
1. When products or procedures being discussed are off-label, unlabelled, experimental, and/or investigational (not US Food and Drug Administration [FDA] approved); and
2. Any limitations on the information presented, such as data that are preliminary or that represent ongoing research, interim analyses, and/or unsupported opinions. Faculty may discuss information about pharmaceutical agents that is outside of FDA-approved labelling. This information is intended solely for CME and is not intended to promote off-label use of these medications. If you have any questions, contact the medical affairs department of the manufacturer for the most recent prescribing information.

TO ENROLL

To enroll in the *Neuroimaging Clinics of North America* Continuing Medical Education program, call customer service at 1-800-654-2452 or sign up online at http://www.theclinics.com/home/cme. The CME program is available to subscribers for an additional annual fee of USD 244.40.

METHOD OF PARTICIPATION

In order to claim credit, participants must complete the following:

1. Complete enrolment as indicated above.
2. Read the activity.
3. Complete the CME Test and Evaluation. Participants must achieve a score of 70% on the test. All CME Tests and Evaluations must be completed online.

CME INQUIRIES/SPECIAL NEEDS

For all CME inquiries or special needs, please contact elsevierCME@elsevier.com.

NEUROIMAGING CLINICS OF NORTH AMERICA

SERIES OF RELATED INTEREST

MRI Clinics of North America
Available at: www.Mri.theclinics.com
PET Clinics
Available at: www.pet.theclinics.com
Radiologic Clinics of North America
Available at: www.Radiologic.theclinics.com

THE CLINICS ARE AVAILABLE ONLINE!
Access your subscription at:
www.theclinics.com

Contributors

CONSULTING EDITOR

SURESH K. MUKHERJI, MD, MBA, FACR
Professor and Chairman, Walter F. Patenge
Endowed Chair, Department of Radiology,
Michigan State University, Chief Medical
Officer and Director of Health Care Delivery,
Michigan State University Health Team, East
Lansing, Michigan, USA

EDITORS

GUL MOONIS, MD
Associate Professor, Department of Radiology,
Director, Head and Neck Imaging, Columbia
University Irving Medical Center, New York,
New York, USA

AMY FAN-YEE JULIANO, MD
Department of Radiology, Massachusetts
Eye and Ear Infirmary, Harvard Medical School,
Boston, Massachusetts, USA

AUTHORS

VANESA CARLOTA ANDREU-ARASA, MD, PhD
Neuroradiology Fellow, Department of
Radiology, Boston Medical Center, Boston
University School of Medicine, Boston,
Massachusetts, USA

ANJA BERNAERTS, MD
Department of Radiology, GZA Hospitals
Antwerp, Wilrijk, Belgium

LARISSA T. BILANIUK, MD
Professor, Department of Radiology,
Perelman School of Medicine at University of
Pennsylvania, Neuro-Radiologist, The
Children's Hospital of Philadelphia,
Philadelphia, Pennsylvania, USA

MARY BETH CUNNANE, MD
Department of Radiology, Assistant Professor,
Harvard Medical School, Staff Radiologist,
Massachusetts Eye and Ear Infirmary,
Massachusetts General Hospital, Boston,
Massachusetts, USA

HUGH D. CURTIN, MD
Department of Radiology, Massachusetts Eye
and Ear Infirmary, Boston, Massachusetts,
USA

BERT DE FOER, MD, PhD
Department of Radiology, GZA Hospitals
Antwerp, Wilrijk, Belgium

KATHRYN E. DEAN, MD
Assistant Professor, Department of
Radiology, Weill Cornell Medicine, New York
Presbyterian Hospital, New York, New York,
USA

AKIFUMI FUJITA, MD, PhD
Associate Professor, Department of Radiology,
Jichi Medical University, School of Medicine,
Shimotsuke, Tochigi, Japan

DANIEL THOMAS GINAT, MD, MS
Department of Radiology, University of
Chicago, Pritzker School of Medicine,
Chicago, Illinois, USA

JUSTIN S. GOLUB, MD, MS
Assistant Professor, Department of
Otolaryngology–Head and Neck Surgery,
Vagelos College of Physicians and Surgeons,
New York Presbyterian/Columbia University
Irving Medical Center, New York, New York,
USA

MAI-LAN HO, MD
Assistant Professor, Department of Radiology,
Mayo Clinic, Rochester, Minnesota, USA

SACHIN JAMBAWALIKAR, PhD
Chief of Medical Physics, Assistant
Professor, Department of Radiology, Columbia
University Medical Center, New York,
New York, USA

AMY FAN-YEE JULIANO, MD
Department of Radiology, Massachusetts Eye
and Ear Infirmary, Harvard Medical School,
Boston, Massachusetts, USA

ANA H. KIM, MD
Department of Otolaryngology–Head and Neck
Surgery, Columbia University Medical Center,
New York, New York, USA

**RAEKHA KUMAR, BSc, MBBS, MRCP,
FRCR**
Specialist Radiology Registrar, Department of
Radiology, Northwick Park and Central
Middlesex Hospitals, London North West
University Healthcare NHS Trust, London,
United Kingdom

JOSHUA E. LANTOS, MD
Assistant Professor, Department of Radiology,
Weill Cornell Medicine, New York Presbyterian
Hospital, New York, New York, USA

KRISTEN LEEMAN, MD
Assistant Professor, Department of Radiology,
Weill Cornell Medicine, New York Presbyterian
Hospital, New York, New York, USA

**RAVI KUMAR LINGAM, BSc(Hon), MB BCh,
MRCP, FRCR, EBiHNR**
Department of Radiology, Northwick Park and
Central Middlesex Hospitals, London North
West University Healthcare NHS Trust,
Consultant Radiologist, Senior Clinical
Lecturer, Imperial College London, London,
United Kingdom

MICHAEL Z. LIU, MS
Associate, Department of Radiology,
Columbia University Medical Center,
New York, New York, USA

GUL MOONIS, MD
Associate Professor, Department of Radiology,
Director, Head and Neck Imaging, Columbia
University Irving Medical Center, New York,
New York, USA

AARON N. PEARLMAN, MD
Associate Professor, Department of
Otolaryngology–Head and Neck Surgery, Weill
Cornell Medicine, New York Presbyterian
Hospital, New York, New York, USA

TIFFANY PENG, MD
Resident, Department of Otolaryngology–Head
and Neck Surgery, Columbia University
Medical Center, Weill Cornell Medicine,
New York Presbyterian Hospital, New York,
New York, USA

APOORVA T. RAMASWAMY, MD
Resident, Department of Otolaryngology–Head
and Neck Surgery, Vagelos College of
Physicians and Surgeons, New York
Presbyterian/Columbia University Irving
Medical Center, New York, New York, USA

NAOKO SAITO, MD, PhD
Associate Professor, Department of Radiology,
Saitama International Medical Center, Saitama
Medical University, Hidaka, Saitama, Japan

OSAMU SAKAI, MD, PhD, FACR
Chief of Neuroradiology, Professor, Departments
of Radiology, Otolaryngology–Head and Neck
Surgery, and Radiation Oncology, Boston
Medical Center, Boston University School
of Medicine, Boston, Massachusetts,
USA

KARUNA V. SHEKDAR, MD
Assistant Professor of Clinical Radiology,
Department of Radiology, Perelman School of
Medicine at University of Pennsylvania,
Neuro-Radiologist, The Children's Hospital
of Philadelphia, Philadelphia, Pennsylvania,
USA

ANNE MARIE SULLIVAN, MD
Department of Radiology, CRA Medical
Imaging, East Syracuse, New York, USA

EDWARD K. SUNG, MD
Assistant Professor, Department of Radiology,
Boston Medical Center, Boston University
School of Medicine, Boston, Massachusetts,
USA

**PHILIP TOUSKA, MBBS, BMedSci (Hons),
FRCR**
Department of Radiology, Guy's and St.
Thomas' Hospitals NHS Foundation Trust,
London, United Kingdom

**RAM VAIDHYANATH, DMRD, DNB, FRCR,
EBiHNR**
Consultant Radiologist, Department of
Radiology, University Hospitals of Leicester,
Honorary Senior Lecturer, Leicester University,
Leicester, United Kingdom

ELIZABETH K. WEIDMAN, MD
Assistant Professor, Department of Radiology,
Weill Cornell Medicine, New York Presbyterian
Hospital, New York, New York, USA

Contents

Temporal bone and ear structure inflammation is commonly due to infection. It can be associated with a variety of complications and postinflammatory sequelae. Where the ear is easily inspected, clinical evaluation suffices. At the deeper aspect of the temporal bone, clinical evaluation is limited. High-resolution computed tomography scanning is suited for temporal bone imaging and is the modality of choice. MR imaging is useful to characterize disease, define the extent and spread of disease, or as a surveillance tool. MR imaging can be used with high-resolution computed tomography scanning to give a comprehensive evaluation of a complex disease process.

Visualization of the morphologic substrate of Ménière disease, the endolymphatic hydrops, can be performed using noncontrast or contrast-enhanced MR imaging techniques. Noncontrast MR imaging uses a heavily T2-weighted sequence; however, its reproducibility remains to be confirmed. Contrast-enhanced MR imaging techniques mainly use a 3-dimensional fluid-attenuated inversion recovery sequence after intratympanic gadolinium administration or after a 4-hour delayed intravenous gadolinium administration. The latter technique is most frequently used and is able to detect and grade Ménière disease. It is a reliable technique with a high diagnostic accuracy, enabling visualization of endolymphatic hydrops.

Many bone dysplasias, some common and others rare, may involve the temporal bone causing conductive, sensorineural, or mixed hearing loss, vestibular dysfunction, or skull base foraminal narrowing, potentially affecting quality of life. Some conditions may affect only the temporal bone, whereas others may be more generalized, involving different regions of the body. High-resolution computed tomography may detect subtle osseous changes that can help define the type of dysplasia, and MR imaging can help define the degree of activity of lesions and potential associated complications.

Mary Beth Cunnane

Although not all patients with tinnitus require imaging, patients with tinnitus and asymmetric hearing loss, additional neurologic findings, or pulsatile tinnitus should be evaluated with an appropriately tailored imaging study. Choice of imaging study should be guided by type of hearing loss and additional physical examination findings, such as middle ear lesion, presence of carotid bruit, or pulsatile tinnitus extinguished by jugular compression.

Mai-Lan Ho

Third window abnormalities are bony defects of the inner ear that enable abnormal communication with the middle ear and/or cranial cavity. Vestibular symptoms include vertigo and nystagmus induced by loud noises or increases in pressure. Auditory symptoms involve "pseudo-conductive" hearing loss with a low-frequency air-bone gap at audiometry, resulting from decreased air and increased bone conduction. High-resolution temporal bone computed tomography is the first-line imaging modality for evaluation of third window pathology and is critical for accurate diagnosis and management. This article reviews the fundamental mechanisms of the third window phenomenon and describes imaging findings and differential diagnosis.

Anne Marie Sullivan, Hugh D. Curtin, and Gul Moonis

The differential diagnosis of a red and/or pulsatile retrotympanic mass includes aberrant internal carotid artery, persistent stapedial artery (PSA), glomus tympanicum, and dehiscent jugular bulb. By recognizing the features of aberrant internal carotid artery and PSA on high-resolution computed tomography, these entities can be assessed by the radiologist. PSA is further classified by type because each type demonstrates a unique set of imaging features in addition to features common to all types. Although rarely encountered, it is important to reliably and consistently detect these anomalies because failure to do so can lead to disastrous surgical outcomes.

Karuna V. Shekdar and Larissa T. Bilaniuk

Temporal bone high-resolution computed tomography (HRCT) and magnetic resonance (MR) imaging are valuable tools in the evaluation of pediatric hearing loss. Computed tomography is important in the evaluation of pediatric conductive hearing loss and is the imaging modality of choice for evaluation of osseous abnormalities. MR imaging is the modality of choice for evaluation of sensorineural hearing loss. A broad spectrum of imaging findings can be seen with hearing loss in children. HRCT and MR imaging provide complementary information and are often used in conjunction in the preoperative evaluation of pediatric candidates for cochlear implantation.

Daniel Thomas Ginat

There is a wide variety of congenital syndromes that can involve the temporal bone. Many of these have overlapping features due to common embryologic abnormalities, such as first and second branchial anomalies. Diagnostic imaging is often important in the workup of hearing deficits related to congenital syndromes. This article reviews the imaging features of selected congenital syndromes with temporal bone abnormalities, including Treacher Collins syndrome, oculo-auriculo-vertebral dysplasia spectrum, Klippel-Feil syndrome, branchio-oto-renal syndrome, Pierre Robin sequence, CHARGE syndrome, Pendred syndrome, Down syndrome, Trisomy 18, Turner syndrome, and neurofibromatosis type 2.

Joshua E. Lantos, Kristen Leeman, Elizabeth K. Weidman, Kathryn E. Dean, Tiffany Peng, and Aaron N. Pearlman

Imaging plays an important role in the evaluation of temporal bone trauma. Certain imaging findings can significantly change patient management or change surgical approach. Precise knowledge of clinical or surgical management can guide the review of imaging to detect these key findings. This article reviews the clinical and imaging findings as well as management of complications from temporal bone trauma, including hearing loss, vertigo, perilymphatic fistula, cerebrospinal fluid leak, facial nerve injury and vascular injury.

Philip Touska and Amy Fan-Yee Juliano

In their variety, temporal bone tumors mirror the complexity of the structure from which they arise. They include more familiar lesions, such as vestibular schwannomas and paragangliomas, and also rarer neoplasms, such as nonvestibular schwannomas, sarcomas, giant cell tumors, Schneiderian papillomas, and endolymphatic sac tumors. Diagnostic imaging is invaluable in evaluating such lesions because they are typically challenging to access surgically and monitor clinically. The ability to differentiate tumors from benign ('don't touch') or indolent lesions can prevent unnecessary morbidity. This article reviews a range of temporal bone neoplasms, focusing on imaging approaches and characteristic imaging findings.

Apoorva T. Ramaswamy and Justin S. Golub

Vestibular schwannomas are the most common tumor of the cerebellopontine angle. The history of their management has driven advances in imaging, lateral skull base surgery, as well as radiosurgery. With these advances, a shift has occurred from life-saving treatment for late-stage disease to quality of life focused management of smaller tumors. The complicated treatment paradigms involving observation, stereotactic radiosurgery and surgery require close communication between the treatment and neuroradiology teams.

Neuro-otologists rely on the expertise and judgment of a skilled neuroradiologist to identify radiographic abnormalities in the complicated regional anatomy of the temporal bone and middle and posterior fossa, and more importantly, to alert the surgeon to potential operative pitfalls. This article highlights some of the common otologic surgical procedures that stress this important dynamic. The surgical perspective on quick and effective clinical decision-making pearls to keep in mind during a thorough radiographic analysis of the ear and lateral skull base is presented.

Temporal bone pathologies are challenging to discern because of their small size and subtle contrast. MR imaging is one of the key modalities in evaluating otologic diseases. Current advancement in MR techniques provide multiparametric information for evaluation of these pathologies. The aim of this article is to review state-of-the-art 3-dimensional morphologic and diffusion sequences for otologic MR imaging.

Foreword

Update on Temporal Bone Imaging with Emphasis on Clinical and Surgical Perspectives

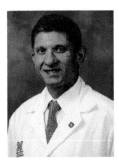

Suresh K. Mukherji, MD, MBA, FACR
Consulting Editor

Imaging of the temporal bone has been a challenging area for radiologists dating back to the days of conventional tomography. Computed tomography and MR imaging have allowed "easier" visualization of the anatomy that we were "pretty sure" we saw on the conventional tomograms. However, the anatomy and pathology continue to challenge, perplex, and, at times, intimidate!

In this issue of *Neuroimaging Clinics*, Drs Juliano and Moonis have created highly organized and state-of-the-art text that covers the spectrum of temporal imaging. The articles cover a variety of temporal anomalies that include congenital, traumatic, infectious, and neoplastic maladies. There are also two articles authored by otologic surgeons that provide important insights on how our interpretations directly impact clinical care.

All the articles are authored by recognized experts in Head and Neck radiology and neuro-otology. The articles are superb, and I am very grateful for the authors' time and expertise for creating such extraordinary contributions.

Finally, I want to personally thank Amy and Gul for accepting our invitation to guest edit this important topic. For those of you who have not had the privilege of meeting them, they are two of the nicest and smartest people I have ever met. I have both known and admired their work since they were Fellows, and the future of Head and Neck radiology is in excellent "hands" with such talented individuals. Thank you so much!

Suresh K. Mukherji, MD, MBA, FACR
Department of Radiology
Michigan State University
Michigan State University Health Team
846 Service Road
East Lansing, MI 48824, USA

E-mail address:
sureshkm@msu.edu

Neuroimag Clin N Am 29 (2019) xv
https://doi.org/10.1016/j.nic.2018.10.002
1052-5149/19/© 2018 Published by Elsevier Inc.

Preface
Hear and Now

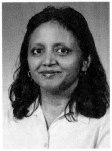 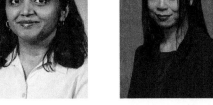

Gul Moonis, MD   Amy Fan-Yee Juliano, MD
Editors

The temporal bone is traditionally considered a challenging area for imaging analysis, especially considering its intricate anatomy containing numerous structures within a small area as well as the wide variety of pathology that occurs there.

In this issue of *Neuroimaging Clinics*, we present up-to-date information relevant to radiologists in a systematic manner, addressing basic anatomy and diagnoses, practical and novel imaging techniques, and clinical entities of which to be aware. In particular, we included among the authors two practicing otologic surgeons, who provide for us important and unique perspectives on the clinical decision-making process and the role of imaging in that. Since vestibular schwannoma is the most common tumor in the temporal bone region, another clinical article addresses the treatment options for this entity. The article on temporal bone trauma is clinically oriented as well.

Leading experts in the field of imaging of temporal bone inflammation, dysplasias, and Meniere disease provide an updated review of these important topics. Tinnitus is an important clinical problem, and a dedicated article regarding this provides a comprehensive review. Third window lesions of the temporal bone have gained interest in recent literature and are an important cause of conductive hearing loss and vertigo. This is addressed in detail in an article dedicated to this topic. An article on arterial anatomy of the temporal bone provides embryologic-imaging correlation. Two articles on imaging of the pediatric temporal bone provide important insights into

this challenging area. The article on temporal bone tumors contains lesser known and less often discussed entities, in addition to the classic common diagnoses encountered routinely. Finally, an article on advanced MR imaging of the temporal bone attempts to demystify the plethora of imaging sequences that can be encountered in general practice.

We are deeply grateful to Dr Mukherji for the opportunity to create this issue. We hope that this collection of articles will serve as useful references for practicing radiologists in both academic and private practice settings. We dedicate this issue to Zo and Ro, who it is hoped will carry on the legacy of BFF-dom from our generation to theirs.

Gul Moonis, MD
Department of Radiology
Columbia University Irving Medical Center
622 West 168th Street, PB-1-301
New York, NY 10032, USA

Amy Fan-Yee Juliano, MD
Department of Radiology
Massachusetts Eye and Ear Infirmary
Harvard Medical School
243 Charles Street
Boston, MA 02114, USA

E-mail addresses:
Gm2640@cumc.columbia.edu (G. Moonis)
amy_juliano@meei.harvard.edu (A.F.-Y. Juliano)

neuroimaging.theclinics.com

Neuroimag Clin N Am 29 (2019) xvii
https://doi.org/10.1016/j.nic.2018.10.001
1052-5149/19/© 2018 Published by Elsevier Inc.

Inflammation of the Temporal Bone

Ravi Kumar Lingam, MB BCh, MRCP, FRCR, EBiHNR[a],*,
Raekha Kumar, BSc, MBBS, MRCP, FRCR[b], Ram Vaidhyanath, DMRD, DNB, FRCR, EBiHNR[c]

KEYWORDS

- Temporal bone • CT • MR imaging • Ear • Inflammation • Otitis • Diffusion weighted
- Cholesteatoma

KEY POINTS

- Temporal bone inflammation is usually due to infection.
- It is associated with a wide variety of complications and postinflammatory sequelae.
- High-resolution computed tomography scanning is the imaging modality of choice for imaging temporal bone and ear infection.
- MR imaging has added value in characterizing disease, defining its extent and spread, and as a surveillance tool.
- Combining the use of computed tomography and MR imaging can give a comprehensive evaluation of a complex inflammatory process.

Inflammation of the temporal bones and ear structures is commonly due to infection. It can be associated with a variety of complications and postinflammatory sequelae. High-resolution computed tomography (HRCT) is ideally suited for imaging the temporal bone by depicting the bony detail well and is the imaging modality of choice. MR imaging is useful to either characterize the disease, define the extent and spread of disease within and beyond the temporal bone, or as a surveillance tool. MR imaging can also be used together with HRCT to give a comprehensive evaluation of a complex disease process.

EXTERNAL EAR INFLAMMATORY DISEASES
Simple External Otitis

Simple external otitis is a common external ear inflammation commonly caused by infection from a variety of pathogens. It is often referred to as swimmer's ear because moisture plays a significant role. Chronic external otitis can also be secondary to allergy (eczema) and, rarely, is associated with first branchial cleft anomalies. Because the external auditory canal is easily and well-examined clinically, imaging is seldom required for the assessment of simple external otitis (Fig. 1). When imaging is used, HRCT is the preferred modality because it can demonstrate reliably the extent of disease, bony involvement, and adjacent middle ear status.[1,2]

Chronic Sclerosing External Otitis

Chronic sclerosing external otitis is an idiopathic condition that clinically presents with intense pruritus with scant discharge. It is often bilateral and begins at the medial end of the canal at the lateral

Disclosure Statement: No disclosures.
[a] Department of Radiology, Northwick Park & Central Middlesex Hospitals, London North West University Healthcare NHS Trust, Imperial College London, Watford Road, London HA1 3UJ, UK; [b] Department of Radiology, Northwick Park & Central Middlesex Hospitals, London North West University Healthcare NHS Trust, Watford Road, London HA1 3UJ, UK; [c] Department of Radiology, University Hospitals of Leicester, Leicester University, Infirmary Square, Leicester LE1 5WW, UK
* Corresponding author.
E-mail address: raviklingam@yahoo.co.uk

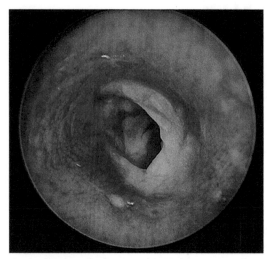

Fig. 1. Otitis externa. Otoendoscopic image of the right external auditory canal demonstrates otorrhea and narrowing secondary to bacterial external otitis (usually *Pseudomonas*).

surface of the tympanic membrane. Over time, the granulation tissue is gradually replaced by a fibrous tissue, causing stenosis and a fibrous plug and hence the synonym medial canal fibrosis. HRCT reflects this process, demonstrating mild soft tissue thickening of the tympanic membrane and medial canal walls in the early stage to soft tissue obliteration of the medial canal lumen against the tympanic membrane in the later stages of the disease.[1] There are no associated bony changes and the adjacent middle ear cleft is not involved (**Fig. 2**).

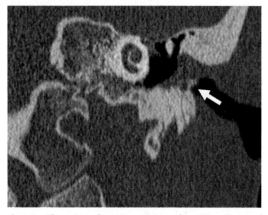

Fig. 2. Chronic sclerosing external otitis. Coronal bone-weighted high-resolution computed tomography shows the left medial bony external auditory canal is obliterated with soft tissue extending to the tympanic membrane (*white arrow*). There is no associated bony erosion.

Necrotizing External Otitis

Clinical

Necrotizing external otitis (malignant external otitis) is a severe infection of the external canal where there is rapid inflammatory spread beyond the confines of the canal into the deep neck spaces, skull base, or temporomandibular joint. It often begins insidiously at the osseous–cartilaginous junction and is often associated with canal bony wall destruction. The typical clinical presentation is severe unilateral otalgia and otorrhea in elderly patients with poorly controlled diabetes and who are not responding to topical treatment. The incriminating organism is commonly *Pseudomonas aeruginosa*. The disease is associated with significant morbidity and often requires intensive and long-term antimicrobial management, regular aural toilet, and close surveillance for secondary complications.[2,3] Complications include cranial nerve palsies (typically VII, IX, X, XII, and IX) from involvement at or around their exit foramina at the skull base,[3] meningeal disease, venous sinus thrombosis, and occasionally internal carotid artery occlusion.[4]

Imaging

Imaging can aid in establishing the diagnosis and in monitoring treatment response. Bone-weighted HRCT is the current initial modality of choice because it can depict well the erosion and destruction of the bony canal and/or adjacent skull base and confirm the diagnosis[4,5] (**Figs. 3 and 4**). Intravenous contrast-enhanced CT scanning/MR imaging can also depict the soft tissue inflammation and spread into the deep neck spaces and intracranially, but MR imaging is preferred owing to its superior soft tissue resolution and capability of depicting bone marrow and intracranial disease.[2] A baseline pretreatment scan against which interval scans can be compared allows complementary imaging assessment of treatment response and in this regard the lack of ionizing radiation confers MR imaging an additional advantage over CT and radionuclide imaging.[2] The use of radionuclide scans (3-phase technetium Tc-99m bone scans, leukocyte scintigraphy, gallium Ga-67 scintigraphy, single-proton emission computed tomography, and PET with fluorodeoxyglucose) is limited by low specificity, high cost, elaborate preparation of the radionuclides, and limited availability.[2]

Imaging features of necrotizing external otitis include:

- Bony canal wall erosion or destruction on HRCT,
- Medial condylar fat space infiltration,

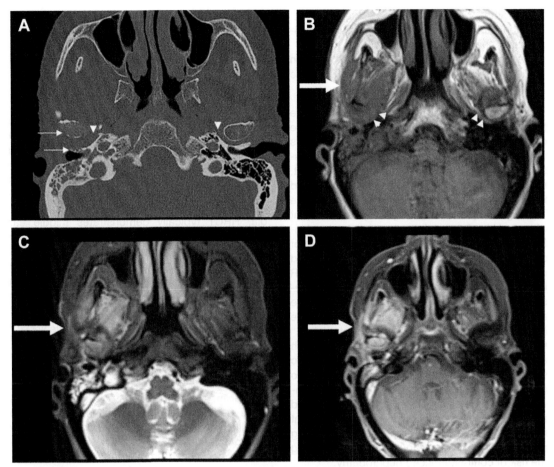

Fig. 3. Necrotizing external otitis with anterior spread. Axial bone-weighted high-resolution computed tomography (HRCT) image (*A*) shows abnormal bony destruction of the anterior wall of the external auditory canal and right mandibular condyle (*thin arrows*). Axial T1-weighted (*B*), axial short T1 inversion recovery (*C*) and fat-saturated T1-weighted postcontrast (*D*) images demonstrate inflammatory soft tissue extending into the right masticator space and right mandibular condyle (*thick arrow*). Right mastoid fluid also noted. Note medial condylar spaces (*arrowheads*).

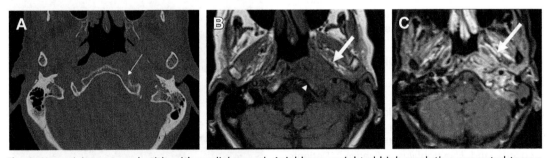

Fig. 4. Necrotizing external otitis with medial spread. Axial bone-weighted high-resolution computed tomography image (*A*) shows subtle bony destruction at the basiocciput (*thin arrow*). Axial T1-weighted (*B*) and fat-saturated T1-weighted postcontrast (*C*) images demonstrate inflammatory soft tissue extending into the left parapharyngeal and retropharyngeal neck spaces (*thick arrow*) with involvement of the basiocciput (*arrowhead*).

20000

- An anterior pattern of deep neck space invasion into temporomandibular joint and masticator space (see **Fig. 3**), and
- A medial pattern of deep neck space invasion into paraphayngeal space and skull base (typically basiocciput; see **Fig. 4**).

On CT or MR imaging, medial condylar space (see **Fig. 3**) infiltration has been proposed as one of the most frequent diagnostic findings in patients with necrotizing external otitis.[4] Abnormal soft tissue in the ear canal, although not always present, resolves early.[4] The deep neck space and bone marrow changes are well-depicted on the T1-weighted (T1W) MR images by replacement of normal high fat signal by intermediate signal inflammatory soft tissue (see **Figs. 3** and **4**). After successful treatment, infratemporal fossa and skull base marrow changes on CT scanning, MR imaging, and radionuclide imaging reverse, but residual changes secondary to granulation tissue and fibrosis/scarring may persist for a long time (more than a year) and not disappear completely.[4] Hence, clinical and microbiological evaluation with an erythrocyte sedimentation rate is essential to supplement imaging findings when deciding to change or stop treatment.[3,4] Recently, diffusion-weighted MR imaging (DWI) has been described as a novel imaging technique to monitor treatment response[5] and has the advantage of not requiring administration of intravenous contrast obviating the risk of contrast-induced nephropathy.

Relapsing Polychondritis

At the pinna of the ear, inflammation of the cartilage can be associated with relapsing polychondritis, an autoimmune disorder that typically spares the external auditory canal but may involve the cartilages of the nose, upper respiratory tract, and peripheral joints. Involvement of the pinna is clinically apparent as a red and tender ear and MR imaging can be used to confirm this finding, detect other involved sites in the head and neck, and monitor treatment response[2] (**Fig. 5**).

MIDDLE EAR INFLAMMATORY DISEASES
Acute Otitis Media

Clinical
Acute otitis media is an acute infection of the middle ear cleft. It is a common childhood disease often related to bacterial infections such as *Streptococcus* and *Haemophilus influenza*.[6] Patients present with a history of headaches, fever, otalgia, otorrhea, and postauricular swelling over several days or weeks. It is principally a clinical diagnosis. There is an erythematous appearance to the

external auditory canal with discharge visualized and postauricular edema. The auricle can also be lateralized (laterally bulging) owing to an underlying collection.[7] Otoscopy often demonstrates a red, bulging tympanic membrane (**Fig. 6**).

Imaging
Imaging is indicated in acute otitis media if there is clinical concern regarding complications or in assessing the extent of infection, including spread into the deep neck spaces and periauricular regions.[8] HRCT provides excellent anatomic detail of the middle ear cleft, including the ossicular chain and facial nerve canal. With otitis media, HRCT typically demonstrates middle ear cleft opacification, usually centered dependently within the mesohypotympanum, with preservation of the bony architecture of the mastoid and ossicular chain.[7] Mastoid fluid is commonly an incidental HRCT finding; hence, acute mastoiditis remains a clinical diagnosis with the presence of pain. Postcontrast HRCT is indicated if there is clinical concern for associated intracranial complications.

Complications of acute otitis media
Coalescent mastoiditis and related abscesses Otitis media can lead to coalescent mastoiditis, a condition wherein there is progressive bony resorption and erosion of the mastoid septae with an associated empyema (**Fig. 7**).[7] This process occurs owing to inflammatory debris and

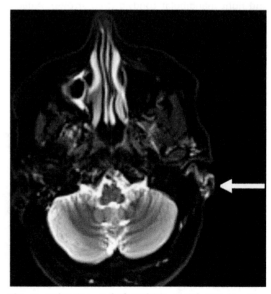

Fig. 5. Relapsing polychondritis. Axial MR imaging short T1 inversion recovery image shows thickening and hyperintense signal in the cartilaginous structures of the pinna of the left ear (*white arrow*).

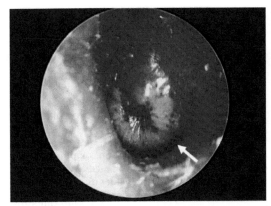

Fig. 6. Acute otitis media. Otoendoscopic image of left tympanic membrane demonstrates acute suppurative otitis media, with edema, erythema and, marked lateral bulging (*white arrow*) secondary to mucopurulent exudate within the middle ear cavity.

granulation tissue blocking the aditus ad antrum leading to poor mastoid drainage. Secondary dehiscence of the mastoid wall can result in extraosseous spread of infection leading to meningitis, cellulitis, and abscess or empyema formation, which requires a postcontrast HRCT with relevant reconstructions for assessment (see **Fig. 7**; **Fig. 8**).

- *Subperiosteal abscess*: Peripherally enhancing, periauricular fluid collection owing to spread via the lateral mastoid cortex. Commonly postauricular in location (see **Fig. 7**).
- *Bezold abscess*: Peripherally enhancing collection related to a mastoid tip defect that subsequently leads to spread of infection inferiorly with inflammatory changes noted around the sternocleidomastoid muscle. Without treatment, this can spread to the larynx and mediastinum.[9]
- *Subdural empyema*: Peripherally enhancing collection in the subdural space located in the middle and/or posterior cranial fossae adjacent to the inflamed mastoid.
- *Brain abscess*: Peripherally enhancing mass located in the temporal lobe or cerebellum adjacent to the inflamed mastoid. MR imaging with contrast (see **Fig. 8**) and DWI can help to confirm the presence of an abscess by demonstrating peripheral enhancement and restricted diffusion respectively.

Venous sinus thrombosis Coalescent mastoiditis can lead to a secondary thrombosis affecting the sigmoid sinus or internal jugular vein adjacent to

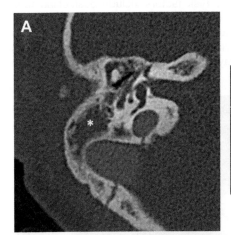

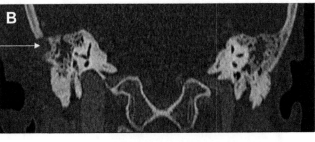

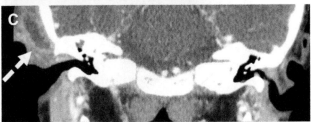

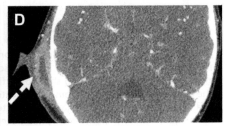

Fig. 7. Acute otitis media. Axial bone-weighted high-resolution computed tomography (*A*) and coronal (*B*) and postcontrast soft tissue weighted coronal (*C*) and axial (*D*) images show soft tissue opacification of the right middle ear cleft (*asterisk*) with coalescent mastoiditis with cortical breach at the lateral mastoid cortex (*B, thin arrow*) and a postauricular inflammatory abscess (*C, D, dashed arrow*).

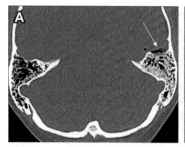
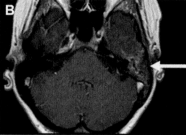
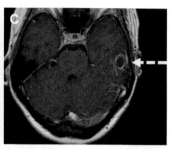

Fig. 8. Acute otitis media with neurologic complications. Axial bone-weighted high-resolution computed tomography image (*A*) shows opacification of the left middle ear cleft in keeping with acute otitis media with pneumocephalus related to breach of the tegmen (*thin arrow*). Axial T1-weighted postcontrast images (*B, C*) demonstrate associated meningeal enhancement (*thick arrow*) with a temporal lobe abscess (*dashed arrow*).

the infection. A postcontrast HRCT in the venous phase is required for appropriate assessment and to demonstrate the extent of thrombus; this feature will be demonstrated as a filling defect (empty delta sign; Fig. 9). Patients are at risk of a secondary venous cerebral infarction and associated haemorrhage.[7]

Petrous apicitis Spread of infection from the middle ear and mastoid into the pneumatized petrous apex can result in petrous apicitis and Gradinego syndrome.

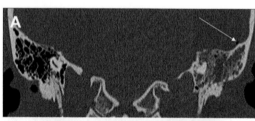

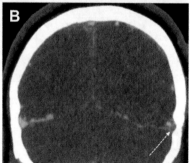

Fig. 9. Acute otitis media with neurologic complications. Coronal bone-weighted high-resolution computed tomography image (*A*) show opacification of the left middle ear cleft in keeping with acute otitis media. There is a locule of gas adjacent to the tegmen tympani (*thin arrow*) indicating pneumocephalus related to breach of the tegmen. Coronal postcontrast venogram (*B*) demonstrates a thrombus within the left transverse sinuses extending into the sigmoid sinus (*dashed arrow*).

Facial nerve palsy Facial nerve palsy is a rare complication of acute otitis media accounting for 5% of cases and is typically associated with complete recovery.[9]

Chronic Otitis Media

Clinical

Chronic otitis media is related to longstanding infection and inflammation of the middle ear cavity, and can include the mastoid (chronic otomastoiditis). It results from repeated bouts of acute infection with unresolved and resistant bacterial infections. Risk factors include eustachian tube dysfunction and traumatic perforation of the tympanic membrane.[6] Patients often present with a chronically discharging ear (usually >6 weeks) and may have conductive hearing loss. On

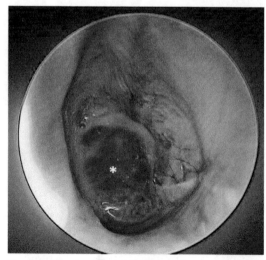

Fig. 10. Chronic otitis media. Otoendoscopic image of left tympanic membrane shows a large aural polyp (*asterisk*) protruding through the tympanic membrane perforation secondary to active mucosal chronic otitis media.

examination, there is perforation of the tympanic membrane (**Fig. 10**).

Imaging

The role of imaging with HRCT is primarily to assess for complications. HRCT demonstrates inflammatory debris and fluid in the middle ear cleft. Granulation tissue can also be present as sequelae of inflammation, which will surround the ossicles without destruction or displacement.[6] The tympanic membrane may also be retracted owing to eustachian tube dysfunction and middle ear atelectasis. In addition, there may be underpneumatization of the mastoid owing to osteoneogenesis leading to thickening of the trabeculae with reduction in air spaces.[7]

Complications and sequelae

Tympanosclerosis Tympanosclerosis refers to foci of calcification and ossification within the middle ear cleft as a healing response to chronic inflammation (**Figs. 11** and **12**). This condition can occur in up to 10% of patients with suppurative chronic otitis media.[10] Patients may present with a severe conductive hearing loss and can have a thick, opaque tympanic membrane on otoscopy.

Tympanosclerosis can involve the:

- Tympanic membrane (myringosclerosis),
- Ossicular surfaces and ligaments (ossicular fixation),
- Crura and footplate of the stapes (ossicular fixation),
- Muscle tendons (stapedius and tensor tympani), and
- Mastoid.

Ossicular fixation Ossicular fixation is a postinflammatory response to chronic otitis media. There are 3 stages of ossicular fixation that can be demonstrated on HRCT:

- *Fibrous:* Soft tissue commonly in the oval window in the peristapedial region (creating a peristapedial tent or elsewhere in the

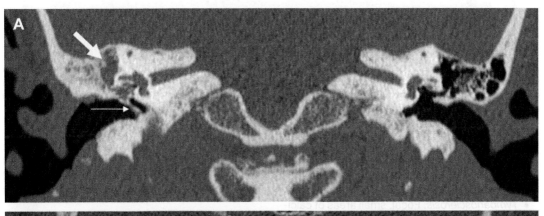
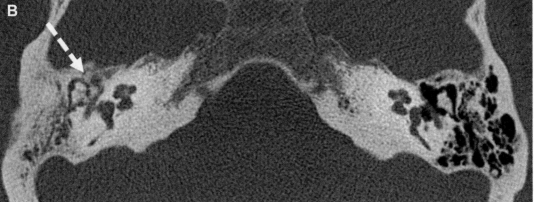

Fig. 11. Chronic otitis media with myringosclerosis/tympanosclerosis. Coronal (*A*) and axial (*B*) bone-weighted high-resolution computed tomography images show a thickened and calcified right tympanic membrane in keeping with myringosclerosis (*thin arrow*) and tympanosclerosis with abnormal nondependent soft tissue at the right epimesotympanum (*dashed arrow*) and mastoid (*thick arrow*) with calcification. The ossicular chain and scutum are intact.

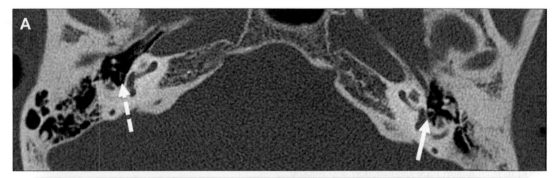

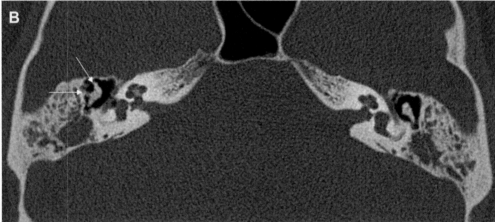

Fig. 12. Tympanosclerosis. Coronal (*A*) and coronal (*B*) bone-weighted high-resolution computed tomography images. (*A*) Hyperdensity of the left stapes (*thick arrow*) in keeping with tympanosclerosis. Normal appearances of the right stapes (*dashed arrow*). (*B*) Ossification of the ligament to the head of malleus and body of incus (*thin arrows*) again demonstrating tympanosclerosis.

epimesotympanum.[1] In the early stages, this finding may be difficult to appreciate on CT. Wide air–bone gaps without ossicular erosion suggest ossicular fixation from fibrous tissue.

- *Tympanosclerosis*: Focal, small areas of calcification can also occur directly related to the ossicular chain (see **Fig. 12**).
- *Osteoneogenesis*: New bone formation, which is rarely seen in the tympanic cavity.

Ossicular erosion Chronic otitis media can lead to an osteitis involving the ossicular chain with an osteoclastic response leading to bony erosion. Patients are more likely to present with a conductive hearing loss. The long and lenticular processes of the incus is most commonly involved owing to a tenuous blood supply, thus, leading to avascular necrosis[11] (**Fig. 13**). HRCT has a 80% sensitivity in assessing ossicular erosion.[10]

Labyrinthitis This condition occurs secondary to chronic middle ear inflammation through fistulization into the bony capsule of the labyrinth. Direct spread can also occur via the oval or round windows.

Facial nerve palsy Facial nerve palsy in chronic otitis media may be a result of osteitis of the facial nerve canal, bony erosion, compression, and inflammation.[12] The facial nerve, particularly at

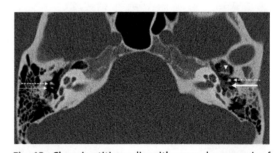

Fig. 13. Chronic otitis media with avascular necrosis of the incus and tympanosclerosis. Axial bone-weighted high-resolution computed tomography image at the incudostapedial joint shows normal appearances of the right malleus and incus (*thin arrow*), but erosion of the lenticular process of the left incus by abnormal soft tissue, indicating avascular necrosis dashed arrow (*thick arrow*). There is a normal manubrium of the malleus (*dashed arrows*). Left-sided tympanosclerosis in the epitympanum (*arrow head*) is present.

the tympanic and mastoid segments, must be imaged carefully on HRCT to assess for canal erosion.

Cholesterol granuloma Cholesterol granuloma is an uncommon and late complication of chronic, recurrent otitis media. The etiology remains uncertain, but recurrent hemorrhages are implicated, causing extensive granulation.[13] Otoscopy demonstrates a blue appearing tympanic membrane. On CT, the mass demonstrates nonspecific smooth expansion within the middle ear cavity, whereas on MR imaging it demonstrates a characteristic high signal on T1W and T2-weighted (T2W) sequences.[14]

ACQUIRED CHOLESTEATOMA
Acquired Middle Ear Cholesteatoma

Clinical
Cholesteatoma is an important complication of chronic otitis media to recognize because it can cause progressive local destruction with otorrhea, hearing loss, and vertigo if left untreated. It is essentially a sac lined with stratified squamous epithelium and filled with keratin debris and usually diagnosed clinically and with otoscopy[15] (Fig. 14). With progression, it can erode the local bony structures and this can be depicted well on HRCT.

Imaging
The following signs on HRCT aid in the clinical diagnosis of middle ear cholesteatoma (Fig. 15):

- Nondependent soft tissue, typically with involvement of the epitympanum and Prussak's space,
- Blunting of the scutum,
- Erosion of the ossicles, typically the malleus and incus, and
- Widening of the mastoid aditus.

HRCT is highly sensitive in detecting bony and ossicular erosion[15] (see Fig. 15; Fig. 16). Although the scutum and ossicles are commonly involved, less frequently, cholesteatoma can erode the facial nerve canal, the tegmen tympani, the lateral semicircular canal, the sigmoid plate, and the posterosuperior external auditory canal. Detection of these complications can steer the surgeon away from further damaging the vulnerable structures and plan necessary repair after clearance of disease. HRCT can also help surgical planning by mapping the extent of disease. This process may be challenging if there is soft tissue opacification of the entire middle ear cleft on HRCT with coexisting fluid and inflammation, and supplementing with nonechoplanar DWI can provide a better surgical map.[16] On MR imaging, cholesteatoma appears as follows.[17,18]

- Intermediate signal on T1W imaging,
- High signal on T2W imaging,
- Nonenhancing or a rim-enhancing on delayed contrast enhanced MR imaging,
- High signal on DWI with high b-values of 800 or 1000 s/mm^2 (Fig. 17), and

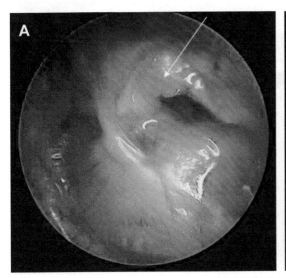
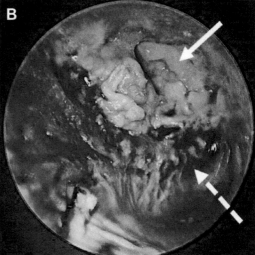

Fig. 14. Cholesteatoma. (A) Otoendoscopic image of left tympanic membrane demonstrates posterosuperior tympanic membrane retraction within keratin visible in the postero-superior quadrant secondary to cholesteatoma (*thin arrow*). (B) Otoendoscopic image of right tympanic membrane demonstrates attic cholesteatoma (*white arrow*) with attic erosion and active chronic otitis media (*dashed arrow*).

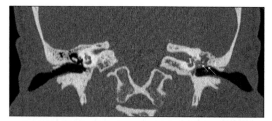

Fig. 15. Middle ear cholesteatoma. Coronal bone-weighted high-resolution computed tomography shows left-sided, abnormal, nondependent soft tissue at the epitympanum with blunting of the scutum (*thin arrow*) and erosion of the body of the incus (*dashed thin arrow*).

- Low signal on the apparent diffusion coefficient (ADC) map.

The high signal of cholesteatoma on DWI is a result of restricted molecular diffusion and the T2 shine through effect.[17] The ADC value of cholesteatoma has also been shown to be significantly lower than that of non-cholesteatomatous tissue and can aid in the qualitative diagnosis of

cholesteatoma.[19] To allow optimal interpretation of DWI images in detecting cholesteatoma[20]:

- Obtain thin slices (<2 mm thick),
- Copy reference the b0 and b1000 images for position and other scanning parameters,
- Reconstruct the ADC map after acquisition, and
- Obtain the corresponding T1W and T2W images and copy reference with DWI for position, slice thickness, and field of view.

Non-echo-planar DWI (single shot and multishot types) is now established as the imaging modality of choice in the detection and management of postoperative cholesteatoma, primarily after canal wall-up mastoidectomy, and offers a noninvasive alternative to traditional second-look or relook surgery.[13,20–22] It performs better than its echo-planar counterpart because it lacks air–bone interface artifact and distortion.[21] A large meta-analysis of 26 studies revealed a high pooled sensitivity and specificity of 91% and 92%, respectively, in detecting cholesteatoma.[13] Its sensitivity is limited by its poor ability to detect cholesteatoma less

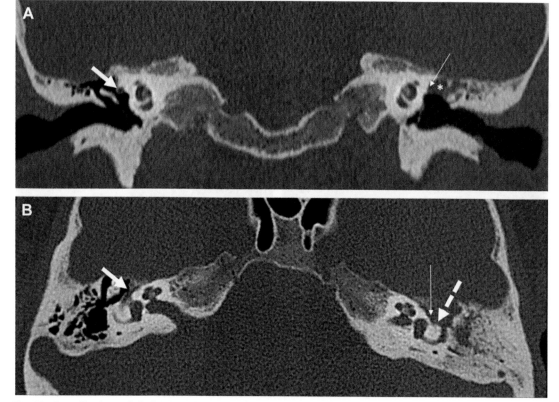

Fig. 16. Complications of cholesteatoma. Coronal (*A*) and axial (*B*) bone-weighted high-resolution computed tomography bone images show left-sided, abnormal, nondependent soft tissue at the epitympanum (*asterisk*) with erosion of the anterior tympanic facial nerve canal (*thin arrows*) and anterior limb of the lateral SCC (*dashed arrow*). Compare with normal right facial nerve canal (*thick arrows*).

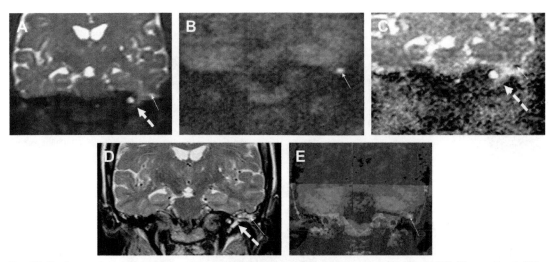

Fig. 17. Postoperative cholesteatoma. Coronal diffusion-weighted MR images b0 (*A*), b1000 (*B*), apparent diffusion coefficient map (*C*) and T2-weighted (*D*) images shows abnormal soft tissue within the epitympanum with a small focus of restricted diffusion in keeping with residual cholesteatoma (*thin arrow*) among noncholesteatomatous soft tissue, which demonstrates facilitated diffusion (*dashed arrow*). To aid surgical planning, coronal fusion high-resolution computed tomography/b1000 (*E*) localizes the focus of the cholesteatoma in relation to bone anatomy at the lateral epitympanum. (A preoperative computed tomography scan was used in this case to avoid further radiation exposure).

than 2 to 3 mm in size or mural cholesteatoma. A negative DWI scan cannot, therefore, exclude a small residual or recurrent cholesteatoma and for DWI to replace second-look surgery, it will require serial scanning over a period of time before discharge.[20,21,23] A myriad of false-positive findings have been described to include nonspecific inflammation, proteinaceous fluid, bone powder, silastic sheets, cholesterol granulomas, and ear canal cerumen. Correlating with T1W images, ADC mapping and follow-up monitoring all can decrease the false-positive rate.[20] DWI also performs well in estimating the size of the cholesteatoma and localizing disease.[24] Anatomic localization of the detected cholesteatoma can also be enhanced by interpreting with T1W and T2W images or by fusing the DWI images with the HRCT images[21] (see **Fig. 17**).

INFLAMMATION OF THE FACIAL NERVE
Clinical

Inflammation of the facial nerve, facial neuronitis, can be a result of infection, vasculitis, or immunologic irritation. The facial nerve contains efferent fibers to the facial muscles and afferent fibers from the tongue, lacrimal gland, and salivary glands and hence clinical signs and symptoms of facial neuronitis includes facial palsy abnormal tearing, reduced taste, hyperacusis, and postauricular pain. The most common cause—idiopathic facial nerve or Bell's palsy—although described as idiopathic, has a strong association with herpes simplex virus infection.[25] In the less common Ramsay-Hunt syndrome secondary to varicella zoster infection, facial neuronitis may be associated with typical vesicular skin rash.

Imaging

Imaging is not routinely indicated unless there is atypical progression of disease or a lack of recovery despite appropriate treatment.[2] The purpose of imaging is to exclude other causes of facial nerve palsy and to positively depict facial nerve inflammation. On MR imaging, parts of the facial nerve can enhance normally and variably, but pathologic enhancement is diagnosed when the intracanalicular and labyrinthine segments are involved (**Fig. 18**).[26] Asymmetric linear enhancement with or without thickening of the tympanic and mastoid segments of the nerve relative to the contralateral side should also be considered abnormal[25] (see **Fig. 18**). In the Ramsay-Hunt syndrome, there is abnormal linear facial nerve enhancement together with enhancement of the vestibular and cochlear nerves.[2,27]

INFLAMMATION OF THE INNER EAR
Labyrinthitis

Clinical
Inflammation of the inner ear (labyrinthitis) is usually secondary to viral infection.[28] Less commonly, it can be due to bacterial infection after meningitis

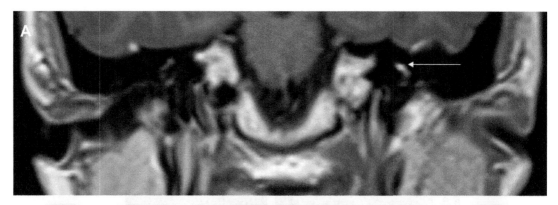

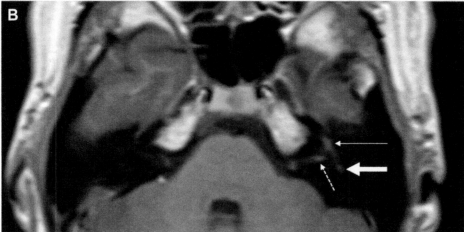

Fig. 18. Bell's palsy. T1-weighted postcontrast MR image with coronal (*A*) and axial (*B*) images showing avid asymmetric smooth enhancement of the left meatal facial nerve (*dashed arrow*) and geniculate ganglion (*thin arrow*). In addition, there is also more asymmetric intense enhancement of the tympanic facial nerve (*thick arrow*).

or otitis media. Patients usually present with acute sensorineural hearing loss, severe vertigo with nausea, vomiting, and gait instability. Labyrinthitis can be classified depending on their route of spread and the causative agent:

- Hematogenic (viral, tuberculosis, syphilis, or autoimmune),
- Meningogenic (bacterial meningitis),
- Tympanic (middle ear infection), or
- Post-traumatic (trauma, surgery).

Imaging

CT and MR imaging show a variable appearance during the different phases of labyrinthitis (**Table 1**). During the acute phase (**Fig. 19**), the only imaging finding is enhancement of the membranous labyrinth.[29] The subacute or fibrous stage is characterized by fibroblastic proliferation of the perilymphatic space. The chronic phase of the disease is referred to as labyrinthitis ossificans and is the result of ossification of the labyrinth[6] (**Fig. 20**). The timing of cochlear implantation is, therefore,

Table 1
Imaging appearance of inner ear during labyrinthitis

	CT	T2W MR Imaging	MR Imaging Postcontrast
Acute labyrinthitis	Normal	Normal high signal	Enhancement (often faint)
Subacute labyrinthitis	Normal	No/low signal	Diffuse or patchy enhancement
Chronic labyrinthitis	High density	No signal	No enhancement

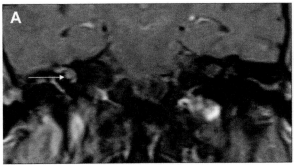

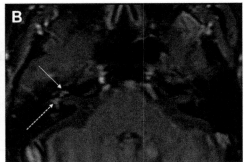

Fig. 19. Acute labyrinthitis. Coronal (*A*) and axial (*B*) fat-saturated T1-weighted postcontrast image shows abnormal enhancement of the right cochlea (*thin arrow*) and right vestibule (*dashed arrow*). Compare with the nonenhancing left inner ear.

critical given the potential for early onset of intra-cochlear fibrosis in patient with labyrinthitis.[30] CT and MR imaging are essential in the workup of a patient with labyrinthitis ossificans before implantation.

INFLAMMATION OF THE PETROUS APEX
Petrous Apex Trapped Fluid

Clinical
The petrous apex is pneumatized in nearly one-third of the population via air cell tracts that directly communicate with the middle ear and mastoid.[31] Hence, infection can spread from the middle ear and mastoid into the petrous apex. Asymptomatic sterile fluid collection can also be trapped in the petrous apex air cells, sometimes resulting from remote middle ear cleft infections (petrous apex effusions).[32]

Imaging
Petrous apex lesions are usually detected inciden-tally on imaging. Many lesions have characteristic CT and MR imaging appearances that can often allow a precise diagnosis (**Table 2**). Because pneumatization is asymmetrical in approximately 4% to 7% of population, normal entities such as

asymmetric bone marrow, pneumatization, and trapped fluid in the petrous apex can cause diag-nostic dilemma. Fluid signal on T1W and T2W MR imaging sequences are characteristic of trap-ped fluid and are not associated with bony erosion on HRCT[2,33,34] (**Fig. 21**).

Petrous Apicitis

Clinical
Infection of the pneumatized petrous apex is termed petrous apicitis and is usually a result of medial extension of acute otomastoiditis.[35] The classic clinical triad of otomastoiditis, sixth cranial nerve palsy, and pain in the distribution of the fifth nerve secondary to petrous apicitis is called Gra-denigo syndrome, although patients rarely have all 3 symptoms.[2,36]

Imaging
HRCT demonstrates opacification of the petrous apex initially and bony destruction during later stages of the disease (**Fig. 22**). MR imaging find-ings include low signal on T1W and high signal on T2W images along with contrast enhancement of the apex.[2] Enhancement of the adjacent meninges and cranial nerves occurs as the

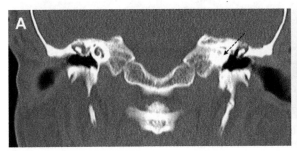

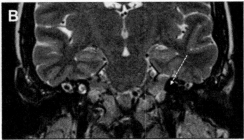

Fig. 20. Labyrinthine ossificans. Coronal (*A*) bone-weighted image shows bony obliteration of the left cochlea in keeping with labyrinthine ossificans (*dashed arrow*). The right bony labyrinth is normal. (*B*) Coronal T2-weighted MR imaging confirms loss of normal T2 signal within the left cochlea (*dashed arrow*).

Table 2
Imaging features of petrous apex lesions

	T1W MR Imaging	T2W MR Imaging	Contrast	Expansion
Trapped fluid	Low	High	No	No
Cholesterol granuloma	High	High	No	Yes
Mucocele	Low	High	No	Yes
Cholesteatoma	Low	High	No	Yes
Petrous apicitis	Low	High	Yes	No

disease extends beyond the petrous apex. This process can also lead to intracranial abscess formation and DWI is helpful in its delineation.

Osteomyelitis of the Petrous Apex

Infection of the nonpneumatized part of the petrous apex, or osteomyelitis of the petrous apex, is rare and usually secondary to necrotizing external otitis or suppurative otitis media.[34] HRCT demonstrates minimal signs initially and bony erosion, destruction, and sclerosis. MR imaging demonstrates signal changes in the petrous apex marrow, adjacent soft tissue involvement, and intracranial extension (**Fig. 23**).

Mucocele of the Petrous Apex

Clinical
Mucocele of the petrous apex is not common and occurs in the pneumatized part of the petrous apex. It is thought to represent a postinflammatory obstruction of air cells. It is usually asymptomatic but, with expansion of the bony boundaries, it can cause pain and/or cranial nerve palsy.

Imaging
On HRCT, mucoceles are well-circumscribed with smooth and sharp margins and are associated with septal erosion. It can be difficult to differentiate mucoceles from petrous apex congenital cholesteatoma. They are typically hypointense on T1W imaging, hyperintense on T2W MR images (**Fig. 24**), and do not typically enhance.[2] DWI can help to differentiate mucoceles from a cholesteatoma; a cholesteatoma typically demonstrates restricted diffusion.

Cholesterol Granuloma

Clinical
Petrous apex cholesterol granuloma is a foreign body giant cell inflammatory reaction to deposition of cholesterol crystals in the petrous apex. Although this lesion can be asymptomatic and incidentally discovered on imaging, it may present clinically with a variety of symptoms.

Imaging
Characteristically, cholesterol granuloma appears as an expansile lesion with high T1W and T2W signal on MR imaging. They often have a distinct

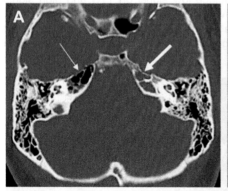
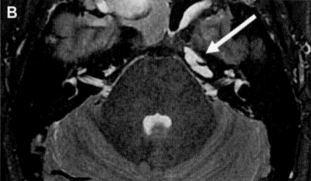

Fig. 21. Trapped fluid in the petrous apex. Axial (*A*) bone-weighted high-resolution computed tomography shows opacification of the left petrous apex with preserved trabeculae (*thick arrow*). Axial (*B*) T2-weighted image showing asymmetric high signal in the left petrous apex (*thick arrow*). Note the pneumatization of the right petrous apex with mild opacification (*thin arrow*). Lack of expansion, bone remodeling, and destruction helps to differentiate trapped fluid from the mucocele and tumor.

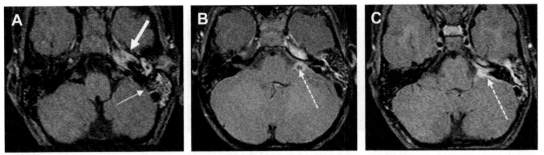

Fig. 22. Petrous apicitis. Gadolinium-enhanced fat suppressed T1-weighted image (*A*) shows enhancement of the left petrous apex (*thick arrow*) as well as in the middle ear and mastoid (*thin arrow*). There is a small, ringlike enhancing lesion (*B*) adjacent to the apex consistent with an abscess as well as dural enhancement (*dashed arrows; C*).

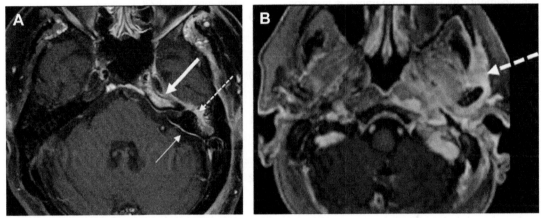

Fig. 23. Osteomyelitis of petrous bone secondary to necrotizing otitis externa. Gadolinium enhanced fat-suppressed T1-weighted image (*A*) showing enhancement of the left petrous apex (*thick arrow*), dura (*thin arrow*), and in the middle ear (*thin dashed arrow*). (*B*) Extensive involvement of the left skull base with involvement of the left masticator space (*thick dashed arrow*).

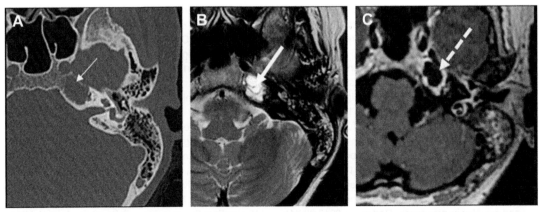

Fig. 24. Mucocele of the petrous apex. Axial (*A*) bone-weighted high-resolution computed tomography image demonstrates expansion of the left petrous apex with loss of trabeculation and thinning of the cortex (*thin arrow*). Corresponding axial T2-weighted image (*B*) shows high signal (*thick arrow*) that was of low signal on T1-weighted image (not shown). There is thin rim enhancement (*C*) after gadolinium administration (*dashed arrow*).

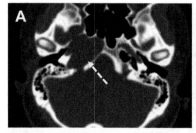 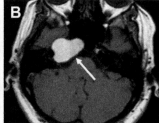 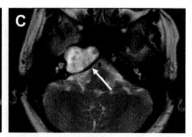

Fig. 25. Cholesterol granuloma. Axial (*A*) bone-weighted high-resolution computed tomography image shows a smooth bony expansile lucent lesion at the petrous apex of the temporal bone on the right (*dashed arrow*). Axial T1-weighted (*B*) and axial T2-weighted (*C*) images demonstrate characteristic T1 and T2 hyperintensity respectively within the petrous apex (*thick arrows*), in keeping with a cholesterol granuloma.

low T2W signal rim owing to hemosiderin deposition and do not typically enhance after contrast enhancement.[2] Its HRCT appearance is less specific and is usually that of an expansile lucent lesion with cortical thinning and trabecular destruction (**Fig. 25**).

ACKNOWLEDGMENTS

The authors would like to thank Mr Surojit Pal, ENT surgeon at LNWUH NHS Trust for providing the clinical images.

REFERENCES

1. Trojanowska A, Drop A, Trojanowski P, et al. External and middle ear diseases: radiological diagnosis based on clinical signs and symptoms. Insights Imaging 2012;3(1):33–48.

2. Lingam RK, Ram V. Magnetic resonance imaging of the ear. In: Saba L, editor. Magnetic resonance imaging handbook: image principles, neck and brain. Boca Raton: CRC Press Taylor & Francis Group; 2016. p. 287–324.

3. Grandis RJ, Branstetter BF, Yu VL. The changing face of malignant (necrotizing) external otitis: clinical, radiological and anatomic correlation. Lancet Infect Dis 2004;4:34–9.

4. Al-Noury K, Lotfy A. Computed tomography and magnetic resonance imaging findings before and after treatment of patients with malignant external otitis. Eur Arch Otorhinolaryngol 2011;268:1727–34.

5. Cherko M, Nash R, Singh A, et al. Diffusion-weighted magnetic resonance imaging as a novel imaging modality in assessing treatment response in necrotizing otitis externa. Otol Neurotol 2016;37(6):704–7.

6. Juliano AF, Ginat DT, Moonis G. Imaging review of the temporal bone: part I. anatomy and inflammatory and neoplastic processes. Radiology 2013;269(1): 17–33.

7. Koch BL, Hamilton BE, Hudgins PA, et al, editors. Diagnostic imaging: head and neck. 3rd edition. Amirsys Publishing, Inc; 2016.

8. Vazquez E, Castellote A, Piqueras J, et al. Imaging of complications of acute mastoiditis in children. Radiographics 2003;23(2):359–72.

9. Lemmerling MM, De Foer B, Verbist BM, et al. Imaging of inflammatory and infectious diseases in the temporal bone. Neuroimaging Clin North Am 2009; 19(3):321–37.

10. Lemmerling MM, De Foer B, VandeVyver V, et al. Imaging of the opacified middle ear. Eur J Radiol 2008; 66(3):363–71.

11. Keskin S, Çetin H, Tore HG. The correlation of temporal bone CT with surgery findings in evaluation of chronic inflammatory diseases of the middle ear. Eur J Gen Med 2011;8(1):24–30.

12. Kim J, Jung GH, Park SY, et al. Facial nerve paralysis due to chronic otitis media: prognosis in restoration of facial function after surgical intervention. Yonsei Med J 2012;53(3):642–8.

13. Lingam RK, Bassett P. A meta-analysis on the diagnostic performance of non - echo-planar diffusion-weighted imaging in detecting middle ear cholesteatoma: 10 years on. Otol Neurotol 2017;38(4): 521–8.

14. Tringali S, Linthicum FH Jr. Cholesterol granuloma of the petrous apex. Otol Neurotol 2010;31(9): 1518–9.

15. Khemani SC, Singh A, Lingam RK, et al. Radiological imaging of cholesteatoma. The Otorhinolaryngologist 2010;3(2):69–78.

16. Majithia A, Lingam RK, Nash R, et al. Staging primary middle ear cholesteatoma with non-echoplanar (half-Fourier-acquisition single-shot turbo-spin-echo) diffusion-weighted magnetic resonance imaging helps plan surgery in 22 patients: our experience. Clin Otolaryngol 2012;37(4):325–30.

17. Khemani S, Singh A, Lingam RK, et al. Imaging of postoperative middle ear cholesteatoma. Clin Radiol 2011;66(8):760–7.

18. De Foer B, Vercruysse JP, Bernaerts A, et al. Middle ear cholesteatoma: non-echo-planar diffusion-weighted MR imaging versus delayed gadolinium-enhanced T1-weighted MR imaging—value in detection. Radiology 2010;255(3):866–72.

19. Lingam RK, Khatri P, Hughes J, et al. Apparent diffusion coefficients for detection of postoperative middle ear cholesteatoma on non-echoplanar diffusion weighted images. Radiology 2013;269(2):504–10.

20. Lingam RK, Nash R, Majithia A, et al. Non-echoplanar diffusion weighted imaging in the detection of post-operative middle ear cholesteatoma: navigating beyond the pitfalls to find the pearl. Insights Imaging 2016;(75):669–78.

21. Lingam RK, Connor SEJ, Casselman JW, et al. MRI in otology: applications in cholesteatoma and Meniere's disease. Clin Radiol 2018;73(1):35–44.

22. Nash R, Wong PY, Kalan A, et al. Comparing diffusion weighted MRI in the detection of post-operative middle ear cholesteatomain children and adults. Int J Pediatr Otorhinolaryngol 2015;79(12): 2281–5.

23. Steens S, Venderink W, Kunst D, et al. Repeated postoperative follow-up diffusion-weighted magnetic resonance imaging to detect residual or recurrent cholesteatoma. Otol Neurotol 2016;37:356–61.

24. Khemani S, Lingam RK, Kalan A, et al. The value of non-echo planar HASTE diffusion-weighted MR imaging in the detection, localisation and prediction of extent of postoperative cholesteatoma. Clin Otolaryngol 2011;36(4):306–12.

25. Gilden DH. Bell's palsy. N Engl J Med 2004;351(13): 1323–31.

26. Martin-Duverneuil N, Sola-Martinez MT, Miaux Y, et al. Contrast enhancement of the facial nerve on MRI: normal or pathological? Neuroradiology 1999; 39:207–12.

27. Iwasaki H, Toda N, Takahashi M, et al. Vestibular and cochlear neuritis in patients with Ramsay Hunt syndrome: a Gd-enhanced MRI study. Acta Otolaryngol 2013;133(4):373–7.

28. Paparella MM, Sugiura S. The pathology of suppurative labyrinthitis. Ann Otol Rhinol Laryngol 1967; 76(3):554–86.

29. Abele TA, Wiggins RH 3rd. Imaging of the temporal bone. Radiol Clin North Am 2015;53(1):15–36.

30. Merkus P, Free RH, Mylanus EAM, et al. Dutch Cochlear Implant Group (CI-ON) consensus protocol on postmeningitis hearing evaluation and treatment. Otol Neurotol 2010;31(8):1281–6.

31. Bruni M, Wong R, Tabor M, et al. Pneumatization patterns of the petrous apex and lateral sphenoid recess. J Neurol Surg B Skull Base 2017;78(06): 441–6.

32. Schmalfuss IM. Petrous apex. Skull Base Imaging; 2018. p. 233–46.

33. Chapman PR, Shah R, Curé JK, et al. Petrous apex lesions: pictorial review. Am J Roentgenol 2011;196: WS26–37.

34. Razek AA, Huang BY. Lesions of the petrous apex: classification and findings at CT and MR imaging. RadioGraphics 2012;32(1):151–73.

35. Gadre AK, Chole RA. The changing face of petrous apicitis-a 40-year experience. Laryngoscope 2017; 128(1):195–201.

36. Vitale M, Amrit M, Arora R, et al. Gradenigos syndrome: a common infection with uncommon consequences. Am J Emerg Med 2017;35(9):1388.e1–2.

Imaging of Ménière Disease

Anja Bernaerts, MD*, Bert De Foer, MD, PhD

KEYWORDS

- MR imaging • Endolymphatic hydrops • Temporal bone disease • Ménière disease • Classification
- Diagnosis

KEY POINTS

- The delayed (4-hour) intravenous gadolinium-enhanced 3D FLAIR MR imaging technique is most frequently used and is able to detect and grade endolymphatic hydrops in patients with Ménière disease with a high sensitivity and specificity.
- The intratympanic gadolinium administrated MR imaging technique is also accurate but has the disadvantage of evaluating only one ear, of being invasive and an off-label use of gadolinium.
- The non-contrast MR imaging technique uses a coronal heavily T2-weighted sequence in which a saccular height greater than 1.6 mm is regarded as pathological.
- Using a 4-stage grading system for vestibular hydrops yields a higher sensitivity without loss of specificity, compared to the currently used 3-stage grading system.
- Cochlear and vestibular perilymphatic enhancement is more pronounced on the affected side in patients with Ménière disease.

INTRODUCTION

Ménière disease (MD) is a chronic disease with a reported estimated prevalence of 17 to 513 patients per 100,000.[1] It is characterized by spontaneous episodic attacks of vertigo, fluctuating low-frequency hearing loss, tinnitus, aural fullness and pressure with a progressive loss of audiovestibular functions.[1,2] More than 150 years ago, Prosper Ménière was the first to recognize the inner ear as the site of origin for this clinical syndrome,[3] instead of being attributed to "apoplectiform cerebral congestion." Hallpike and Cairns[4] pointed out the endolymphatic hydrops (EH) as the pathologic counterpart for MD. EH is a condition characterized by distension of the structures filled with endolymph. The cochlear duct, the saccule, the utricle and ampullae contain endolymph, and a change in the volume of these structures is tightly correlated with the symptoms of MD, as observed on temporal bone analysis.[5]

Anatomically, the endolymphatic space is normally the smallest component of the inner ear fluid compartments. Within the cochlea, the smaller scala media (or cochlear duct) occupies around 8% to 26% of the cochlear fluid spaces on MR imaging. It is surrounded by the perilymphatic space.[6]

Within the vestibule, endolymphatic spaces comprise the saccule and utricle occupying 20% to 41% of the fluid spaces on MR imaging, again enclosed by the larger perilymphatic compartment.[6]

The perilymph is similar in composition to extracellular fluid, but the endolymph is unique in that it has a higher concentration of potassium than sodium. The formation and homeostasis of the membranous labyrinth is not completely clear, but the endolymphatic sac seems to play a role in reabsorbing the endolymph.[6]

The causal relationship between EH and MD is not fully understood and seems to be complex.

Disclosure of Conflict of Interest: There are no potential conflicts of interest, relevant relationships, or financial interests to report regarding this article.
Department of Radiology, GZA Hospitals Antwerp, Oosterveldlaan 24, Wilrijk 2610, Belgium
* Corresponding author.
E-mail address: anja.bernaerts@gza.be

Neuroimag Clin N Am 29 (2019) 19–28
https://doi.org/10.1016/j.nic.2018.09.002

EH may result from a number of processes, such as viral infection, trauma, autoimmune disorders, and electrolyte imbalance.[6] Moreover, EH does not necessarily result in symptoms of MD, and EH is not present in all patients diagnosed with MD. For example, EH can also be found in patients with superior canal dehiscence and large vestibular aqueduct syndrome,[7] or in patients with sudden sensorineural hearing loss.[8,9] In the clinical literature, however, a strong correlation exists between the degree of MR imaging EH and impairment of hearing function and saccule function.[10,11] The diagnosis of MD is based on a combination of the patient's symptoms, and the results of the clinical examination and functional tests.

In 1995, the American Academy of Otolaryngology–Head and Neck Surgery established a specific set of criteria for the diagnosis of MD (Table 1).[12] In this classification, the disease is divided into certain (with postmortem histologic confirmation), definite, probable, and possible categories.

Recently, the classification committee of the Bárány society formulated simplified diagnostic criteria for MD, jointly with several national and international organizations[13] (Table 2). This proposed classification is similar to the American Academy of Otolaryngology–Head and Neck Surgery 1995 criteria; however, it includes only 2 categories: definite MD and probable MD. The diagnosis of definite MD is based on clinical criteria and requires the observation of an episodic vertigo syndrome associated with audiometrically documented low- to medium-frequency sensorineural hearing loss and fluctuating aural symptoms (hearing, tinnitus, and/or fullness) in the affected ear. The duration of the vertigo episodes is limited to a period between 20 minutes and 12 hours. Probable MD is a broader concept defined by episodic vestibular symptoms (vertigo or dizziness) associated with fluctuating aural symptoms occurring in a period from 20 minutes to 24 hours.

Recent developments of high-resolution MR imaging of the inner ear have now enabled us to visualize in vivo EH in patients with suspected MD. Imaging of EH mainly relies on the fact that contrast only penetrates the perilymphatic

---

Table 1
The 1995 American Academy of Otolaryngology–Head and Neck Surgery guidelines for diagnosis of Ménière disease

Certain	Definite Ménière's disease, plus histopathologic confirmation of hydrops
Definite	Two or more definitive spontaneous episodes of vertigo of ≥20 min Audiometrically documented hearing loss on ≥1 occasion Tinnitus or aural fullness in the treated ear Other causes excluded
Probable	One definitive episode of vertigo Audiometrically documented hearing loss on ≥1 occasion Tinnitus or aural fullness in the treated ear Other causes excluded
Possible	Episodic vertigo of the Ménière type without documented hearing loss or Sensorineural hearing loss, fluctuating or fixed, with disequilibrium but without definitive episodes Other causes excluded

From Committee on Hearing and Equilibrium. Committee on hearing and equilibrium guidelines for the diagnosis and evaluation of therapy in Ménière disease. American Academy of Otolaryngology - Head and Neck Foundation, Inc. Otolaryngol Head Neck Surg 1995;113(3):181–5.

Table 2
Amended 2015 criteria for diagnosis of Ménière disease

Definite	Two or more spontaneous episodes of vertigo, each lasting 20 min to 12 h Audiometrically documented low to midfrequency sensorineural hearing loss in 1 ear, defining the affected ear on ≥1 occasion before, during, or after 1 of the episodes of vertigo Fluctuating aural symptoms (hearing, tinnitus, or fullness) in the affected ear Not better accounted for by another vestibular diagnosis
Probable	Two or more episodes of vertigo or dizziness, each lasting 20 min to 24 h Fluctuating aural symptoms (hearing, tinnitus, or fullness) in the affected ear Not better accounted for by another vestibular diagnosis

From Goebel JA. 2015 equilibrium committee amendment to the 1995 AAO-HNS guidelines for the definition of Ménière's disease. Otolaryngol Head Neck Surg 2016;154(3):403–4.

compartment passing the blood–perilymph barrier, thus causing a negative contrast with the nonenhancing endolymphatic spaces (**Fig. 1**).

In this article, we discuss the different MR techniques that are able to detect and visualize EH. These techniques include a noncontrast technique using a heavily T2-weighted sequence and 2 contrast-enhanced techniques, the intratympanically administered gadolinium and the intravenously administered gadolinium technique.

MR IMAGING METHODS FOR THE VISUALIZATION OF ENDOLYMPHATIC HYDROPS

The data on the use of noncontrast MR imaging techniques in the evaluation of patients with MD in literature are limited. It has been reported a long time ago that the fluid-containing structures of the inner ears can be visualized using high-resolution 3-dimensional (3D) Fourier transform MR imaging sequences such as constructive interference in steady state.[14] So far, to the best of our knowledge, only 2 articles have documented and evaluated the saccule measurement on coronal reformations of either an axial high-resolution T2-weighted 3D fast imaging using steady-state acquisition[15] or a constructive interference in steady state sequence.[16] Both heavily T2-weighted sequences were performed on a 3T machine. Because this is a noncontrast technique, both works were able to include normal, healthy volunteers as a control group.

In this technique, the height and width of the saccule in the vestibule are measured in patients with definite MD and compared with the so-called normal ear in the MD patients as well as the normal control group in 1 study[16] and with the normal control group in the other work.[15] It is reported that, in patients with MD, the EH causes an augmentation of the height and width of the saccule. The saccule can be detected as a small, oval, hypointense lesion in the vestibule on a coronal reconstruction. Overall, the height of the saccule in patients with MD is reported to be greater than 1.6 mm (**Fig. 2**).

One of these papers[16] reports a high specificity but a low sensitivity using this technique. The advantage of this technique is that it requires no contrast administration. The disadvantage of this technique is that it only evaluates vestibular hydrops; cochlear hydrops is not evaluated with

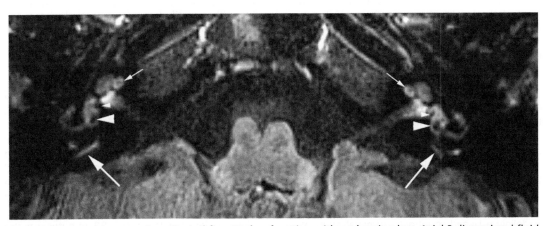

Fig. 1. A 48-year-old woman investigated for attacks of vertigo without hearing loss. Axial 3-dimensional fluid-attenuated inversion recovery (FLAIR) image of both ears 4 hours after intravenous administration of a double dose of gadolinium, at the level of the lower part of the vestibule. There is bilateral enhancement of the cochlea, the vestibule, the semicircular canals, and the internal auditory canal. Note that the enhancement of the membranous labyrinth can be regarded as symmetric. In the bilateral cochlea, the cochlear duct can be seen as a small hypointense line (*small arrows*). The cochlear duct is part of the endolymphatic space and does not enhance, in contrast with the surrounding enhancing perilymphatic space. There are no signs of a dilated cochlear duct, so there are no signs of a cochlear hydrops. In the bilateral vestibules, the saccule (*small arrowhead*) and utricle (*large arrowhead*) can nicely be discriminated. Both the saccule and utricle are part of the endolymphatic spaces and do not enhance, in contrast with the surrounding perilymphatic space. Note that the saccule is the smallest structure of both and is located anterior, inferior, and medial in the vestibule. There are no signs of vestibular hydrops. The vestibular aqueduct is visible on both sides with a symmetric enhancement (*large arrows*). This examination can be regarded as normal. There are no signs of a cochlear and/or vestibular hydrops. The enhancement of the membranous labyrinth as well as the vestibular aqueduct is symmetric. The enhancement in the fundus of the internal auditory canal is seen in all cases.

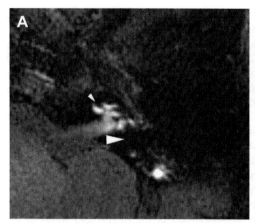 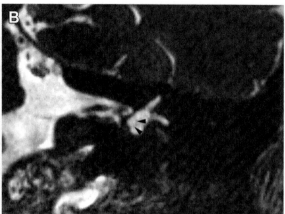

Fig. 2. (*A*) A 79-year-old man, clinically categorized based on the 2015 Bárány society criteria as definite Ménière disease. Cropped axial 3D FLAIR image of the left ear, 4 hours after intravenous administration of a double dose of gadolinium, at the level of the lower part of the vestibule. Note the complete fusion of the nonenhancing enlarged saccule and utricle without any surrounding residual contrast (*large arrowhead*), apart from some limited amount of contrast at the anterior and inferior delineation of the vestibule. The nonenhancing dilated saccule and utricle completely compress the enhancing perilymphatic space. No residual enhancing perilymphatic space can be seen in this case, confirming the presence of the highest grade of a vestibular endolymphatic hydrops grade 2 according to the 3-stage grading system by Baráth and colleagues.[21] In the cochlea, the dilated cochlear duct or scala media causes a complete obliteration of the scala vestibuli (*small arrowhead*), representing a cochlear endolymphatic hydrops grade 2. Note that there is also some enhancement in the fundus of the internal auditory canal. This is seen in all patients on delayed gadolinium enhanced 3D FLAIR imaging. The patient was treated with an endolymphatic sac decompression surgery. (*B*) The same patient as in (*A*). Coronal reformation of the left ear of a submillimeter 3D constructive interference in steady state (CISS) sequence, at the level of the internal auditory canal, and the vestibule. Anterior, inferior, and medially in the vestibule, a small linear hypointense line running in a craniocaudal direction can be seen (*arrowheads*) delineating the saccule. Measurement of the height of the saccule was 2.2 mm, compatible with a vestibular endolymphatic hydrops. The normal height of the saccule on a coronal reformation of a 3D CISS sequence is 1.6 mm according to Venkatasamy and colleagues[15] and Simon and associates.[16] Note that, with this technique, evaluation of the cochlea is not possible.

this technique. Moreover, the reliability and reproducibility of measuring such small anatomic structures remains to be confirmed.

The contrast-enhanced hydrops MR imaging essentially exist out of 2 different contrast techniques. The first technique consists of imaging of the membranous labyrinth after an intratympanically gadolinium-based contrast medium administration. The second technique uses an intravenous gadolinium-based contrast administration with subsequent delayed MR imaging.

The first application of intratympanic administration of gadolinium was done in guinea pigs in which it was demonstrated that intratympanically administrated gadolinium was shown to be distributed throughout the perilymphatic space of the labyrinth, whereas the endolymphatic compartment remained impermeable.[17] In the images obtained, the scala media (cochlear duct, endolymphatic space) was visualized as a filling defect. In 2007, Nakashima and colleagues[18] reported the clear visualization of EH in patients with MD by intratympanic injection of a

gadolinium-based contrast medium using a 3D fluid-attenuated inversion recovery (FLAIR) sequence on a 3T machine.[18]

In most studies, the tympanic membrane is punctured with a thin needle after applying local anesthetic with injection of a 8-fold diluted solution. Other studies used a 5-fold or a 16-fold dilution. The total amount of fluid injected varies between 0.3 and 0.6 mL. Patients are asked to lay still for about 30 minutes on the contralateral side. Scanning is typically performed after 24 hours.[19] It is said that intratympanic gadolinium disappears from the labyrinth after 6 to 7 days. The intratympanic administration of gadolinium is considered an off-label use of gadolinium.[19]

Intratympanically administered drugs are thought to be absorbed mainly through the round window membrane. Individual differences in the permeability of the round window membrane after intratympanic gadolinium administration have been reported.[19] Recently, absorption through the annular ligament of the oval window membrane has been suggested as an alternative route for intratympanically administrated drug distribution, although this route can be blocked by the significant EH in the vestibule.[19]

Compared with the intratympanic route of gadolinium administration, the intravenous administration has the advantage of being able to evaluate and compare both ears at the same time, independent of oval or round window permeability and allowing an assessment of the blood–perilymph barrier. Moreover, it is an approved use of gadolinium.[6,19]

Various protocols with standard single (0.2 mL/kg body with gadolinium diethylenetriamine penta-acetic acid [Gd-DTPA]), double dose and triple dose gadolinium administration have been described to demonstrate EH in the cochlea and vestibule of patients with MD.[6,19] In humans, intravenously injected gadolinium not only accumulates in the perilymphatic space, but also in the fluid in the anterior portion of the eye, the subarachnoid space surrounding the optic nerve, Meckel's cave, and the fundus of the internal auditory canal (see **Fig. 1**).[6,19]

Different time intervals after intravenously administrated gadolinium have also been tested. The time interval between the intravenous administration of gadolinium and imaging has been shown to influence the degree of perilymphatic enhancement, with a 4-hour delay resulting in a maximum contrast enhancement with the perilymph of both symptomatic and asymptomatic ears.[19]

A high-resolution MR imaging sequence with an as high as possible signal-to-noise ratio is required to demonstrate the lower concentration of gadolinium in the perilymph after intravenous injection as compared with intratympanic injection. To have the highest signal-to-noise ratio and to optimize the image quality, a 3T magnet is required with a dedicated head coil and a high number of receive channels. Initially, an optimized 3D FLAIR sequence with inversion-recovery turbo spin echo was used, but also heavily T2-weighted 3D FLAIR sequences were used. Most of these sequences are long so patient immobilization to avoid motion degradation is crucial.[6,19]

Various techniques have been described to enhance the visualization of either the perilymphatic or the endolymphatic compartment and to suppress the signal of surrounding structures such as bone and air. Positive perilymph or positive endolymph images can be acquired by varying the inversion time of the 3D FLAIR sequence. For example, by shortening the inversion time of the 3D FLAIR, the signal of the perilymph is suppressed, increasing the signal from the endolymph while the signal from the surrounding bone and air remains low.[6,19] These sequences could then be visually compared with high-resolution heavily T2-weighted cisternographic sequences. Naganawa and colleagues[19] developed a series of sequences and postprocessing techniques for MR imaging in patients with MD. For example, a subtraction of a positive endolymph image from a positive perilymph image was termed a HYDROPS image (hybrid of the reversed image of the positive endolymphatic signal and native image of the positive perilymph signal), demonstrating anatomic information of the various inner ear compartments in one image series. However, such postprocessing to decrease temporal bone signal is not necessarily required, and less time-consuming 3D FLAIR–based techniques have also proven to be successful.[6,19]

DIAGNOSTIC IMAGING CRITERIA FOR MÉNIÈRE'S DISEASE

Various semiquantitative grading criteria have been proposed. Nakashima and colleagues[20] divided EH grades into none, mild, and significant. Cochlear hydrops was observed as a dilated scala media with mild cochlear hydrops being reported when the scala media remained smaller than the compressed scala vestibuli and significant cochlear hydrops being reported when the scala media was larger than the scala vestibuli.

The ratio of the endolymphatic space was compared with the whole vestibular fluid space with mild vestibular hydrops being defined as a ratio of 34% to 50% and severe vestibular hydrops being greater than 50% of the vestibule.[20]

Baráth and colleagues[21] defined the normal study as a barely visible nonenhancing cochlear duct in the enhancing scala vestibuli and scala tympani (**Fig. 3**). Grade 1 cochlear hydrops is defined as mild dilation of the nonenhancing cochlear duct into the scala vestibuli with partial obstruction of the scala vestibuli (**Fig. 4**). In grade 2 cochlear hydrops, the scala vestibuli is uniformly obstructed by the maximally distended cochlear duct (**Fig. 5**).[21]

In the vestibule—in normal cases—one can clearly discriminate the nonenhancing saccule and utricle in the enhancing vestibule. The saccule is the smallest of both structures and is located anterior, inferior, and medial in the vestibule (see **Fig. 1**; **Fig. 6**). A grade 1 vestibular hydrops presents as a distention of the endolymphatic space of the saccule or utricle or both, with the enhancing perilymphatic space still visible along the periphery of the bony vestibule (**Fig. 7**). In a grade 2 vestibular hydrops, the saccule

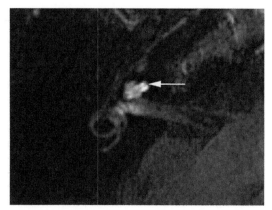

Fig. 3. A 63-year-old man investigated for vertigo, gait instability, and hearing loss, clinically confined to the right ear. Cropped axial 3D FLAIR image of the right ear, 4 hours after intravenous administration of a double dose of gadolinium, at the level of the mid turn of the cochlea. Note the clear delineation of the enhancing scala vestibuli and scala tympani (perilymphatic space) in between the nonenhancing cochlear duct or scala media (endolymphatic space), which can be seen as a very thin, hypointense line (*arrow*). These are normal findings. There is no cochlear hydrops. Compare with Figs. 4 and 5.

diseased ears had EH on MR imaging, whereas 78% of the clinically normal ears had no EH on MR imaging. However, 22% of clinically normal ears showed EH on MR imaging and 10% of ears with a clinical diagnosis of MD did not show EH.[21]

Other classification systems exist and comparing all these grading systems with each other remains difficult. For example, compared with the Nakashima classification,[20] the Baráth classification[21] apparently has a higher threshold as the Baráth mild classification seems to equal the Nakashima significant grade.

In a more recent study, the semiquantitative grading systems were questioned; the authors noted that saccular abnormalities were much more common than those of the utricle on temporal bone sections. They proposed the inversion of the saccule to utricle ratio (SURI) on an oblique sagittal section as a marker of EH. The saccule to utricle inversion was only found in patients with MD (50%) and was felt to be a more reliable approach than conventional semiquantitative methods for distinguishing subjects with MD from healthy subjects.[22] However, in this classification system, only vestibular hydrops is evaluated and it is more elaborate than visual semiquantitative assessment because it requires the acquisition of oblique sagittal reconstructions.

Our own date from a recent study (Bernaerts A, Vanspauwen R, Blaivie C, et al. Delayed intravenous contrast-enhanced 3D FLAIR MR

and utricle are extremely distended without any visible surrounding enhancing perilymphatic space (Fig. 8).[21]

By using this technique and classification, Baráth and colleagues[21] found a high interobserver agreement. Ninety percent of clinically

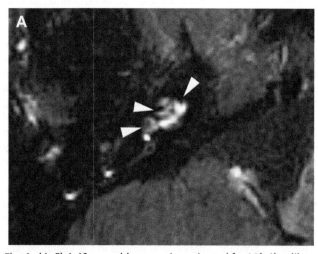

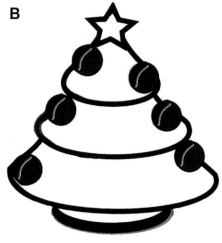

Fig. 4. (*A, B*) A 46-year-old woman investigated for Ménière-like symptoms confined to the right ear. (*A*) Cropped axial 3D FLAIR image of the right ear, 4 hours after intravenous administration of a double dose of gadolinium, at the level of the mid turn of the cochlea. The nonenhancing dilated cochlear duct (*arrowheads*) can be seen as a small nonenhancing nodule bulging into the enhancing scala vestibuli. Cochlear hydrops grade 1. There remains some enhancing scala vestibuli visible. Compare with Figs. 3 and 5. The image in (*A*) can be compared to a X-mass tree (the enhancing scala vestibuli and scala tympani) with X-mass balls (the nodular enlarged nonenhancing scala media or cochlear duct) in it.

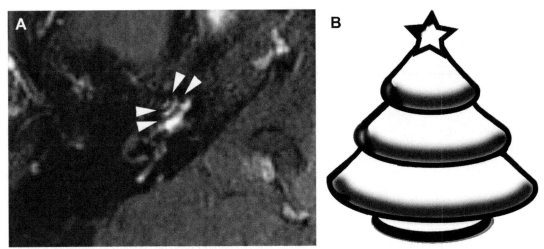

Fig. 5. (*A, B*) A 53-year-old woman with known right-sided definite Ménière disease according to the 2015 Bárány society criteria. (*A*) Cropped axial 3D FLAIR image of the right ear, 4 hours after intravenous administration of a double dose of gadolinium, at the level of the mid turn of the cochlea. The enlarged scala media or cochlear duct is completely pushing away the scala vestibuli and can be seen as bandlike hypointensities (*arrowheads*) in the mid and apical turn of the cochlea. Compare with **Figs. 3** and **4**. The image in (*A*) can be compared to a X-mass tree (the enhancing scala vestibuli) with X-mass garlands (the linear enlarged nonenhancing scala media or cochlear duct) in it.

imaging in patients with Ménières's disease: new diagnostic criteria. Submitted for publication) with delayed gadolinium enhanced 3D FLAIR MR imaging in 148 patients (296 ears) also confirms that adding an extra low-grade vestibular hydrops to the Baráth classification, in which the saccule –normally the smallest of the 2 vestibular sacs- has become equal or larger than the utricle -but not yet confluent-

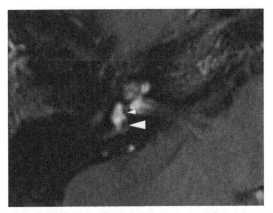

Fig. 6. A 58-year-old woman investigated for vertigo and dizziness. She had no hearing loss. Cropped axial 3D FLAIR image of the right ear, 4 hours after intravenous administration of a double dose of gadolinium, at the level of the lower part of the vestibule. The saccule (*small arrowhead*) and utricle (*large arrowhead*) can nicely be discriminated. Note that the saccule is the smallest structure and is located anterior, inferior, and medial in the vestibule. There are no signs of a vestibular hydrops. The saccule and utricle are filled with endolymph and do not enhance. This property makes them clearly visible against the background of the enhancing perilymphatic space in the vestibule. These are considered normal findings.

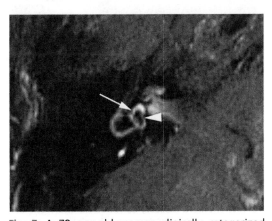

Fig. 7. A 78-year-old woman clinically categorized based on the 2015 Bárány society criteria as having definite Ménière disease confined to the right ear. Cropped axial 3D FLAIR image of the right ear, 4 hours after intravenous administration of a double dose of gadolinium, at the level of the lower part of the vestibule. Note the enlargement of the saccule and utricle (*arrowhead*), which have become confluent but still are surrounded by perilymphatic contrast enhancement (*arrow*). According to the Baráth classification (3-stage grading system), this is a grade 1 vestibular hydrops. However, using our 4-stage grading system, this is a grade 2 vestibular hydrops.

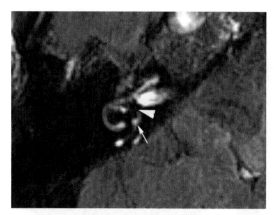

Fig. 8. A 53-year-old woman with known right-sided definite Ménière disease according to the 2015 Bárány society criteria. Same patient as in Fig. 5. Cropped axial 3D FLAIR image of the right ear, 4 hours after intravenous administration of a double dose of gadolinium, at the level of vestibule. Note the enlargement of saccule and utricle which are confluent, without any surrounding contrast (*arrowhead*). There is only some contrast visible in the base of the posterior semicircular canal (*arrow*). In the Baráth classification—using the 3-stage grading system—this is considered a grade 2 vestibular hydrops. Using our 4-stage grading system, this is a grade 3 vestibular hydrops.

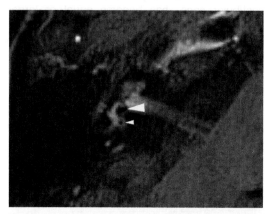

Fig. 9. A 49-year-old woman clinically categorized based on the 2015 Bárány society criteria as having definite Ménière disease, confined to the right ear. Cropped axial 3D FLAIR image of the right ear, 4 hours after intravenous administration of a double dose of gadolinium at the level of the lower part of the vestibule. Note the enlargement of the saccule (*large arrowhead*) compared with the utricle (*small arrowhead*). Normally, the saccule is the smallest of the 2 structures in the vestibule. In this patient, the saccule is enlarged but not yet touching the utricle. In the Baráth classification—using the 3-stage grading system—this finding is regarded as normal. However, this finding should be regarded -according to our study- as a mild form of vestibular hydrops and should be considered abnormal: vestibular hydrops grade 1 in our 4-stage grading system.

significantly increases the sensitivity without loss of specificity for the diagnosis of definite MD (Figs. 9 and 10). By adding this extra low-grade vestibular hydrops, the classification for vestibular hydrops goes from a 3-stage grading system[21] to a 4-stage grading system, resulting in a higher accuracy of MR imaging in detecting MD (see Fig. 10). It should be stressed that the evaluation of vestibular hydrops has to be performed on the most caudal slice through the vestibule because the saccule is located anterior, inferior, and medial in the vestibule (see Figs. 6–10).

Our data indicate that further large-scale studies with correlation to clinical and other technical investigations are required to fine tune the MR imaging grading system in patients with MD to come to a more accurate classification system in optimal correlation with clinical findings and other technical investigations in patients with MD.[20–23]

EH has also been reported in the so-called normal ear of patients with MD. Reported numbers vary from 10%[23] to 22%.[21] Probably, this is related to the fact that MD is part of a continuous spectrum with various patterns of disease evolution and progression. These figures could also correlate with the reported incidence of 35% of patients who develop bilaterality of the condition within 10 years after onset of the disease.[23]

It has already been described that the disruption of the blood–perilymph barrier results in an asymmetrical enhancement of the membranous labyrinth in patients with MD.[21,24,25] The enhancement in patients with MD is reported to be more pronounced on the affected side.[21] Our study confirms this asymmetrical perilymphatic enhancement in patients with MD (Fig. 11). Moreover, our data show that adding this perilymphatic enhancement criterion to the EH criteria augments the specificity while maintaining the sensitivity.

A clinical diagnosis of MD is often difficult due to its varying and fluctuating symptoms. The increasing number of publications on delayed gadolinium-enhanced 3D FLAIR in the radiologic literature illustrates the increasing role of the application of this specific MR imaging technique in the diagnosis of patients with MD. Although the MR imaging demonstration and grading of EH does not feature in current clinical diagnostic criteria, it is likely that further technological developments and validation of this technique will result in it becoming a useful diagnostic tool, which probably will influence therapeutic decisions and the evaluation of therapeutic success in MD.

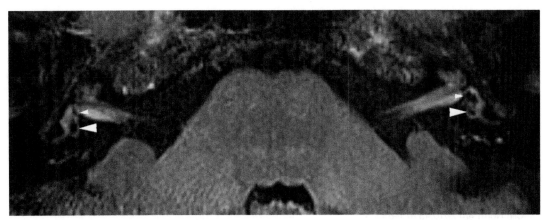

Fig. 10. A 67-year-old woman clinically categorized based on the 2015 Bárány society criteria as probable Ménière disease, confined to the left ear. Axial 3D FLAIR image of both ears, 4 hours after intravenous administration of a double dose of gadolinium at the level of the lower part of the vestibule. On the right side, the saccule (*small arrowhead*) and the utricle (*large arrowhead*) can be separately discriminated. The saccule is located anterior to the utricle and is the smallest of the 2 structures in the vestibule; this finding is normal. On the left side, the saccule (*small arrowhead*) is enlarged and is bigger than the utricle (*large arrowhead*). Note, however, that the saccule and utricle are not yet confluent. In the Baráth classification—using the 3-stage grading system—this finding is regarded as normal. However, this finding should be regarded -according to our study- as a mild form of vestibular hydrops and should be considered abnormal: vestibular hydrops grade 1 in our 4-stage grading system. Compare the abnormal vestibular hydrops grade 1 on the left side with the normal situation on the right side.

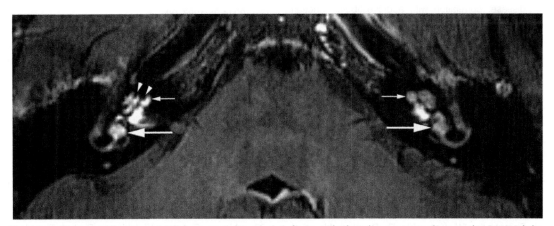

Fig. 11. A 51-year-old woman with known right-sided definite Ménière disease according to the 2015 Bárány society criteria. Axial 3D FLAIR image of both ears, 4 hours after intravenous administration of a double dose of gadolinium at the level of the vestibule. There is enlargement of the scala media/cochlear duct in the right ear (*arrowheads*) bulging into the scala vestibuli: cochlear hydrops grade 1. Note that the perilymphatic enhancement of the cochlea (*small arrows*) is more pronounced on the right side compared with the left side. Although there are no signs of vestibular hydrops—the saccule and utricle still can be discriminated separately—the perilymphatic enhancement of the vestibule (*large arrows*) is also more pronounced on the right side than on the left side. The more pronounced enhancement of the perilymphatic spaces on the affected side of patients with Ménière disease can be regarded - according to our study- as highly sensitive and specific for Ménière disease. It is caused by disturbance of the blood–perilymph barrier.

REFERENCES

1. Nakashima T, Pyykkö I, Arroll MA, et al. Menière's disease [review]. Nat Rev Dis Primers 2016;2:16028.
2. Sajjadi H, Paparella MM. Meniere's disease. Lancet 2008;372:406–14.
3. Menière P. Maladies de l'oreille interne offrant des symptomes de la congestion cerebral apoplecti-forme. Gaz Med (Paris) 1861;16:88.
4. Hallpike CS, Cairns H. Observations on the pathology of Ménière's syndrome: (section of otology). Proc R Soc Med 1938;31:1317–36.
5. Salt AN, Plontke SK. Endolymphatic hydrops: pathophysiology and experimental models. Otolaryngol Clin North Am 2010;43:971–83.
6. Lingam RK, Connor SEJ, Casselman JW, et al. MRI in otology: applications in cholesteatoma and Ménière's disease. Clin Radiol 2018;73:35–44.
7. Sone M, Yoshida T, Morimoto K, et al. Endolymphatic hydrops in Superior canal dehiscence and large vestibular aqueduct syndromes. Laryngoscope 2016;126:1446–50.
8. Okazaki Y, Yoshida T, Sugimoto S, et al. Significance of endolymphatic hydrops in ears with unilateral sensorineural hearing loss. Otol Neurotol 2017;38:1076–80.
9. Attyé A, Eliezer M, Medici M, et al. In vivo imaging of saccular hydrops in humans reflects sensorineural hearing loss rather than Menière's disease symptoms. Eur Radiol 2018;28:2916–22.
10. Gürkov R, Flatz W, Louza J, et al. In vivo visualization of endolymphatic hydrops in patients with Menière's disease: correlation with audiovestibular function. Eur Arch Otorhinolaryngol 2011;268:1743–8.
11. Gürkov R, Flatz W, Louza J, et al. In vivo visualized endolymphatic hydrops and inner ear functions in patients with electrocochleographically confirmed Menière's disease. Otol Neurotol 2012;33:1040–5.
12. AAO – HNS Committee on hearing and equilibrium guidelines for the diagnosis and evaluation of therapy in Menière's disease. American Academy of Otolaryngology – Head and Neck Foundation, Inc. Otolagynol Head Neck Surg 1995;113:181–5.
13. Lopez-Escamez JA, Carey J, Chung WH, et al. Diagnostic criteria for Menière's disease. J Vestib Res 2015;25.
14. Casselman JW, Kuhweide R, Deimling M, et al. Constructive interference in steady state-3DFT MR imaging of the inner ear and cerebellopontine angle. AJNR Am J Neuroradiol 1993;14:59–69.
15. Venkatasamy A, Veillon F, Fleury A, et al. Imaging of the saccule for the diagnosis of endolymphatic hydrops in Meniere disease, using a three-dimensional T2-weighted steady state free precession sequence: accurate, fast, and without contrast material intravenous injection. Eur Radiol Exp 2017;1:14.
16. Simon F, Guichard JP, Kania R, et al. Saccular measurements in routine MRI can predict hydrops in Menière's disease. Eur Arch Otorhinolaryngol 2017;274:4113–20.
17. Zou J, Pyykö I, Bretlay P, et al. In vivo visualization of endolymphatic hydrops in guinea pigs: magnetic resonance imaging evaluation at 4.7 tesla. Ann Otol Rhinol Laryngol 2003;112:1059–65.
18. Nakashima T, Naganawa S, Sugiura M, et al. Visualization of endolymphatic hydrops in patients with Menière's disease. Laryngoscope 2007;117:415–20.
19. Naganawa S, Nakashima T. Visualization of endolymphatic hydrops with MR imaging in patients with Ménière's disease and related pathologies: current status of its methods and clinical significance. Jpn J Radiol 2014;32:191–204.
20. Nakashima T, Naganawa S, Pyykö I, et al. Grading of endolymphatic hydrops using magnetic resonance imaging. Acta Otolaryngol Suppl 2009;560:5–8.
21. Baráth K, Schuknecht B, Naldi AM, et al. Detection and grading of endolymphatic hydrops in Meniere disease using MR imaging. AJNR Am J Neuroradiol 2014;35:1387–92.
22. Attyé A, Eliezer M, Boudiaf N, et al. MRI of endolymphatic hydrops in patients with Menière's disease: a case-controlled study with a simplified classification based upon saccular morphology. Eur Radiol 2017;27:3138–46.
23. Huppert D, Strupp M, Brandt T. Long-term course of Menière's disease revisited. Acta Otolaryngol 2010;130:644–51.
24. Pakdaman MN, Ishiyama G, Ishiyama A, et al. Blood-Labyrinth barrier permeability in Menière disease and idiopathic sudden sensorineural hearing loss: findings on delayed postcontrast 3D-FLAIR MRI. AJNR Am J Neuroradiol 2016;37:1903–8.
25. Ishiyama G, Lopez IZ, Ishiyama P, et al. The blood labyrinthine barrier in the human normal and Menière's disease macula utriculi. Sci Rep 2017;7(1):253.

Otosclerosis and Dysplasias of the Temporal Bone

Vanesa Carlota Andreu-Arasa, MD, PhD[a],
Edward K. Sung, MD[a], Akifumi Fujita, MD, PhD[b],
Naoko Saito, MD, PhD[c], Osamu Sakai, MD, PhD[a,d,e,*]

KEYWORDS

- Bone dysplasia - Otosclerosis - Fibrous dysplasia - Paget disease - Osteogenesis imperfecta
- Osteopetrosis

KEY POINTS

- Otosclerosis is a bone disorder that results in abnormal bone remodeling with areas of demineralization and dense bone replacement adjacent to the oval window (fenestral otosclerosis) and/or more extensive involvement of the otic capsule (retrofenestral/cochlear otosclerosis).
- Fibrous dysplasia is a congenital disorder that results in marrow fibrosis, abnormal matrix production, and stimulation of osteoclastic reabsorption.
- Paget disease is a chronic disorder characterized by excessive bone formation by osteoclasts, with an early osteolytic stage, an intermediate stage with reabsorption and sclerosis, and a late sclerotic stage.
- Osteogenesis imperfecta is caused by an error in collagen formation that manifests in the temporal bone, with proliferation of undermineralized, thickened bone and microfractures, and shares similar temporal bone imaging findings with otosclerosis.
- Osteopetrosis is characterized by decreased osteoclast activity, resulting in defective bone reabsorption leading to thick and dense bones.

INTRODUCTION

Numerous bone diseases and dysplasias may affect the temporal bone, resulting in auditory and/or vestibular dysfunction. Otosclerosis only involves the temporal bone, whereas other dysplasias may affect other areas of the body. Depending on the affected region, patients may present with conductive, sensorineural, or mixed hearing loss, or neuropathies from cranial nerve compression, which can have tremendous impact on quality of life.

High-resolution computed tomography (CT) is sensitive for detecting subtle osseous changes, making it the initial imaging modality of choice,

[a] Department of Radiology, Boston Medical Center, Boston University School of Medicine, 820 Harrison Avenue, FGH 3rd Floor, Boston, MA 02118, USA; [b] Department of Radiology, Jichi Medical University, School of Medicine, 3311-1 Yakushiji, Shimotsuke, Tochigi 329-0498, Japan; [c] Department of Radiology, Saitama International Medical Center, Saitama Medical University, 1397-1 Yamane, Hidaka, Saitama 350-1298, Japan; [d] Department of Otolaryngology–Head and Neck Surgery, Boston Medical Center, Boston University School of Medicine, 820 Harrison Avenue, FGH 3rd Floor, Boston, MA 02118, USA; [e] Department of Radiation Oncology, Boston Medical Center, Boston University School of Medicine, 820 Harrison Avenue, FGH 3rd Floor, Boston, MA 02118, USA
* Corresponding author. Department of Radiology, Boston Medical Center, Boston University School of Medicine, 820 Harrison Avenue, FGH 3rd Floor, Boston, MA 02118.
E-mail address: osamu.sakai@bmc.org

Neuroimag Clin N Am 29 (2019) 29–47
https://doi.org/10.1016/j.nic.2018.09.004
1052-5149/19/© 2018 Elsevier Inc. All rights reserved.

whereas MR imaging is useful to assess the membranous labyrinth and bone marrow to evaluate vascularity or activity of the disease, and for potential cranial nerve involvement.

OTOSCLEROSIS

Otosclerosis or otospongiosis is a multifactorial bone disorder, with genetic and environmental causes, that results in abnormal bone remodeling and reabsorption, new bone deposition, and vascular proliferation.[1] Typical presentation is within the second to fourth decades of life. Otosclerosis more frequently affects white persons and women, and is bilateral in 80% to 85% of cases.[2] Clinical prevalence of otosclerosis is estimated to be 0.3% to 0.4%, although histologic otosclerosis is significantly higher at 2.5% to 12%.[1]

Pathology

The temporal bone uniquely has persistence of the primary endochondral (nonlamellar) bone that forms the middle layer of the otic capsule, between the inner endosteal layer and outer periosteal layer. This middle layer is partly calcified in the near-term fetus but is rapidly replaced by bone. Endochondral ossification progresses around the otic capsule, occurring last in the region of the fissula ante fenestram; thus, this site is most predisposed to contain persistent fibrocartilage even into adulthood. In otosclerosis, there is an otospongiotic phase where the lamellar bone around the vessels of the otic capsule is resorbed, creating perivascular spaces, which become filled with osteoclasts. Subsequently, new bone is deposited, larger in volume than the initially resorbed portion, which is converted into lamellar bone.[1]

The most common area of involvement in otosclerosis is the fissula ante fenestram, anteromedial to the oval window, which is an embryologic remnant of embryonic cartilage and connective tissue that runs from the oval window to the cochleariform process where the tensor tympani tendon turns laterally toward the malleus. Otosclerosis may also involve the rest of the otic capsule in 49% to 60%, the round window niche in 30%, and the stapes footplate in 12% to 15% of cases.[1]

Clinical Presentation

Conductive hearing loss (CHL) is almost always present, and there may be mixed hearing loss (MHL) with a sensorineural component depending on location and extent of disease, whereas isolated sensorineural hearing loss (SNHL) is extremely rare. The clinical findings of fenestral otosclerosis are characteristic, including progressive CHL up to about 50 to 60 dB, absence of stapedial reflexes, normal tympanic membrane, and no evidence of middle ear inflammation. At otoscopic inspection, the promontory may have a faint pink tinge corresponding to the prominent vascularity of the disease, the so-called Schwartze sign.[3] In the presence of these clinical findings, imaging may not be necessary to make the diagnosis of otosclerosis. However, superior semicircular canal bone dehiscence may mimic otosclerosis clinically,[4] in which case CT imaging can help to differentiate between these two entities.

The clinical diagnosis of otosclerosis may be challenging when the patient presents with SNHL or MHL secondary to cochlear or retrofenestral involvement. The mechanism of SNHL is not well understood, but could be caused by involvement of the cochlear endosteum and spiral ligament, with release of proteolytic enzymes that cause hyalinization by collagen deposition.[5]

Diagnostic Imaging

The role of imaging is to confirm the clinical diagnosis, assess the extent of disease, and exclude other conditions that may have similar clinical findings. High-resolution CT is the modality of choice, which can detect subtle bone findings. Previous large cohort studies have shown excellent correlation between the degree of hearing loss and the severity of CT imaging findings.[6] Recently, cone-beam CT has gained popularity, theoretically providing higher spatial resolution with lower radiation dose, with reports of good correlation to intraoperative findings.[7] Techniques using thin axial sections of 0.5 to 0.625 mm and overlapped reconstructions with coronal and oblique reformats are helpful to localize subtle demineralization and evaluate the oval window, stapes footplate, and round window niche.

Various CT grading systems have been proposed. Symons and Fanning have recently published a CT grading system with correlation to implant performance: grade 1, solely fenestral with either spongiotic or sclerotic lesions; grade 2, patchy localized cochlear disease (with or without fenestral involvement) to the basal cochlear turn (grade 2A), middle/apical turns (grade 2B), or both (grade 2C); and grade 3, diffuse confluent cochlear involvement. This grading system has excellent interobserver and intraobserver agreement.[5]

MR imaging with high-resolution temporal bone sequences is useful to assess the membranous labyrinth and bone marrow to evaluate vascularity or activity of the disease,[3] and for potential cranial nerve involvement. Assessment of the membranous labyrinth is particularly important before placement of a cochlear implant.

Fenestral otosclerosis
Demineralization typically occurs in the area of the fissula ante fenestram, just anteromedial to the oval window (**Fig. 1**). The cochlear promontory, round window niche, and facial nerve canal may also be involved. The disease may extend to involve the entire footplate of the stapes and the annular ligament, which can lead to mechanical fixation of the stapedovestibular joint, resulting in CHL (**Fig. 2**). Complete obliteration of the oval window occurs in 2% of cases (**Fig. 3**), and may be associated with secondary torsional subluxation of the incus. Otosclerosis may also present as isolated round window involvement.[2]

Early disease is visualized as a small area of demineralization anteromedial to the oval window that represents spongiotic bone replacing the normal dense bone. Other areas of the otic capsule should be carefully evaluated to assess the extent of disease. Some authors have found correlation between the location and size of the demineralized focus and the degree of CHL.[2] With more pronounced disease, proliferation of the demineralized bone is seen, which narrows the oval window, and thickens and fixes the stapes footplate. Furthermore, obliteration of the round window niche may occur (**Fig. 4**). If this occurs, stapes surgery is likely to be less successful and hearing improvement may be minimal.[3]

Nonactive mature otosclerosis manifests as sclerotic foci approaching the same density as the rest of the otic capsule. Irregular outline of the capsule with endosteal and periosteal scalloping may be noted as an indirect finding. Nonactive, mature otosclerotic changes of the oval window margins and within the staples footplate are more easily identified, seen as complete obliteration of the oval window, referred to as obliterative fenestral otosclerosis. This has been classified into three types: type 1, massive thickening of the entire footplate that fills the oval window niche; type 2, bony overgrowth at the margins of the oval window; and type 3, combination of footplate thickening and marginal overgrowth.[3]

The round window is a particularly important region to scrutinize, because disease in this location is subtle.[8] Ossicular integrity should also be assessed and reported, to help increase the success of surgery. Although uncommon, lateral ossicular fixation may be seen in otosclerosis, which manifests as a bony web between the malleus or incus and the attic wall.[3] Involvement of the facial nerve canal should also be evaluated, because bone dehiscence with exposure of the facial nerve may complicate surgery. Because of the high incidence of bilateral disease, the contralateral temporal bone should also be carefully evaluated, even in the absence of symptoms. MR imaging is not the routine modality used for diagnosing fenestral otosclerosis, but can identify foci of enhancement within the areas of demineralization, indicative of active disease (**Fig. 5**).

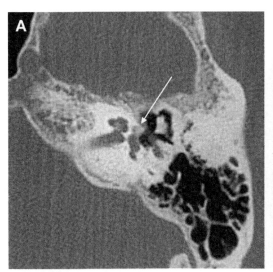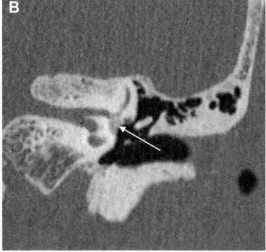

Fig. 1. Fenestral otosclerosis in a 66-year-old woman with conductive hearing loss. Axial (*A*) and coronal (*B*) CT images demonstrate a small area of demineralization anterior to the footplate of the stapes, in the region of fissula ante fenestram (*arrows*).

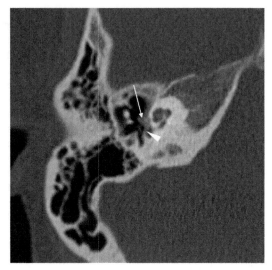

Fig. 2. Fenestral otosclerosis in a 41-year-old woman with conductive hearing loss. Axial CT image demonstrates a small area of demineralization in the region of the fissula ante fenestram with proliferation of demineralized bone (*arrow*) resulting in impingement and thickening of the stapes footplate (*arrowhead*).

Cochlear (retrofenestral or labyrinthine) otosclerosis

Cochlear otosclerosis is less common, and is nearly always seen in conjunction with fenestral otosclerosis.[2] Patients normally present with MHL, and sometimes with pulsatile tinnitus.

Demineralized spongiotic vascular bone appears around the cochlear capsule, and may extend around the vestibule, semicircular canals, and internal auditory canal (IAC). Involvement of the cochlear endosteum and spiral ligament may lead to release of proteolytic enzymes as the possible cause of SNHL. There may be correlation between the area of involvement (apical vs basal turn) and the type of frequency loss in SNHL (low vs high frequency, respectively). Some authors associate the extent of the disease with the early versus late onset and severity of the SNHL.[2]

CT findings in cochlear otosclerosis are usually much less subtle than in fenestral otosclerosis, with extensive demineralization seen around the cochlea in a ring-like fashion, referred to as the "double ring" or "fourth ring of Valvassori" (**Figs. 6** and **7**).[2] It may abut the lumen of the labyrinth or be separated from it by normal or sclerotic bone. A cavitary lucency anterior to and extending up to the IAC may be seen (**Fig. 8**).[9] Typical findings from fenestral otosclerosis are also almost always present concurrently. The chronic or sclerotic phase may not show any manifestation on CT other than a subtle periosteal thickening, because lesions undergo remineralization and may become indistinguishable from normal otic capsule bone.

MR imaging may demonstrate a ring of perichlear and perilabyrinthine intermediate signal on T1- and T2-weighted images, and enhancement in the active phase caused by contrast pooling in the numerous blood vessels found in active otospongiotic foci (see **Figs. 7** and **8**).[3] Enhancement of otospongiotic lesions correlates with the demineralized areas on CT. In some locations

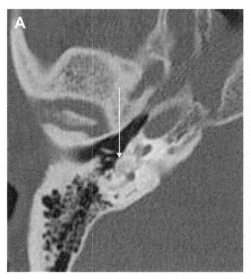

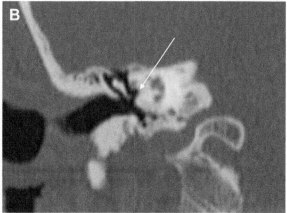

Fig. 3. Fenestral otosclerosis with oval window obliteration in a 66-year-old woman with bilateral conductive hearing loss. Axial (*A*) and coronal (*B*) CT images show an area of mature otosclerosis appearing as a large sclerotic focus, causing obliteration of the oval window (*arrows*).

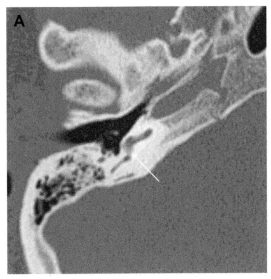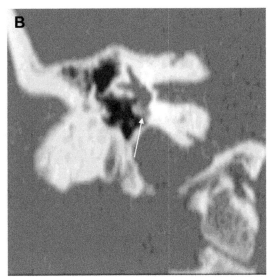

Fig. 4. Fenestral otosclerosis with round window obliteration in a 32-year-old woman with profound conductive hearing loss. Axial (*A*) and coronal (*B*) CT images demonstrate prominent overgrowth of the demineralized otosclerotic focus obstructing the round niche (*arrows*).

where partial volume averaging can present diagnostic challenges on CT (eg, the lateral wall of the labyrinth), MR imaging may show findings better than CT.[10] MR imaging is also useful for assessment of the membranous labyrinth before cochlear implant surgery,[11] where loss of the normal high signal on T2-weighted images may indicate fibrosis or bone deposition.

Treatment

Otosclerosis is treated medically with fluorides, which may prevent or arrest hearing loss by limiting bony changes.[12] Treatment with third-generation bisphosphonates has been recently shown to stabilize or prevent progression in otosclerosis-related SNHL.[13]

Surgical management is the mainstay treatment of fenestral otosclerosis, including stapedectomy (removal of stapes) or stapedotomy (footplate fenestration) usually combined with placement of a stapes prosthesis to restore ossicular chain continuity (**Figs. 9** and **10**). Successful surgical correction of CHL is achieved in up to 94.2% of patients.[14] Oval window narrowing with less than 1.4-mm height is associated with increased risk of technical difficulties at surgery.[15]

Severe complications from stapedial surgery, such as displacement of the prosthesis, perilymphatic fistula, labyrinthitis, or reparative granulomas extending into the vestibule, range from 0.2% to 3%.[16] CT can evaluate the integrity and positioning of the prosthesis, ossicular

necrosis, or resorption,[17] and the presence of air in the vestibule; whereas MR imaging can evaluate for fibrotic changes and granulation tissue.

Recurrent or persistent CHL after stapes surgery occurs in up to 5.8% of cases,[14] usually a result of prosthesis migration or dislocation (**Figs. 11** and **12**).[18] The "lateralized piston syndrome" is characterized by lateral piston extrusion out of the oval window, and is associated with incus necrosis caused by pressure on the incus.[19]

Cochlear implantation may be complicated by cochlear ossification. A high proportion of patients with cochlear implants may experience facial nerve stimulation by the distal electrodes,[20] thought to be caused by reduced electrical resistance of otospongiotic bone located between the cochlea and the facial nerve canal. Postoperative evaluation of the cochlear implant is performed with radiographs or CT, with a recent study showing that cone-beam CT is comparable to conventional CT in localization of the electrodes with lower radiation.[21]

Differential Diagnosis

Fenestral otosclerosis has a limited differential diagnosis. A cochlear cleft is a small nonosseous space in the otic capsule commonly seen in children, which is mistaken for fenestral otosclerosis (**Fig. 13**). Tympanosclerosis with fixation of the stapes footplate as a sequelae of chronic otitis media may present clinically with CHL similar

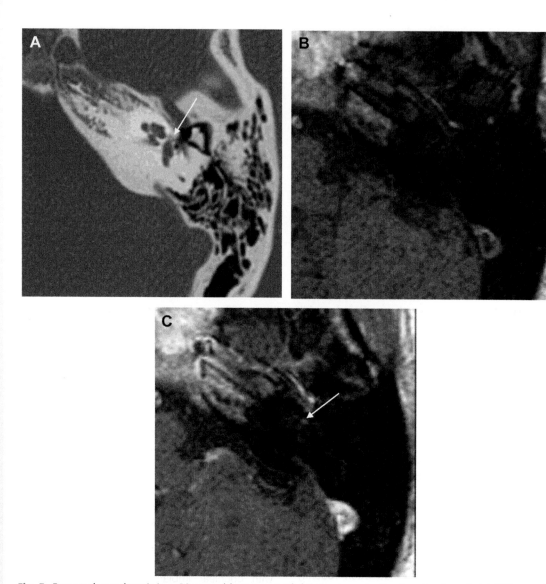

Fig. 5. Fenestral otosclerosis in a 29-year-old woman with bilateral conductive hearing loss. Axial CT image (*A*) demonstrates a focus of demineralization anterior to the footplate of the stapes, in the region of fissula ante fenestram (*arrow*). Axial precontrast (*B*) and postcontrast (*C*) T1-weighted MR images demonstrate a focus of enhancement corresponding to the area of demineralization on CT (*arrow*).

to otosclerosis, but is differentiated on CT. Osteogenesis imperfecta (OI) may demonstrate findings similar to fenestral otosclerosis.

The primary differential diagnosis of cochlear otosclerosis is OI caused by the nearly identical presentation, but OI often demonstrates more extensive demineralization along the otic capsule. Paget disease (PD), ankylosing spondylitis, rheumatoid arthritis, and otosyphilis may also show similar imaging findings to otosclerosis, but usually have some other systemic manifestations. Labyrinthitis ossificans as a sequela of a previous infectious or inflammatory process could also mimic otosclerosis.

VARIOUS BONE DYSPLASIAS THAT AFFECT TEMPORAL BONES
Fibrous Dysplasia

Fibrous dysplasia (FD) is a benign disorder that causes marrow fibrosis, abnormal matrix production, and stimulation of osteoclastic reabsorption. Whether osteoclasts or osteoblasts predominate depends on the phase of the disease. The estimated prevalence is 1 to 2 per 30,000 people, more commonly affecting children and young adults.[22] The craniofacial bones are affected in 46% of cases, with temporal bone involvement occurring in only 24% of these cases.[22] FD is classified into three subgroups: (1) monostotic (70%);

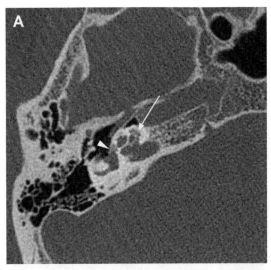

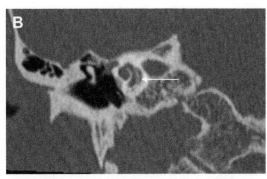

Fig. 6. Cochlear otosclerosis in a 36-year-old woman with mixed hearing loss. Axial (*A*) and coronal (*B*) CT images show pronounced demineralization surrounding and abutting the cochlea (*arrows*). Note an area of demineralization in the region of fissula ante fenestram (*arrowhead*).

(2) polyostotic (27%); and (3) McCune-Albright syndrome, in which FD is associated with endocrinopathies and skin hyperpigmentation (3%).[23]

Clinical manifestations vary depending on the extent and location of disease. The most common symptoms include headache and hearing loss, more commonly CHL. Hearing loss could be the result of narrowing or stenosis of the external auditory canal (EAC) or IAC, and facial paresis caused by facial canal involvement.[24]

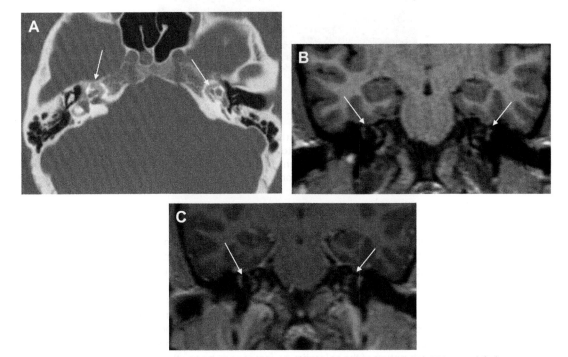

Fig. 7. Cochlear otosclerosis in a 34-year-old woman with bilateral hearing loss. Axial CT image (*A*) demonstrates extensive demineralization (*arrows*) surrounding the cochleae bilaterally. Coronal T1-weighted MR image (*B*) demonstrates intermediate signal in the region around the cochleae (*arrows*) corresponding to the demineralization on CT. Postcontrast T1-weighted MR image (*C*) demonstrates mild enhancement of the lesions (*arrows*).

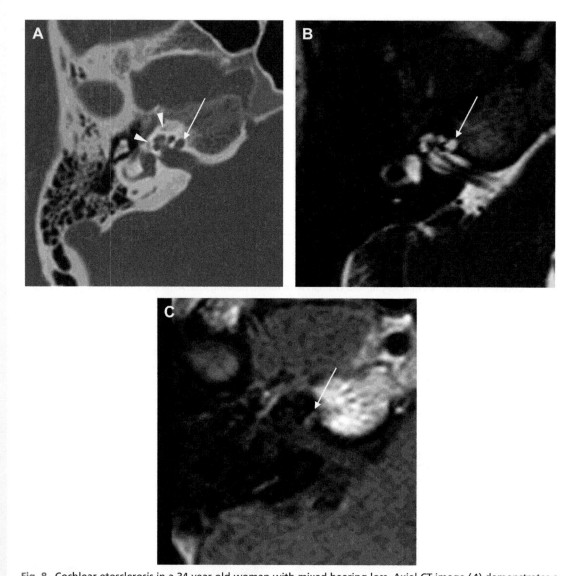

Fig. 8. Cochlear otosclerosis in a 34-year-old woman with mixed hearing loss. Axial CT image (*A*) demonstrates a cavitary lucency (*arrow*) anterior to and extending up to the IAC, which is separated from the cochlea by dense bone. There is also ground-glass lucency around the cochlea (*arrowheads*). Axial high-resolution T2-weighted MR image (*B*) demonstrates fluid signal in the cavitary lesion (*arrow*). Postcontrast (*C*) T1-weighted MR image demonstrates mild enhancement within the lesion (*arrow*).

Radiologically, there are three forms of FD, including pagetoid (56%), sclerotic (23%), and cystic (21%) patterns. Pagetoid pattern presents with regions of bony expansion and mixed areas of lucency and sclerosis. Sclerotic pattern presents with homogenously dense areas and bony expansion. Cystic pattern presents with oval cystic lesions with sclerotic borders.[23] A mixed form can also be present, with a combination of the sclerotic and cystic patterns.

CT features of FD depend on the quantity of bone and fibrous tissue, and the degree of mineralization. The margins between normal and abnormal bone are difficult to delineate. The cortex is usually preserved but may be thinned, whereas the matrix is filled with fibrous tissue and disorganized bony trabeculae. The most common CT presentation in the temporal bone is the sclerotic form, with homogenously increased density, loss of normal trabecular pattern, and increased bone thickness (**Figs. 14** and **15**). Obstruction of the EAC is common and may result in infection, keratosis obturans, and cholesteatomas (seen in 40% of cases).[23] FD that is initially

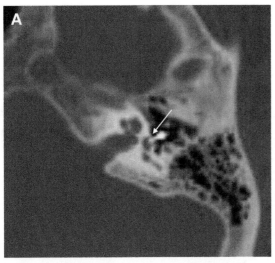

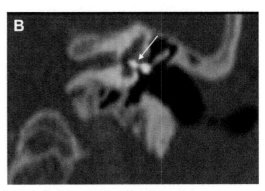

Fig. 9. Fenestral otosclerosis, status post stapedotomy and piston prosthesis placement in a 59-year-old woman. Axial (*A*) and coronal (*B*) CT images demonstrate a piston prosthesis with its medial tip at the oval window (*arrows*).

limited to the mastoid or middle ear may extend to the cochlea and labyrinth in a later stage. In cystic FD, the lytic process can erode the vestibule or posterior semicircular canal and may result in vertigo and hearing loss.[24] Facial weakness or SNHL may be the result of cranial nerve compression.[24]

MR imaging is useful to assess the soft tissue and fibrous components, and to evaluate the effect of these lesions on adjacent structures, such as the cranial nerves. MR imaging characteristics of FD are variable, with low-to-intermediate T1 and low-to-high T2 signal intensity, small regions of T2 hyperintensity that may represent cystic regions, and variable enhancement pattern.[25]

Treatment
Conservative treatment of choice is bisphosphonates, although the therapeutic efficacy of these agents remains uncertain. In patients with IAC or EAC involvement, canaloplasty may be needed. In patients with middle ear and mastoid cavity involvement, tympanomastoidectomy may be needed to manage complications, such as cholesteatoma.

Differential diagnosis
When FD involves the petrous apex, the MR imaging findings could potentially be difficult to differentiate from low-grade chondrosarcoma, atypical chordoma, or intraosseous meningioma, and therefore CT evaluation is critical in avoiding misdiagnoses. PD may be also confused with FD, but is usually bilateral, seen in older patients, and presents with predominance of lucencies and small number of sclerotic areas.

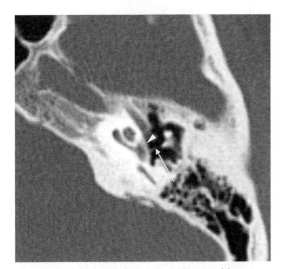

Fig. 10. Fenestral otosclerosis in a 32-year-old woman. She had undergone a stapedectomy, with subsequent progression of disease with increased ossification, requiring revision surgery. Axial CT image demonstrates focal osseous proliferation impinging the footplate (*arrowhead*). A linear thin prosthesis (*arrow*) is placed after laser stapedectomy, which is in contact with long process of the incus and extending to the footplate.

Paget Disease

PD, or osteitis deformans, is a chronic bone disorder characterized by excessive bone formation by osteoclasts, resulting in widened diploic spaces, thickened cortex, and coarsened trabeculae. The estimated prevalence is 3% to 11%, with an

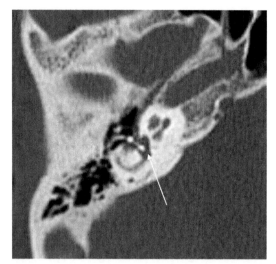

Fig. 11. Fenestral otosclerosis, status post stapedectomy and prosthesis placement in a 46-year-old woman. Axial CT image demonstrates a stapes prosthesis with medial displacement and excessive penetration into the vestibule (*arrow*).

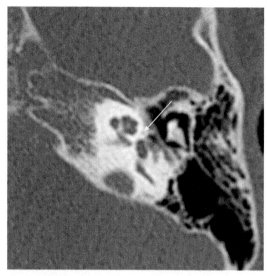

Fig. 13. Cochlear cleft in a 4-year-old girl who was scanned for right otitis media (*not shown*). Axial CT image demonstrates a subtle focal lucency anterior to the oval window (*arrow*), in the region of the fissula ante fenestram.

increased frequency with advancing age.[26,27] Men are slightly more frequently affected than women, and polyostotic disease presentation is more common than monostotic disease.

Different etiologies have been proposed including inherited factors, endocrine or vascular

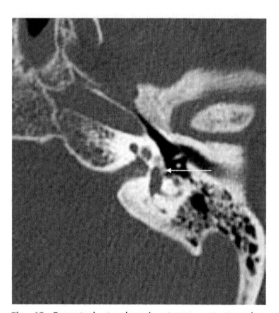

Fig. 12. Fenestral otosclerosis, status post stapedectomy and prosthesis placement in a 54-year-old woman with persistent conductive hearing loss after prosthesis placement. Subluxation of the stapes prosthesis is seen with respect to the oval window without vestibular penetration (*arrows*).

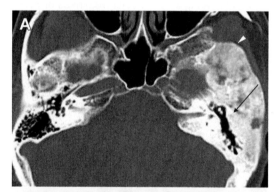

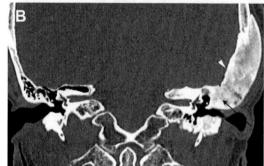

Fig. 14. Fibrous dysplasia in a 61-year-old woman with left temporal swelling and headache. Axial (*A*) and coronal (*B*) CT images show ground-glass opacity and bony expansion that causes narrowing of the middle ear cavity and sclerosis of the mastoid air cells (*arrows*). Note the preserved cortex (*arrowheads*).

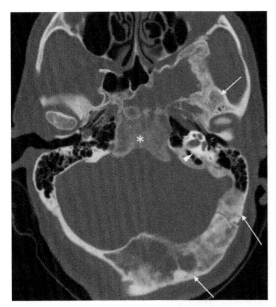

Fig. 15. Fibrous dysplasia in a 43-year-old woman with headaches. Axial CT image demonstrates bony expansion and internal mixed densities involving the left occipital and temporal bones (*arrows*) and more homogeneous ground-glass density of the clivus (*asterisk*). Note the left otic capsule is spared (*arrowhead*).

disease, and infections. The pathophysiology is characterized by increased bone turnover caused by osteoclastic bone resorption (osteolytic stage) followed by osteoclastic repair (osteoclastic-osteoblastic stage).[27] Normal bone is replaced by primitive woven or abnormal lamellar bone and fibrovascular tissue, resulting in soft and porous bone that may be unstable, deform under stress, and susceptible to fracture. Malignant transformation to osteosarcoma is rare.

In PD with temporal bone involvement, the most common presenting symptom is hearing loss (85%), and other symptoms may include headache and tinnitus.[26] Hearing loss is usually bilateral, progressive, and with predominantly high-frequency sensorineural component and a low-frequency conductive loss.[27] Some patients have shown ossicular fixation, such as at the stapes footplate resulting in CHL.[27] The disease may affect the EAC and middle ear through increased ossicular mass or fusion with distortion/obliteration of the round or oval window. Other potential mechanisms for SNHL include damage to the cochlear hair cells and compression of the auditory nerves.

Imaging findings depend on the stage of the disease. In the early stage of PD, the skull demonstrates predominantly well-defined lytic lesions (Fig. 16). In the temporal bone, demineralization

begins at the petrous pyramids where there is the greatest amount of marrow deposition, and progresses inferiorly and laterally. Areas of resorption tend to advance from the periphery of the otic capsule to the central areas. In the early stage, the otic capsule shows a blurry, washed-out appearance (Fig. 17).[27] In the intermediate stage, osteolytic and osteoblastic areas coexist with trabecular and cortical thickening. In this stage, the temporal bone shows thinning of the otic capsule and ground-glass opacities. In the late stage, enlargement of the bone with diffuse expansion of the calvarium is seen with lesions having a "cotton-wool" appearance, reflecting sclerotic areas on a background of osteolytic lesions. The stapes footplate can be thickened and bone enlargement may result in foraminal and canal narrowing and obliteration of the mastoid air cells.[27]

MR imaging findings also correlate with the stage of the disease. Depending on the phase, PD lesions may show decreased T1 and elevated T2 signal, representing increased vascularity (see Fig. 17).[27] Because of the hypervascular nature of the disease, enhancement is seen mostly in the areas of bone expansion.

Treatment
Patients with PD may be treated with bisphosphonates or calcitonin. Bisphosphonates reduce the increased rate of bone turnover,[27] whereas calcitonin inactivates the osteoclasts and therefore reduces bone reabsorption. Dynamic contrast-enhanced MR imaging may be useful for

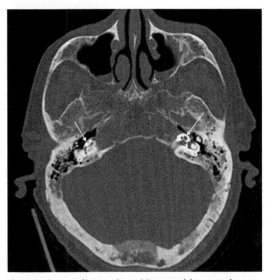

Fig. 16. Paget disease in a 90-year-old man who was brought to the emergency department after a fall. Axial CT image demonstrates mild expansion of the skull and skull base with patchy sclerosis. Note the otic capsules are spared (*arrows*).

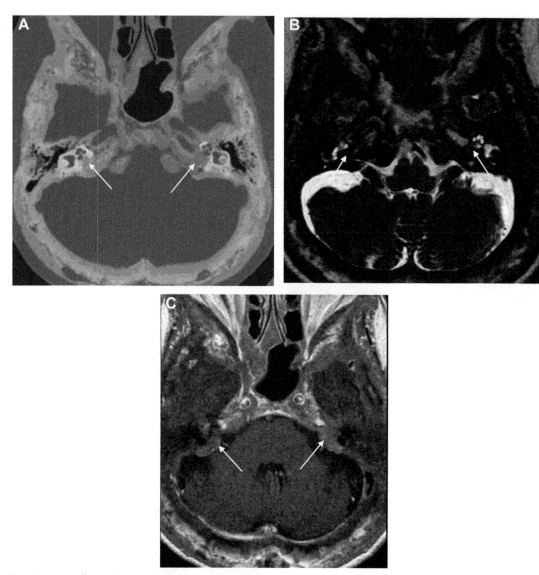

Fig. 17. Paget disease in a 78-year-old woman with vertigo and left pulsatile tinnitus. Axial CT image (*A*) demonstrates expansile heterogeneous bone throughout the skull and skull base, including the temporal bones. Note obliteration of the IACs (*arrows*). Axial high-resolution T2-weighted image (*B*) demonstrates effacement of the CSF signal in the IACs (*arrows*). Axial postcontrast T1-weighted image (*C*) demonstrates hypervascularity of the lesions (*arrows*).

monitoring treatment.[28] Hearing aids including bone-anchored hearing aid or cochlear implantation may be used.

Differential diagnosis

Several diseases may be included in the differential diagnosis for PD. FD presents as predominant ground-glass opacities replacing the normal temporal bone with fibro-osseous tissue, but, unlike PD, FD rarely involves the otic capsule. Osteopetrosis demonstrates a uniform dense involvement of the mastoid air cells and does not result in increased bone volume. Otosclerosis lesions are symmetric, whereas PD lesions are usually asymmetric.

Osteogenesis Imperfecta

OI is a rare heritable genetic disorder with heterogeneous penetrance that affects the connective tissue, resulting from an error in type 1 collagen formation. It presents with osteopenia and abnormal bone fragility, defective dentition, blue coloration of the sclera, ligamentous laxity, and hearing loss.[29] The initial Sillence classification

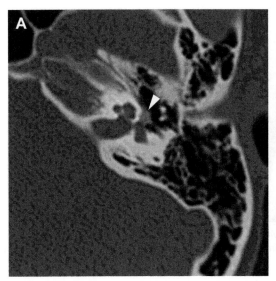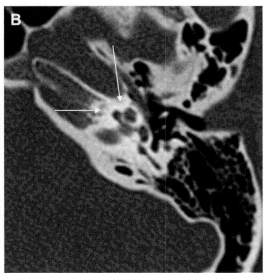

Fig. 18. Osteogenesis imperfecta in a 22-year-old woman with mixed hearing loss. Axial CT images (*A*, *B*) demonstrate demineralization in the region of the fissula ante fenestram (*arrowhead*) and around the cochlea (*arrows*).

described four major types (Sillence types I-IV) in 1979, but in 2009 the International Nomenclature Group for Constitutional Disorders of the Skeleton classified OI into five different groups based on phenotype alone, similar to the Sillence classification. Type 1 is the most common and mildest form that reflects decreased production of type I collagen. Patients present with fractures, deafness after childhood, hyperflexibility, and blues sclera. Type 2 is the most severe form with death in utero or shortly after birth caused by multiple fractures. Type 3 presents with bone deformities and fractures, short stature, dentinogenesis imperfecta, and blue sclera. Type 4 has variable severity, with some patients manifesting normal sclera and dentin, and with minimal bone fragility. Type 5 presents with calcification of the interosseous membranes and/or hypertrophic callus.[30]

In OI, there is thickening and undermineralization of the bones, with numerous and large vascular spaces.[29] OI is characterized by generalized osteopenia, cortical thinning and diminished trabeculae, deformity of long bones, and multiple fractures. Microfractures have been found in the otic capsule, anterior process and handle of the malleus, and the stapes crura,[29] resulting in CHL. There is also a possibility of increased susceptibility to otitis media with effusion.[31] OI may also manifest with SNHL, which is thought to be the consequence of atrophy of the cochlear hair cells and stria vascularis, in addition to bone formation within the otic capsule.

Temporal bone CT findings of OI are similar to those of otosclerosis, but are usually more extensive, reflecting proliferation of undermineralized

thickened bone around the otic capsule with microfractures, hemorrhage, and reparative fibrovascular tissues (**Figs. 18** and **19**). The thickened bone extends through the labyrinth causing narrowing of the middle ear cavity, and therefore the oval window becomes narrowed and the stapes crura appear subsequently embedded in dysplastic bone.[3] In addition, fractures result in dehiscence of the stapes arch, fixation of the stapes footplate, or atrophy of the long process of the incus, causing CHL. Postcontrast MR imaging often shows symmetric, focal, or band-like, enhancing pericochlear areas that correspond to the demineralization on CT, similar to otosclerosis, representing proliferating areas of undermineralized bone or the associated inflammation (see **Fig. 19**). High-resolution T2-weighted imaging may show irregularities of the labyrinth and cochlea, reflecting spongiotic foci.[29]

Treatment

Bisphosphonates may improve quality of life of patients with OI.[32] Patients with CHL from ossicular fracture or stapes footplate fixation are surgically treated through stapedectomy and prosthesis placement. Bone-anchored hearing aid is an alternative treatment of patients with CHL and unilateral hearing impairment. Treatment of SNHL in patients with OI is similar to patients without OI, and includes cochlear implants.

Differential diagnosis

Temporal bone imaging findings of OI are similar to those of otosclerosis, but often more extensive. PD is more common in older patients, with lack

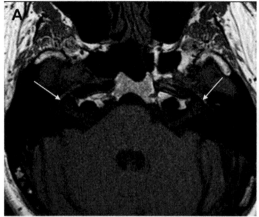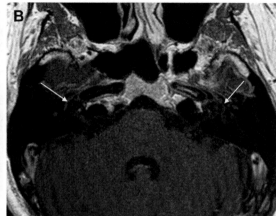

Fig. 19. Osteogenesis imperfecta in a 35-year-old man with a history of bilateral sensorineural hearing loss. Axial precontrast (*A*) and postcontrast (*B*) T1-weighted MR images show mild symmetric pericochlear enhancement (*arrows*).

of prominent hypertrophic bone around the stapes and oval window.

Osteopetrosis

Osteopetrosis is a heterogeneous group of heritable skeletal disorders characterized by decreased osteoclast activity, resulting in defective absorption of the primary spongiosa, which leads to bone thickening. The affected bones although appearing dense are fragile and susceptible to fractures.

Osteopetrosis is inherited in two models: autosomal-dominant osteopetrosis (ADOP; type I and II), a benign form that appears in young adults; and autosomal-recessive osteopetrosis (AROP), a more severe form that occurs in infancy. ADOP type I manifests with dense sclerosis of the spine and calvarium, sparing the skull base and temporal bone, with strong bones and infrequent fractures. In patients with ADOP type II, sclerosis involves the spine and skull base, sparing the calvarium, and fractures are frequent with minimal trauma.[33]

Clinical manifestations of osteopetrosis result from the consequences of bone overgrowth. Eustachian tube obstruction, otitis media, and cranial nerve deficits may be seen. IAC and EAC narrowing and ossicular fixation may be present. SNHL may be caused by cochlear nerve compression or decreased cochlear blood supply.

On imaging, osteopetrosis manifests differently depending on the type. ADOP type I shows sclerosis of the skull without involvement of the spine, and long bone deformity. ADOP type II shows sclerosis of the skull base, little involvement of the calvarium, and thickening of the vertebrae. AROP shows generalized dense bone with

striations as a result of alternating areas of mature and sclerotic bone.[3] In AROP, temporal bone CT demonstrates poor pneumatization of the mastoid bone that is filled with osteoporotic bone. There is narrowing of the EAC and thickening of the stapes, causing CHL. The IAC appears small, narrowed, and flared in a "trumpet shape," with sclerotic changes in the otic capsule.[3] MR imaging demonstrates calvarial thickening and sclerosis with decreased marrow space and is useful to evaluate consequences of bony overgrowth (Fig. 20).

Treatment
Patients can undergo surgical decompression of the IAC when there is compression of the facial or vestibulocochlear nerves, although there has been no clear evidence of success of this treatment. Patients with profound hearing loss may benefit from cochlear implantation (Fig. 21).[34]

Differential diagnosis
The differential diagnosis for osteopetrosis includes PD, because it is characterized by bone formation, but also by bone reabsorption, which may help distinguish them. FD demonstrates expansion of marrow space with heterogeneous density or signal. Fluorosis also demonstrates severe diffuse bony sclerosis, but often with a different history.

Camurati-Engelmann Disease

Camurati-Engelmann disease or progressive diaphyseal dysplasia is a rare autosomal-dominant inherited bone metabolic disorder characterized by hyperostosis of long bones and skull. In milder cases, there is diaphyseal involvement,

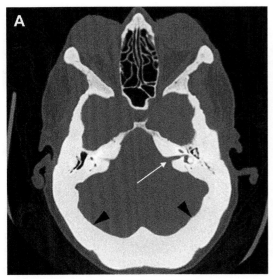

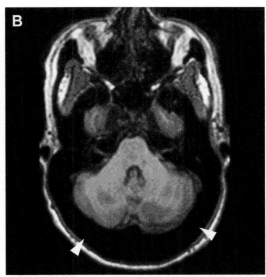

Fig. 20. Osteopetrosis in a 60-year-old woman. Axial CT image (*A*) shows diffusely increased bone density through the entire skull and skull base (*arrowheads*), including the temporal bones, resulting in narrowing of the IACs (*arrow*) and obliteration of the mastoid air cells bilaterally. Axial T1-weighted MR image (*B*) demonstrates diffuse sclerosis of the skull base with loss of normal bone marrow signal (*arrowheads*) and mass effect on intracranial structures.

whereas severe cases involve hyperostosis and sclerosis of the skull base and calvarium. The severe hyperostosis may lead to compression of the brain, brainstem, cranial nerves, and vessels going through the skull base foramina, with variable symptoms depending on the affected structures.[35]

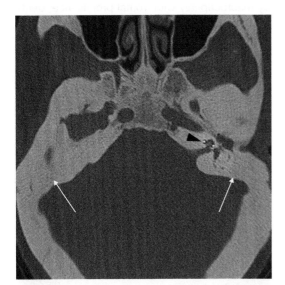

Fig. 21. Osteopetrosis in a 72-year-old woman with profound mixed hearing loss. Axial CT image demonstrates diffusely increased bone density with poor formation of the mastoid air cells (*arrows*) and narrowed tympanic cavities. A cochlear implant is placed on the left (*arrowhead*).

CT demonstrates extensive hyperostosis and thickening of the skull base (**Fig. 22**). The middle ear may be encased by sclerotic bone, and marked foraminal narrowing may be seen.[3] MR imaging demonstrates T1 and T2 low signal in the skull base and calvarium reflecting the diffuse sclerosis, and may demonstrate cranial nerve compression, particularly of cranial nerves II, VII, and VIII.[36]

Craniodiaphyseal Dysplasia

Craniodiaphyseal dysplasia is a rare syndrome characterized by massive and progressive hyperostosis of the craniofacial bones and diaphyseal expansion of the tubular bones. Pathogenesis is unknown and hereditary and sporadic cases have been reported.[37] Clinical manifestations are seen as a consequence of the massive sclerosis of the skull that may lead to intracranial hypertension; direct compression of the brain, brainstem, and spinal cord; and foraminal narrowing. The marked sclerosis of the skull and neural foraminal narrowing is best demonstrated on CT. The paranasal sinuses and mastoid air cells are not developed. MR imaging may show hyperostosis and the complications resulting from compression of various structures.[38]

Craniometaphyseal Dysplasia

Craniometaphyseal dysplasia is an autosomal inherited disease,[37] characterized by maxillofacial, calvarial, and skullbase bone overgrowth

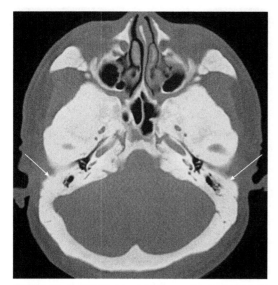

Fig. 22. Camurati-Engelmann disease in a 44-year-old man with headache and hearing loss. Axial CT image shows thickening and sclerosis of the entire skull base, with narrowing of the tympanic cavities and poorly formed mastoid air cells (*arrows*). (*Courtesy of Dr Kenichi Nagasawa.*)

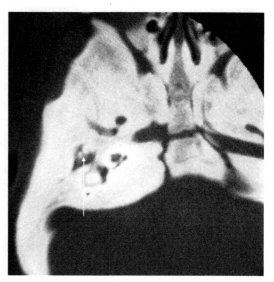

Fig. 23. Craniometaphyseal dysplasia in a 2-year-old boy. Axial CT image through the right temporal bone demonstrates marked thickening and severe diffuse sclerosis of the skull base. Note the marked narrowing of the tympanic cavity with impingement of the malleus and incus (*arrow*). (*Courtesy of Dr Noriko Aida.*)

that results in facial deformities and metaphyseal widening of the tubular bones. CHL or MHL is common, whereas the labyrinth is usually unaffected.[39] CT demonstrates the sclerosis of the frontal and occipital bones, and hyperostosis of the skull base that results in obliteration and poor pneumatization of the mastoid air cells, and narrowing of the skull base foramina (**Fig. 23**).[40]

Frontometaphyseal Dysplasia (Gorlin-Cohen Syndrome)

Frontometaphyseal dysplasia is a rare hereditary X-linked dominant craniotubular disorder characterized by supraorbital hyperostosis, hypertelorism, broad nasal bridge, and micrognathia.[41] CT demonstrates remarkable craniofacial deformities with sclerosis mainly of the frontal, temporal, and parietal bones, which result in bulging of the forehead and temporoparietal regions (**Fig. 24**). The inner table of the skull appears irregular with a gyral pattern.[42] Mastoid air cells are poorly developed.

Metaphyseal Dysplasia (Pyle Disease)

Metaphyseal dysplasia is a rare autosomal-recessive inherited disease[37] characterized by expansion of the metaphyseal regions of the long bones, especially the lower extremities. Mild sclerosis of the calvarium and skull base has been reported in association with this dysplasia.

Because there is only mild involvement of the skull, some investigators do not consider Pyle disease as a craniotubular dysplasia.[3]

Craniometadiaphyseal Dysplasia

Craniometadiaphyseal dysplasia is characterized by macrocephaly with frontal prominence, dental

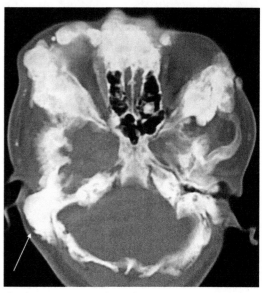

Fig. 24. Frontometaphyseal dysplasia in a 21-year-old man. Axial CT image shows pronounced sclerosis and irregularly shaped osseous proliferation involving the skull base, including the temporal bones (*arrow*).

hypoplasia, and increased bone fragility. Radiologic features include prominent wormian bones in the temporal and parietal regions, thin frontal and anterior parietal bones, and biparietal and occipital protuberances.[43] Diaphyseal widening of the long tubular bones and decreased metaphyseal flaring have also been reported.[44]

Dysosteosclerosis

Dysosteosclerosis is a rare autosomal-recessive inherited disease[37] that presents in early childhood. It is thought to be a form of osteopetrosis with additional features of platyspondyly, metaphyseal osteosclerosis, and red-violet macular skin atrophy. Clinical features include small stature, with limbs disproportionately shortened in comparison with the trunk, and tendency for fractures. There is thickening and sclerosis of the skull base and calvarium, with frontal and biparietal bossing and narrowed chin.[3,40]

Oculo-Dento-Osseous Dysplasia

Oculo-dento-osseous dysplasia is an autosomal-dominant inherited disorder characterized by a narrow nose with hypoplastic alae, microcornea, and syndactyly and/or camptodactyly.[37] Sclerosis of the skull and skull base have been described. The mandible appears enlarged with a widened alveolar ridge and hypoplastic coronoid processes.[40]

Hereditary Hyperphosphatemia

Hereditary hyperphosphatemia or juvenile PD is an autosomal-recessive condition characterized by swelling, fracture and bending of the limbs, and enlargement of the calvarium during early infancy. Initial common presentation is fever and bone pain, whereas later on there is enlargement of the calvarium, and multiple fractures and deformities. Headache and hypertension are common, and there is progressive MHL. On CT, the skull demonstrates "cotton ball patches" as seen in PD with thickening, but decreased bone trabeculation and decreased density of the skull base. Facial bones are usually spared.[40]

Pyknodysostosis (Maroteaux-Lamy Syndrome)

Pyknodysostosis is an autosomal-recessive inherited disorder of the primary spongiosa caused by abnormal expression of a proteinase of the osteoclasts that is required for the degradation of collagen.[37] Characteristic clinical features are dwarfism, pectus excavatum, acro-osteolysis, and hypoplasia of the facial bones.[45]

On imaging, there is generalized osteosclerosis with preservation of the medullary canal of long bones. The skull base can also be sclerotic, with delayed closure of sutures, presence of wormian bones, and lack of pneumatization of the paranasal sinus.[46,47]

Osteopathia Striata (Vorhoeve Syndrome)

Osteopathia striata, or striated skeleton, is a rare inherited disease of the secondary spongiosa. The inheritance pattern is autosomal dominant or sporadic.[37] This condition is characterized by dense linear striations in the diaphyses and metaphyses of tubular bones. Radiologically, there is sclerosis of the skull that may lead to cranial nerve palsies, stenosis of the IAC and EAC, and small underdeveloped paranasal sinus and mastoid air cells (Fig. 25).[46] The long bones and iliac wings appear combed, precipitating the name osteopathia striata.[40] The striations appear parallel to the long axis of the bones, especially in areas of rapid growth.[47]

Generalized Cortical Hyperostosis (Van Buchem Syndrome)

Generalized cortical hyperostosis, or endosteal hyperostosis, is an inherited autosomal-recessive disease that presents in childhood, characterized by increased cortical thickness of the long bones and axial skeleton, skull base, calvarium, and mandible. Narrowing of the skull base foramina

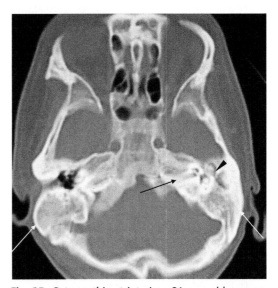

Fig. 25. Osteopathia striata in a 21-year-old woman. Axial CT image shows moderate diffuse sclerosis causing poor formation of the mastoid air cells (*white arrows*), narrowing of the tympanic cavity (*arrowhead*), and stenosis of the IAC (*black arrow*).

with facial nerve palsy and deafness has been described. Tubular bones demonstrate diaphyseal thickening.[47]

SUMMARY

Otosclerosis is a common disease causing hearing loss, but multiple bone dysplasias, some common and others rare, may have a similar clinical presentation. High-resolution CT can detect subtle osseous anomalies and MR imaging can evaluate potential complications in each condition, helping the radiologist narrow or define the diagnosis.

REFERENCES

1. Quesnel AM, Ishai R, McKenna MJ. Otosclerosis: temporal bone pathology. Otolaryngol Clin North Am 2018;51(2):291–303.
2. Purohit B, Hermans R, Op de Beeck K. Imaging in otosclerosis: a pictorial review. Insight Imaging 2014;5(2):245–52.
3. Sakai O, Curtin HD, Hasso AN, et al. Otosclerosis and dysplasias of the temporal bone. In: Som PM, Curtin HD, editors. Head and neck imaging. 5th edition. Philadelphia: Mosby; 2011. p. 1231–61.
4. Merchant SN, Rosowski JJ, McKenna MJ. Superior semicircular canal dehiscence mimicking otosclerotic hearing loss. Adv Otorhinolaryngol 2007;65: 137–45.
5. Lee TC, Aviv RI, Chen JM, et al. CT grading otosclerosis. AJNR Am J Neuroradiol 2009;30(7):1435–9.
6. Naumann IC, Porcellini B, Fisch U. Otosclerosis: incidence of positive findings on high-resolution computed tomography and their correlation to audiological test data. Ann Otol Rhinol Laryngol 2005; 114:709–16.
7. Karpishchenko SA, Zubareva AA, Filimonov VN, et al. The potential of cone beam computed tomography of the temporal bones in the patients presenting with otosclerosis. Vestn Otorinolaringol 2016;81(4):10–3.
8. Juliano AF, Ginat DT, Moonis G. Imaging review of the temporal bone: Part II. Traumatic, postoperative, and noninflammatory nonneoplastic conditions. Radiology 2015;276(3):655–72.
9. Pipin KJ, Muelleman TJ, Hill J, et al. Prevalence of internal auditory canal diverticulum and its association with hearing loss and otosclerosis. AJNR Am J Neuroradiol 2017;38(11):2167–71.
10. Sakai O, Curtin HD, Fujita A, et al. Otosclerosis: computed tomography and magnetic resonance findings. Am J Otolaryngol 2000;21:116–8.
11. Valvassori GE. Imaging of otosclerosis. Otolaryngol Clin North Am 1993;26(3):359–71.
12. Causse JR, Causse JB, Uriel J, et al. Sodium fluoride therapy. Am J Otol 1993;14:482–90.
13. Jan TA, Remenschneider AK, Halpin C, et al. Third-generation bisphosphonates for cochlear otosclerosis stabilizes sensorineural hearing loss in long-term follow-up. Laryngoscope Investig Otolaryngol 2017;2(5):262–8.
14. Vincent R, Sperling N, Oates J, et al. Surgical findings and longterm hearing results in 3,050 stapedotomies for primary otosclerosis: a prospective study with the Otology-Neurotology Database. Otol Neurotol 2006;27(Suppl 2):S25–47.
15. Ukkola-Pons E, Avache D, Pons Y, et al. Oval window niche height: quantitative evaluation with CT before stapes surgery for otosclerosis. AJNR Am J Neuroradiol 2013;34(5):1082–5.
16. Ayache D, Lejeune D, Williams MT. Imaging of postoperative senorineural complications of stapes surgery: a pictorial essay. Adv Otorhinolaryngol 2007; 65:308–13.
17. Whetstone J, Nguyen A, Nguyen-Huynh A, et al. Surgical and clinical confirmation of temporal bone CT findings in patients with otosclerosis with failed stapes surgery. AJNR Am J Neuroradiol 2014;35(6): 1195–201.
18. Lesinski SG. Causes of conductive hearing loss after stapedectomy or stapedotomy: a prospective study of 279 consecutive surgical revisions. Otol Neurotol 2002;23:281–8.
19. Lagleyre S, Calmels MN, Escude B, et al. Revision stapes surgery: the "lateralized piston syndrome. Otol Neurotol 2009;30:1138–44.
20. Rotteveel LJ, Proops DW, Ramsden RT, et al. Cochlear implantation in 53 patients with otosclerosis: demographics, computed tomographic scanning, surgery, and complications. Otol Neurotol 2004;25:943–52.
21. Razafindranaly V, Truy E, Pialat JB, et al. Cone beam CT versus multislice CT: radiologic diagnostic agreement in the postoperative assessment of cochlear implantation. Otol Neurotol 2016;37(9): 1246–54.
22. Lustig LR, Holliday MJ, McCarthy EF, et al. Fibrous dysplasia involving the skull base and temporal bone. Arch Otolaryngol Head Neck Surg 2001; 127(10):1239–47.
23. Kimitsuki T, Komune S. Asymptomatic fibrous dysplasia of the temporal bone. J Laryngol Otol 2015;129(Suppl 2):S42–5.
24. Brown EW, Megarian CA, McKenna MJ, et al. Fibrous dysplasia of the temporal bone: imaging findings. AJR Am J Roentgenol 1995;164(3):679–82.
25. Jee WH, Choi KH, Choe BY, et al. Fibrous dysplasia: MR imaging characteristics with radiopathologic correlation. AJR Am J Roentgenol 1996;167(6):1523–7.
26. Deep NL, Besch-Stokes JG, Lane JI, et al. Paget's disease of the temporal bone: a single-institution contemporary review of 27 patients. Otol Neurotol 2017;38(6):907–15.

27. Hullar TE, Lustig LR. Paget's disease and fibrous dysplasia. Otolaryngol Clin North Am 2003;36(4): 707–32.

28. Libicher M, Kasperk C, Daniels M, et al. Dynamic contrast-enhanced MRI in Paget's disease of bone-correlation of regional microcirculation and bone turnover. Eur Radiol 2008;18(5):1005–11.

29. Alkadhi H, Rissmann D, Kollias S. Osteogenesis imperfecta of the temporal bone: CT and MR imaging in Van der Hoeve-de Kleyn syndrome. AJNR Am J Neuroradiol 2004;25(6):1106–9.

30. Thomas IH, DiMeglio LA. Advances in the classification and treatment of osteogenesis imperfecta. Curr Osteoporos Rep 2016;14(1):1–9.

31. Pillion P, Shapiro J. Audiological findings in osteogenesis imperfecta. J Am Acad Audiol 2008;19(8): 595–601.

32. Marginean O, Tamasanu RC, Mang N, et al. Therapy with pamidronate in children with osteogenesis imperfecta. Drug Des Devel Ther 2017;11:2507–15.

33. Cure JK, Key LL, Goltra DD, et al. Cranial MR imaging of osteopetrosis. AJNR Am J Neruoradiol 2000; 21(6):1110–5.

34. Szymanski M, Zaslawska K, Trojanowska A, et al. Osteopetrosis of temporal bone treated with cochlear implant. J Int Adv Otol 2015;11(2):173–5.

35. Yen JK, Bourke RS, Popp AJ, et al. Camurati-Englemann disease (progressive hereditary craniodiaphyseal dysplasia). Case report. J Neurosurg 1978; 48(1):138–42.

36. Uezato S, Dias G, Inada J, et al. Imaging aspects of Camurati-Engelmann diseases. Rev Assoc Med Bras (1992) 2016;62(9):825–7.

37. Vanhoenacker FM, De Beuckeleer LH, Van Hyl W, et al. Sclerosing bone dysplasias: genetic and radioclinical features. Eur Radiol 2000;10(9):1423–33.

38. Marden F, Wippold F II. MR imaging features of craniodiaphyseal dysplasia. Pediatr Radiol 2004;34(2): 167–70.

39. Sun GH, Samy RN, Tinkle BT, et al. Craniometaphyseal dysplasia-induced hearing loss. Otol Neurotol 2011;32(2):e9–10.

40. Gorlin RJ. Craniotubular bone disorders. Pediatr Radiol 1994;24(6):392–406.

41. Ganigara A, Nishtala M, Chandrika YR, et al. Airway management of a child with frontometaphyseal dysplasia (Gorlin Cohen syndrome). J Anaesthesiol Clin Pharmacol 2014;30(2):279–80.

42. Ehrenstein T, Maurer J, Liokumowitsch M, et al. CT and MR findings in frontometaphyseal dysplasia. J Comput Assist Tomogr 1997;21(2):218–20.

43. Santolaya JM, Hall CM, García-Miñaur S, et al. Craniometadiaphyseal dysplasia, wormian bone type. Am J Med Genet 1998;77(3):241–5.

44. Langer LO Jr, Brill PW, Afshani E, et al. Radiographic features of craniometadiaphyseal dysplasia, wormian bone type. Skeletal Radiol 1991;20:37–41.

45. De Vernejoul MC. Sclerosing bone disorders. Best Pract Res Clin Rheumatol 2008;22(1):71–83.

46. Ihde LL, Forrester DM, Gottsegen CJ, et al. Sclerosing bone dysplasias: review and differentiation from other causes of osteosclerosis. Radiographics 2011;31(7):1865–82.

47. Greenspan A. Sclerosing bone dysplasias-a target site approach. Skeletal Radiol 1991;20(8):561–83.

Imaging of Tinnitus

Mary Beth Cunnane, MD

KEYWORDS

- Pulsatile tinnitus • Dural AVF • Idiopathic intracranial hypertension • Sigmoid wall abnormalities

KEY POINTS

- Primary nonpulsatile tinnitus does not require imaging evaluation.
- Tinnitus with asymmetric hearing loss should be evaluated by imaging. If the hearing loss is conductive, then temporal bone CT is recommended. If the hearing loss is sensorineural, MR imaging is recommended.
- Pulsatile tinnitus should be evaluated by imaging. If there is a retrotympanic mass, then imaging should be performed to evaluate for paragangioma. Otherwise MR imaging/angiography and CTA have both been used to evaluate pulsatile tinnitus.

Tinnitus is a condition in which patients hear a sound that is not present in the external world. Up to 25% of the population experiences tinnitus, but only 8% experience frequent tinnitus and only about 3% of adults experience severe tinnitus.[1,2] Tinnitus is characterized as pulsatile or nonpulsatile. Pulsatile tinnitus is often synchronous with the patient's heartbeat and may be subjective (heard only by the patient) or objective (heard by both the patient and an examiner listening with a stethoscope). Nonpulsatile tinnitus is continuous and may be described as a ringing, hissing, or roaring.

Primary nonpulsatile tinnitus does not have a recognizable cause. It is frequently accompanied by hearing loss, and risk factors include increasing age, noise exposure, hypertension, and anxiety.[1] Secondary nonpulsatile tinnitus is tinnitus that occurs as a symptom of an underlying disorder, such as middle ear disease, otospongiosis, and vestibular schwannoma.

All patients with tinnitus should have a thorough history and physical examination and audiometry to identify associated hearing loss.[3] In their Clinical Practice Guideline on Tinnitus, the American Academy of Otolaryngology makes a strong recommendation against imaging for patients with tinnitus alone.[3] Imaging is only recommended for patients whose tinnitus is unilateral, pulsatile, associated with asymmetric hearing loss, or associated with additional neurologic symptoms. Patients with additional neurologic symptoms (including cranial neuropathy, dizziness, or vertigo) should have imaging directed toward their associated neurologic symptoms (Fig. 1). This article considers the remaining patients with asymmetric hearing loss and pulsatile tinnitus.

UNILATERAL TINNITUS AND TINNITUS WITH ASYMMETRIC HEARING LOSS

Patients whose tinnitus is associated with asymmetric hearing loss should undergo imaging that is tailored to the type of hearing loss. For example, patients with conductive hearing loss should have computed tomography (CT) of the temporal bones. Many disorders that result in conductive hearing loss, including otitis media, superior semicircular canal dehiscence, and otosclerosis, may cause tinnitus. Frequently treatment of the hearing loss also improves tinnitus. For example, a patient with otosclerosis may experience improvement in hearing and tinnitus with stapedectomy.[4,5]

Tinnitus with asymmetric sensorineural hearing loss can be a presentation of retrocochlear pathology, such as vestibular schwannoma (Fig. 2). More than 50% of patients with vestibular schwannoma complain of tinnitus at presentation and most of

Department of Radiology, Massachusetts Eye and Ear Infirmary, Massachusetts General Hospital, Harvard Medical School, 243 Charles Street, Boston, MA 02114, USA
E-mail address: marybeth_cunnane@meei.harvard.edu

Neuroimag Clin N Am 29 (2019) 49–56
https://doi.org/10.1016/j.nic.2018.09.006
1052-5149/19/© 2018 Elsevier Inc. All rights reserved.

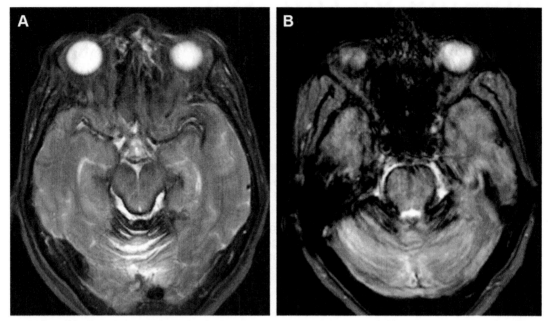

Fig. 1. This patient presented with tinnitus, hearing loss, and vertigo. Because of the sensorineural hearing loss and the additional neurologic symptom of vertigo, MR imaging of the brain and temporal bones was performed. Axial T2-weighted image at the level of the midbrain (*A*) and axial susceptibility-weighted image at the level of the pons (*B*) show linear susceptibility effect, consistent with hemosiderin, coating the surface of the brainstem and the cerebellar folia in this patient with superficial siderosis.

these patients also have asymmetric sensorineural hearing loss.[6] The yield of MR imaging evaluation in these patients is not high, as fewer than 5% have a vestibular schwannoma,[7] but these patients are important to identify early so that they are managed without developing more severe symptoms, such as facial nerve dysfunction, trigeminal neuralgia, and hydrocephalus.[6]

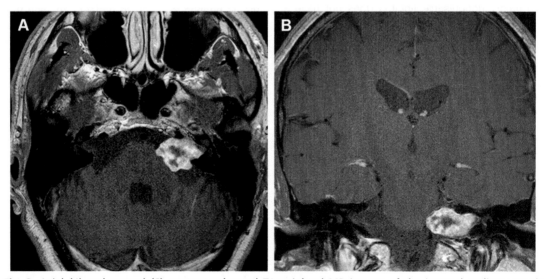

Fig. 2. Axial (*A*) and coronal (*B*) contrast-enhanced T1-weighted MR images of the internal auditory canals demonstrate a 2-cm partially cystic enhancing mass in the left internal auditory canals. The patient presented with left-sided ringing tinnitus and asymmetric sensorineural hearing loss. Pathology of the lesion confirmed vestibular schwannoma.

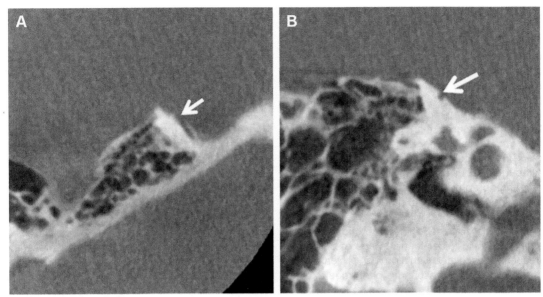

Fig. 3. Axial (*A*) and Stenvers (*B*) views from a CT of the right ear demonstrate dehiscence of the superior semicircular canal (*arrows*).

PULSATILE TINNITUS UNRELATED TO VESSEL ABNORMALITIES

Many causes of pulsatile tinnitus relate directly to abnormal flow in vessels within the head and neck. However, there are other causes of pulsatile tinnitus. Systemic conditions that increase blood flow, such as anemia,[8] thyrotoxicosis, and pregnancy, may all result in bilateral tinnitus.[9] Eustachian tube dysfunction and middle ear myoclonus[10] may also be perceived as pulsatile tinnitus. Vascular tumors frequently present with pulsatile tinnitus, most commonly paragangliomas, such as glomus tympanicum and glomus jugulare.[11,12] Superior semicircular canal dehiscence may result in pulsatile tinnitus because it leads to enhanced bone conduction and increased perception of somatosounds, including blood flow (Fig. 3).[13]

A thorough history and physical examination should identify patients with causes of pulsatile tinnitus that are not related to abnormal vessels within the head and neck. If imaging is indicated, it should be tailored to the diagnosis of the suspected underlying problem, such as thyroid ultrasound in thyrotoxicosis, contrast-enhanced MR imaging or CT of the temporal bone in paraganglioma, and noncontrast CT of the temporal bone for superior semicircular canal dehiscence. Once nonvascular etiologies have been eliminated, the clinician should consider arterial and venous causes of pulsatile tinnitus.

ARTERIAL CAUSES OF PULSATILE TINNITUS

Pulsatile tinnitus, which does not resolve with ipsilateral jugular vein compression, may have an arterial cause. Arterial causes of pulsatile tinnitus include carotid atherosclerotic disease, dural arteriovenous fistulas (AVFs), carotid dissection, fibromuscular dysplasia (FMD), and aberrant internal carotid artery (ICA).[11,12,14,15]

Dural AVFs are abnormal communications between meningeal arteries and dural venous sinuses or subarachnoid veins, which exist between the dural leaflets.[16] Pulsatile tinnitus results from increased arterial flow within the transverse or sigmoid sinuses. This tinnitus can frequently be heard by the examiner when auscultating the mastoid region with a stethoscope.

Dietz and coworkers[17] reported the findings of dural AVFs on MR imaging/MR angiography (MRA), which include increased number and size of extracranial vessels, prominent transosseous collaterals, abnormal flow in the dural venous sinuses or other venous structures, transverse sinus stenosis, and abnormal calvarial signal in the bone overlying the fistula (Fig. 4). CT angiography (CTA) can also be used to screen for dural AVFs in patients with pulsatile tinnitus. Similar to MRA, CTA demonstrates asymmetrically enlarged feeding vessels and prominent transcalvarial vascular channels. In addition, CTA may show a shaggy appearance to the tentorium or draining dural venous sinus.[18]

Dural AVFs may have dural drainage, cortical venous drainage, or a combination of the two. Cortical venous reflux confers an increased risk of intracranial hemorrhage and neurologic complications, such as seizures, and is therefore important to recognize on imaging studies. In general patients who present with pulsatile tinnitus rather than intracranial hemorrhage have a more benign long-term outcome than patients who present with intracranial hemorrhage; however, assessment for cortical venous reflux is still prudent.[19] Although this has classically been done via catheter angiography, time-resolved MRA is a promising noninvasive technique for accurate classification of dural AVFs.[20]

Atherosclerotic disease of the carotid is typically seen in patients older than the age of 50 and is frequently associated with a bruit on clinical examination.[14] Carotid ultrasound is performed to evaluate for extracranial atherosclerotic disease. However, CTA or MRA is better than ultrasound at depicting intracranial carotid stenoses, which could also lead to tinnitus.[21]

FMD is much less common that carotid atherosclerotic disease, but pulsatile tinnitus is frequent in these patients, occurring as a presenting symptom in 27.5%.[22] FMD is best identified with CTA or MRA, which may depict the "beads on a string" appearance of alternating narrowing and dilation of the vessel. Arterial dissection and intracranial aneurysms may also be seen as manifestations of FMD.[23]

Carotid dissection and intracranial aneurysms can also rarely present with pulsatile tinnitus, and for this reason, vascular imaging in patients with pulsatile tinnitus should include the entire circle of Willis.

Normal arterial variants that may result in tinnitus include aberrant ICA[24] and persistent stapedial artery. Patients with an aberrant carotid artery demonstrate absence of the normal vertical segment of the carotid and enlargement of the inferior tympanic and caroticotympanic arteries. CT shows a soft tissue density in the middle ear, in contiguity with the carotid canal, with dehiscence of the lateral bony wall of the carotid canal (**Fig. 5**).[25] Persistent stapedial artery is present in about 0.05% of the population.[26] CT of the temporal bone demonstrates enlargement of the facial nerve canal. It is associated with absence of foramen spinosum, and often with an aberrant ICA.[27]

VENOUS CAUSES OF PULSATILE TINNITUS

Venous causes of pulsatile tinnitus are suspected when compression of the jugular vein causes resolution of the patient's pulsatile tinnitus. This category includes high-riding jugular bulb, transverse sinus stenosis, dural vein thrombosis, and sigmoid wall diverticulum and sigmoid wall dehiscence.

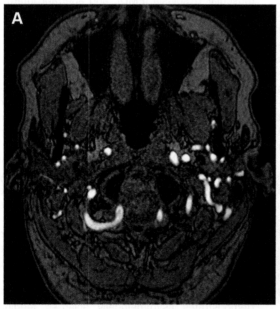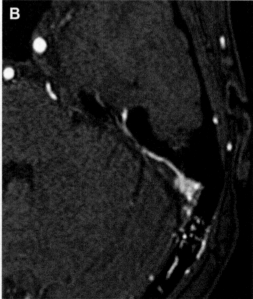

Fig. 4. Axial time-of-flight MR angiography source images demonstrate an increase in the number and size of left external carotid artery branches (*A*), with large vessels surrounding the mastoid tip, involving the parapharyngeal space and surrounding the mandible. A magnified view of the region of the sigmoid notch (*B*) demonstrates flow-related enhancement, consistent with arterial flow, in the sigmoid sinus. Multiple transosseous collaterals are also identified.

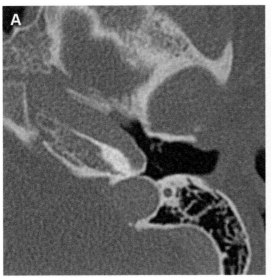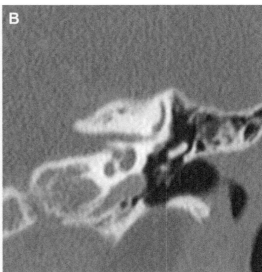

Fig. 5. Axial (*A*) and coronal (*B*) images from a noncontrast temporal bone CT demonstrate enlargement of the inferior tympanic artery, which turns in the middle ear to connect to the petrous segment of the ICA. The aberrant ICA extends into the middle ear cavity, well beyond the cochlear promontory (*B*).

High jugular bulb has been proposed to be associated with pulsatile tinnitus. It has been variously described as extending to the level of the cochlea, inferior bony annulus, or the internal auditory canal.[28] Depending on the definition used, the incidence ranges from 6% to 22% of temporal bones and is more common on the right.[29–33] In a study of 3285 patients who underwent temporal bone CT for a variety of indications, 730 patients (22%) were identified with high jugular bulb, and approximately 50% of these complained of tinnitus. In a subgroup of 26 patients with dehiscent jugular bulb, 57.7% complained of tinnitus (Fig. 6).[29]

Sigmoid wall dehiscence and diverticulum have also been associated with pulsatile tinnitus, and have been treated via endovascular and external approaches with resolution of tinnitus (Fig. 7).[34–37]

Idiopathic intracranial hypertension (IIH) is another important cause of venous tinnitus. The mechanism by which IIH causes pulsatile tinnitus is not well understood, but it has been theorized that increased intracranial pressure leads to narrowing of the transverse sinuses. Narrowing of the transverse sinuses then results in turbulent flow, which is perceived as tinnitus (Fig. 8). In a large clinical series of patients with pulsatile tinnitus, IIH was the most commonly identified cause.[14]

More recently it has been suggested that sigmoid wall dehiscence or diverticulum may also be associated with IIH, because there is considerable overlap in the demographic description of patients with IIH and patients with sigmoid wall dehiscence or diverticulum. In both cases, most patients are female, are overweight or have recently gained weight, and are of reproductive age. It is hypothesized that the turbulent flow seen in the transverse sinus stenosis of patients with IIH causes a jet effect on the sigmoid sinus, resulting in remodeling and dehiscence.[35]

Just as many patients with high jugular bulbs do not complain of tinnitus, Lansley and colleagues[38] have presented findings that suggest that IIH patients without tinnitus were just as likely as IIH patients with tinnitus to demonstrate findings of transverse sinus stenosis and sigmoid wall anomalies. Because sigmoid wall abnormalities are a more recently recognized cause of pulsatile tinnitus, it is likely that further research will help clarify the relationship between sigmoid wall abnormalities, IIH, and tinnitus.

APPROACH TO EVALUATION

The American College of Radiology Appropriateness Criteria for tinnitus recommend CTA of the head and neck, computed tomography venography (CTV) of the head, and CT of the temporal bone as "Usually Appropriate" for the evaluation of pulsatile tinnitus. MR imaging of the temporal bones with contrast and MRA of the head are also deemed "Usually Appropriate."[39] The literature on pulsatile tinnitus is heterogeneous, and the most commonly detected causes of pulsatile tinnitus vary widely between series. Sismanis[14] reported that the most common cause of pulsatile tinnitus was IIH, whereas Sonmez and colleagues[40] report more cases of arterial stenosis

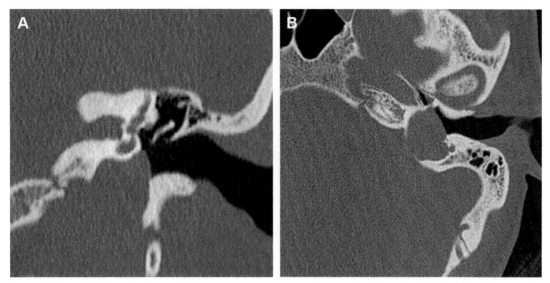

Fig. 6. (*A*) Coronal CT image through the temporal bone demonstrates a high jugular bulb that is well above the inferior bony annulus. (*B*) Axial image shows that there is dehiscence of the bony covering of the jugular bulb anteriorly.

and AVFs. The series of Mattox and Hudgins[41] and Dong and coworkers[42] both feature sigmoid wall dehiscence and diverticulum as prominent causes of pulsatile tinnitus. Hofmann and colleagues[43] pooled data from six series of patients to assess the relative frequency of causes of pulsatile tinnitus. In the pooled data, the most common category was "unknown," followed by arterial stenosis, IIH, venous anatomic variants/anomalies, and dural AVFs.

Given the difficulty in determining the statistically most likely cause of tinnitus, it seems prudent to select the imaging study based on clinical findings. In patients with objective tinnitus and a negative otoscopic examination, MRA or CTA could be used to evaluate for dural AVF and atherosclerotic disease. In patients whose tinnitus resolves with venous pressure, CTA/CTV could be used to evaluate for venous sinus stenosis, high jugular bulb, and sigmoid wall anomalies. Using this approach, most treatable causes of pulsatile tinnitus should be able to be detected radiologically, providing guidance for further treatment.

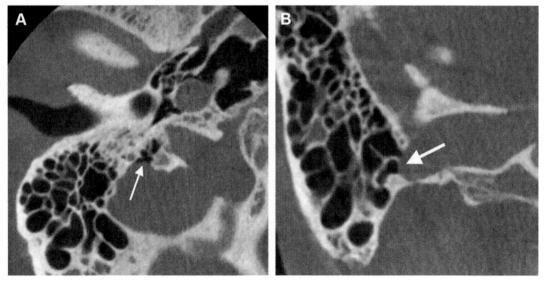

Fig. 7. Axial (*A*) and coronal (*B*) CT images through the sigmoid notch demonstrate dehiscence of the bone overlying the sigmoid sinus (*arrows*) in this patient who presented with pulsatile tinnitus.

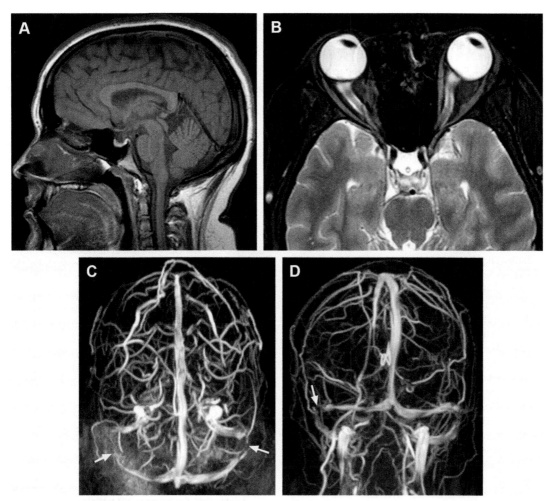

Fig. 8. Sagittal T1-weighted MR image (*A*) in this woman of reproductive age shows flattening of the pituitary gland. Axial T2-weighted MR image (*B*) demonstrates flattening of the posterior globes reflecting papilledema. Magnetic resonance venogram shown in axial (*C*) and coronal (*D*) maximum intensity projection demonstrates narrowing of the distal transverse sinuses (*arrows*).

REFERENCES

1. Shargorodsky J, Curhan GC, Farwell WR. Prevalence and characteristics of tinnitus among US adults. Am J Med 2010;123(8):711–8.
2. Kim HJ, Lee HJ, An SY, et al. Analysis of the prevalence and associated risk factors of tinnitus in adults. PLoS One 2015;10(5):e0127578.
3. Tunkel DE, Bauer CA, Sun GH, et al. Clinical practice guideline: tinnitus. Otolaryngol Head Neck Surg 2014;151(2 Suppl):S1–40.
4. Oliveira CA. How does stapes surgery influence severe disabling tinnitus in otosclerosis patients? Adv Otorhinolaryngol 2007;65:343–7.
5. Rajati M, Poursadegh M, Bakhshaee M, et al. Outcome of stapes surgery for tinnitus recovery in otosclerosis. Int Tinnitus J 2012;17(1):42–6.
6. Stucken EZ, Brown K, Selesnick SH. Clinical and diagnostic evaluation of acoustic neuromas. Otolaryngol Clin North Am 2012;45(2):269–84, vii.
7. Choi KJ, Sajisevi MB, Kahmke RR, et al. Incidence of retrocochlear pathology found on MRI in patients with non-pulsatile tinnitus. Otol Neurotol 2015; 36(10):1730–4.
8. Sunwoo W, Lee DY, Lee JY, et al. Characteristics of tinnitus found in anemia patients and analysis of population-based survey. Auris Nasus Larynx 2018;45(6):1152–8.
9. Levine SB, Snow JB Jr. Pulsatile tinnitus. Laryngoscope 1987;97(4):401–6.
10. Badia L, Parikh A, Brookes GB. Management of middle ear myoclonus. J Laryngol Otol 1994;108(5):380–2.
11. Remley KB, Coit WE, Harnsberger HR, et al. Pulsatile tinnitus and the vascular tympanic membrane: CT, MR, and angiographic findings. Radiology 1990;174(2):383–9.
12. Sismanis A, Smoker WR. Pulsatile tinnitus: recent advances in diagnosis. Laryngoscope 1994;104(6 Pt 1):681–8.

13. Ward BK, Carey JP, Minor LB. Superior canal dehiscence syndrome: lessons from the first 20 years. Front Neurol 2017;8:177.

14. Sismanis A. Pulsatile tinnitus. A 15-year experience. Am J Otol 1998;19(4):472–7.

15. Waldvogel D, Mattle HP, Sturzenegger M, et al. Pulsatile tinnitus: a review of 84 patients. J Neurol 1998; 245(3):137–42.

16. Elhammady MS, Ambekar S, Heros RC. Epidemiology, clinical presentation, diagnostic evaluation, and prognosis of cerebral dural arteriovenous fistulas. Handb Clin Neurol 2017;143:99–105.

17. Dietz RR, Davis WL, Harnsberger HR, et al. MR imaging and MR angiography in the evaluation of pulsatile tinnitus. AJNR Am J Neuroradiol 1994;15(5):879–89.

18. Narvid J, Do HM, Blevins NH, et al. CT angiography as a screening tool for dural arteriovenous fistula in patients with pulsatile tinnitus: feasibility and test characteristics. AJNR Am J Neuroradiol 2011;32(3):446–53.

19. Zipfel GJ, Shah MN, Refai D, et al. Cranial dural arteriovenous fistulas: modification of angiographic classification scales based on new natural history data. Neurosurg Focus 2009;26(5):E14.

20. Farb RI, Agid R, Willinsky RA, et al. Cranial dural arteriovenous fistula: diagnosis and classification with time-resolved MR angiography at 3T. AJNR Am J Neuroradiol 2009;30(8):1546–51.

21. Emery DJ, Ferguson RD, Williams JS. Pulsatile tinnitus cured by angioplasty and stenting of petrous carotid artery stenosis. Arch Otolaryngol Head Neck Surg 1998;124(4):460–1.

22. Olin JW, Froehlich J, Gu X, et al. The United States registry for fibromuscular dysplasia: results in the first 447 patients. Circulation 2012;125(25):3182–90.

23. Varennes L, Tahon F, Kastler A, et al. Fibromuscular dysplasia: what the radiologist should know: a pictorial review. Insights Imaging 2015;6(3):295–307.

24. Botma M, Kell RA, Bhattacharya J, et al. Aberrant internal carotid artery in the middle-ear space. J Laryngol Otol 2000;114(10):784–7.

25. Romo LV, Casselman JW, Robson CD. Congenital anomalies of the temporal bone. In: Som PM, Curtin HD, editors. Head and Neck Imaging. Volume 1. St. Louis (MO): Mosby; 2011. p. 1097–166.

26. Moreano EH, Paparella MM, Zelterman D, et al. Prevalence of facial canal dehiscence and of persistent stapedial artery in the human middle ear: a report of 1000 temporal bones. Laryngoscope 1994;104(3 Pt 1):309–20.

27. Silbergleit R, Quint DJ, Mehta BA, et al. The persistent stapedial artery. AJNR Am J Neuroradiol 2000; 21(3):572–7.

28. Manjila S, Bazil T, Kay M, et al. Jugular bulb and skull base pathologies: proposal for a novel classification system for jugular bulb positions and microsurgical implications. Neurosurg Focus 2018;45(1):E5.

29. Sayit AT, Gunbey HP, Fethallah B, et al. Radiological and audiometric evaluation of high jugular bulb and dehiscent high jugular bulb. J Laryngol Otol 2016; 130(11):1059–63.

30. Atilla S, Akpek S, Uslu S, et al. Computed tomographic evaluation of surgically significant vascular variations related with the temporal bone. Eur J Radiol 1995;20(1):52–6.

31. Overton SB, Ritter FN. A high placed jugular bulb in the middle ear: a clinical and temporal bone study. Laryngoscope 1973;83(12):1986–91.

32. Wadin K, Thomander L, Wilbrand H. Effects of a high jugular fossa and jugular bulb diverticulum on the inner ear. A clinical and radiologic investigation. Acta Radiol Diagn (Stockh) 1986;27(6):629–36.

33. Woo CK, Wie CE, Park SH, et al. Radiologic analysis of high jugular bulb by computed tomography. Otol Neurotol 2012;33(7):1283–7.

34. Eisenman DJ. Sinus wall reconstruction for sigmoid sinus diverticulum and dehiscence: a standardized surgical procedure for a range of radiographic findings. Otol Neurotol 2011;32(7):1116–9.

35. Eisenman DJ, Raghavan P, Hertzano R, et al. Evaluation and treatment of pulsatile tinnitus associated with sigmoid sinus wall anomalies. Laryngoscope 2018. [Epub ahead of print].

36. Liu Z, Chen C, Wang Z, et al. Sigmoid sinus diverticulum and pulsatile tinnitus: analysis of CT scans from 15 cases. Acta Radiol 2013;54(7):812–6.

37. Wang GP, Zeng R, Liu ZH, et al. Clinical characteristics of pulsatile tinnitus caused by sigmoid sinus diverticulum and wall dehiscence: a study of 54 patients. Acta Otolaryngol 2014;134(1):7–13.

38. Lansley JA, Tucker W, Eriksen MR, et al. Sigmoid sinus diverticulum, dehiscence, and venous sinus stenosis: potential causes of pulsatile tinnitus in patients with idiopathic intracranial hypertension? AJNR Am J Neuroradiol 2017;38(9):1783–8.

39. Expert Panel on Neurologic I, Kessler MM, Moussa M, et al. ACR Appropriateness Criteria((R)) tinnitus. J Am Coll Radiol 2017;14(11S):S584–91.

40. Sonmez G, Basekim CC, Ozturk E, et al. Imaging of pulsatile tinnitus: a review of 74 patients. Clin Imaging 2007;31(2):102–8.

41. Mattox DE, Hudgins P. Algorithm for evaluation of pulsatile tinnitus. Acta Otolaryngol 2008;128(4): 427–31.

42. Dong C, Zhao PF, Yang JG, et al. Incidence of vascular anomalies and variants associated with unilateral venous pulsatile tinnitus in 242 patients based on dual-phase contrast-enhanced computed tomography. Chin Med J (Engl) 2015;128(5):581–5.

43. Hofmann E, Behr R, Neumann-Haefelin T, et al. Pulsatile tinnitus: imaging and differential diagnosis. Dtsch Arztebl Int 2013;110(26):451–8.

Third Window Lesions

Mai-Lan Ho, MD

KEYWORDS

- Labyrinthine fistula • Semicircular canal • Third window • Tullio • Vestibular aqueduct

KEY POINTS

- Third window abnormalities are bony defects of the inner ear that enable abnormal communication with the middle ear and/or cranial cavity.
- Vestibular symptoms include vertigo and nystagmus induced by loud noises (Tullio phenomenon) or increases in external auditory canal pressure (Hennebert sign).
- "Pseudo-conductive" hearing loss manifests as a low-frequency air-bone gap resulting from decreased air and increased bone conduction.
- Semicircular canal dehiscence is the most common third window lesion, in which there is deficient bone covering the semicircular canal. High-resolution computed tomography (CT) with multiplanar reformats (Pöschl and Stenvers views) is critical for diagnosis.
- Additional causes of third window pathology include infection, inflammation, neoplasia, trauma, surgery, congenital malformations, and bone dyscrasias.

INTRODUCTION

Third window abnormalities are bony defects of the inner ear that enable abnormal communication with the middle ear and/or cranial cavity. Normally, the inner ear and middle ear are entrained via the oval (first) window and round (second) window membranes. Loss of acoustic energy through a third window yields a "pseudo-conductive" hearing loss with low-frequency air-bone gap, as evidenced by decreased air and increased bone conduction on audiometry.[1,2] Vestibular dysfunction causes vertigo and nystagmus in response to loud noises or increases in pressure (Tullio and Hennebert signs).[3,4] High-resolution temporal bone computed tomography (CT) is the first-line imaging modality for evaluation of third window pathology and is crucial for accurate diagnosis and management.[2,5,6] In this article, the authors review the fundamental mechanisms of the third window phenomenon and describe key imaging findings and differential diagnosis based on anatomic location as well as cause.

NORMAL ANATOMY AND IMAGING TECHNIQUE

The mammalian inner ear is anatomically defined by the bony labyrinth, a hollow periosteum-lined structure within the temporal bone, and consists of hearing (cochlear) and balance (vestibular) organs. Sodium-rich perilymph fills the bony labyrinth and demonstrates negative electrical potential relative to potassium-rich endolymph within the membranous labyrinth. Environmental stimuli induce pressure waves within the perilymph and subsequently endolymph, stimulating cochlear and vestibular receptor cells that yield our perceptions of sound and movement. Multiple vestibular structures cooperate in the perception of balance, containing polarized hair cells that respond to fluid motion in various directions. Two otolithic organs within the vestibule are responsible for detecting linear acceleration. The saccule is located anteriorly, near the cochlea, and senses horizontal acceleration. The utricle is located posteriorly, near the semicircular canals, and senses

Disclosure Statement: No disclosures.
Department of Radiology, Mayo Clinic, 200 First Street Southwest, Rochester, MN 55905, USA
E-mail address: mailanho@gmail.com

Neuroimag Clin N Am 29 (2019) 57–92
https://doi.org/10.1016/j.nic.2018.09.005

vertical acceleration. The superior (anterior), lateral (horizontal, external), and posterior semicircular canals also interconnect with the vestibule to detect angular acceleration in 3 orthogonal planes. The ductus utriculosaccularis (utriculosaccular duct) connects the utricle and saccule and drains through the endolymphatic duct into the endolymphatic sac, a blind-ending pouch along the posterior petrous face adjacent to dura mater (Fig. 1A).[7]

Sound conduction relies on the presence of 2 physiologic windows between the fluid-filled inner ear and air-filled middle ear. The oval window (first window) is a membrane that directly contacts both the stapes footplate and the vestibule of inner ear and is contiguous with perilymph in the scala vestibuli (vestibular duct) of cochlea. The round window (second window) covers the cochlea and is contiguous with perilymph in the scala tympani (tympanic duct) of cochlea (Fig. 1B). The scala vestibuli and scala tympani merge into the helicotrema at the cochlear apex, forming a functionally incompressible column of perilymphatic fluid. Along the remainder of the cochlea, these 2 compartments are separated by endolymph-filled scala media (cochlear duct). The organ of Corti lies on the basilar membrane within the scala media and also contains hair cells capable of mechanotransduction into electrochemical activity. Stereocilia vibrate in proportion to the differential acoustic energy across the length of the basilar membrane, which results in mechanical opening of voltage-dependent channels and depolarization of the hair cells by endolymph. Subsequent release of neurotransmitters triggers transmission of electrical impulses through the cochlear nerve into the brain, enabling perception of sound (Fig. 1C).[7–10]

The inner ear also communicates with the cranial cavity through various bony fossae, which create contiguity between the perilymphatic and subarachnoid spaces. These physiologic openings include the cochlear aqueduct, which transmits the fibrous periotic duct; vestibular aqueduct, which carries the membranous endolymphatic duct and epithelium-lined perilymphatic duct; and multiple small neurovascular foramina. Normally, these bony channels are relatively long and thin in cross-section and therefore do not result in clinically significant dissipation of acoustic energy. Nevertheless, it appears that these additional bony communications can provide near-normal bone conduction hearing when both the oval and the round windows are closed.[11] They can also become of functional importance when abnormally enlarged.[1,2]

Third window lesions are defined as abnormal communications of the inner ear with adjacent spaces, namely the middle ear or cranial cavity (Box 1). The most common example is semicircular canal dehiscence, but abnormalities involving the vestibule and scala vestibuli side of the cochlea can produce a similar effect. Defects in the bony labyrinth enable dissipation of acoustic energy away from the cochleovestibular system into middle ear, dura mater, and/or vascular structures, altering perceptions of sound and balance.[1,2]

Fig. 2 demonstrates the mechanics of air and bone conduction in the presence of normal and third window anatomy. Air-transmitted sound vibrates the tympanic membrane and auditory ossicles and is subsequently transmitted through the oval window into scala vestibuli. Displacement of cochlear perilymph results in equal and opposite motion of the round window, producing a pressure differential across the basilar membrane. The presence of a third window directs acoustic vibrations in other directions away from the oval window, decreasing the total energy delivered to the round window. As a result, the pressure gradient across the basilar membrane is lowered, and there is decreased perception of air-conducted sound.[1,2,9]

Bone-transmitted sounds vibrate the entire temporal bone, including the oval and round windows. Unequal impedance of these 2 membranes results in differential outward motion, creating a pressure difference across the basilar membrane. At low frequencies, the round window vibrates outward to a greater degree than does the oval window. Third window lesions located between the oval and round windows shunt away acoustic energy, decreasing the outward motion of the oval window. This mechanism artifactually increases the pressure gradient across the basilar membrane, heightening the perception of bone-conducted sound.[1,2,9,10]

Clinically, patients with third window pathology present with stereotypical symptoms of vestibular activation, including directional vertigo, nystagmus, oscillopsia, dizziness, imbalance, and/or nausea. Tullio phenomenon refers to induction of vestibular symptoms by everyday loud noises, such as traffic or shouting. Hennebert sign is caused by increases in pressure to a sealed external auditory canal, as can occur with nose-blowing, swallowing, or lifting of heavy objects.[3,4] Additional symptoms are related to bony hyperacusis with autophony produced by dural oscillations, pulsatile tinnitus due to vascular vibrations, and diplacusis from differential air and bone conduction. Patients demonstrate a mixed or "pseudo-conductive" hearing loss, with a characteristic air-bone gap at audiometry that reflects increased bone and decreased air conduction. This phenomenon occurs most significantly at lower sound frequencies (<1 kHz), for which

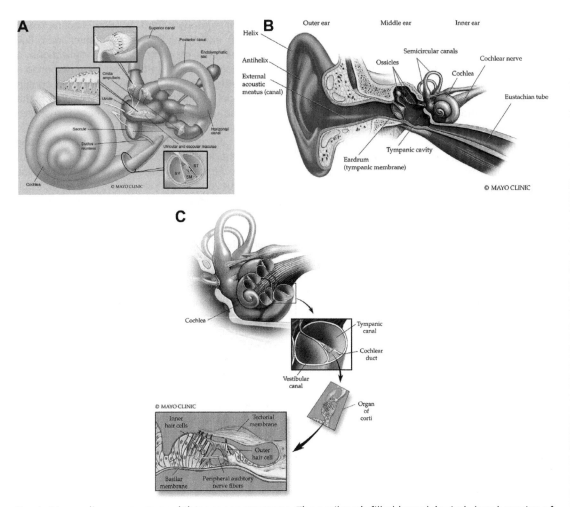

Fig. 1. Mammalian ear anatomy. (*A*) Inner ear structures. The perilymph-filled bony labyrinth (*gray*) consists of the cochlea, which detects sound, and vestibular structures, which coordinate balance. Sodium-rich perilymph fills the bony labyrinth and demonstrates negative electrical potential relative to potassium-rich endolymph within the membranous labyrinth (*blue*). Within the cochlea, the scala vestibuli (SV) is contiguous with the oval window, and scala tympani (ST) is continuous with round window. The scala vestibuli and scala tympani merge into the helicotrema at the cochlear apex, forming a functionally incompressible column of perilymphatic fluid. Along the remainder of the cochlea, these 2 compartments are separated by endolymph-filled scala media (SM). Two otolithic organs within the vestibule are responsible for detecting linear acceleration. Multiple vestibular structures cooperate in the perception of balance. The saccule is located anteriorly, near the cochlea, and senses horizontal acceleration. The utricle is located posteriorly, near the semicircular canals, and senses vertical acceleration. The superior, lateral, and posterior semicircular canals are also interconnected with the vestibule and detect angular acceleration in 3 orthogonal planes. (*B*) The mammalian ear consists of external, middle, and inner ear structures. Sound conduction relies on the presence of 2 physiologic windows between the fluid-filled inner ear and air-filled middle ear. The oval window (first window) is a membrane that directly contacts both the stapes footplate and the vestibule of inner ear and is contiguous with perilymph in the scala vestibuli (vestibular duct) of cochlea. The round window (second window) covers the cochlea and is contiguous with perilymph in the scala tympani (tympanic duct) of cochlea. (*C*) The scala vestibuli and scala tympani merge into the helicotrema at the cochlear apex, forming a functionally incompressible column of perilymphatic fluid. Along the remainder of the cochlea, these 2 compartments are separated by endolymph-filled scala media (cochlear duct). The organ of Corti lies on the basilar membrane within the scala media and contains hair cells capable of mechanotransduction into electrochemical activity. Stereocilia vibrate in proportion to the differential acoustic energy across the length of the basilar membrane. The vibration results in mechanical opening of voltage-dependent channels and depolarization of the hair cells by endolymph. Subsequent release of neurotransmitters triggers transmission of electrical impulses through the cochlear nerve into the brain, enabling perception of sound.

Box 1
Third window lesions

What the referring physician needs to know

- Third window abnormalities are bony defects of the inner ear that enable abnormal communication with the middle ear and/or cranial cavity.
- Clinically, patients present with vertigo and nystagmus induced by loud noises (Tullio phenomenon) or increases in pressure (Hennebert sign).
- On audiometry, there is a characteristic "pseudo-conductive" hearing loss with low-frequency air-bone gap resulting from decreased air and increased bone conduction.
- High-resolution temporal bone CT is the first-line imaging modality for evaluation of third window pathology and is critical for accurate diagnosis and management.

Differential diagnosis by location

- Superior semicircular canal
- Posterior semicircular canal
- Lateral semicircular canal
- Vestibule
- Vestibular aqueduct
- Cochlea (scala vestibuli)

Differential diagnosis by cause

- Idiopathic
- Infection/inflammation
- Cholesteatoma
- Neoplasia
- CSF hypertension
- Trauma
- Surgery
- Congenital malformations
- Bone dyscrasias

electromyography. Third window lesions shunt acoustic energy and generate greater local fluid displacement, resulting in larger deflections of vestibular sensors with a hyperactive response in the affected vestibular organ. VEMP can confirm directional vestibular hyperexcitability with higher response amplitudes and decreased response thresholds.[12–20]

For imaging evaluation of third window lesions, CT of the temporal bones is recommended with 0.5- to 1-mm collimation. Multidetector helical technique enables rapid acquisition of isotropic data with generation of 3dimensional multiplanar reformats. Coronal and sagittal reconstructions aid in precise localization of inner ear pathology. Dedicated oblique reformats are especially useful in visualizing the semicircular canals and diagnosing dehiscence. The Stenvers view is an oblique coronal reconstruction along the long axis of the petrous temporal bone. Images are parallel to the posterior semicircular canal and perpendicular to the superior and lateral semicircular canals. The Pöschl view is an oblique sagittal reconstruction perpendicular to the Stenvers plane. Images are parallel to the superior semicircular canal and cochlea and perpendicular to the posterior and lateral semicircular canals (**Fig. 3**).[5,6,21] MR imaging does not play a primary role in evaluation of third window lesions, but can provide additional characterization of bone marrow and soft tissue abnormalities, perilymphatic fluid composition, and cranial nerve integrity.[22,23]

IMAGING FINDINGS/PATHOLOGY
Superior Semicircular Canal Dehiscence

Semicircular canal dehiscence refers to extreme thinning and/or loss of the bony roof of the semicircular canal. The condition is idiopathic, although both congenital and acquired causes have been proposed: bone rarefaction/underpneumatization, barotrauma or direct mechanical trauma, and cerebrospinal fluid (CSF)/vascular pulsations. Superior semicircular canal dehiscence is the most common and well researched form.[24–27] CT imaging can yield false positives and overestimations of dehiscence, because of the limited spatial resolution in areas of extreme bone thinning. In young patients, it can also be difficult to visualize overlying bone because the optic capsule is incompletely ossified, mimicking dehiscence. Greater specificity is achieved using Pöschl views parallel and Stenvers views perpendicular to the plane of the superior semicircular canal to confirm a true dehiscence.[28–33] The location, approximate size, and morphology of the bony defect can be useful information for clinicians. Focal dehiscence

acoustic energy is more readily dissipated. At higher sound frequencies, there is little or no air-bone gap, because a minority of the total acoustic energy is shunted away to the third window. Tympanometry and acoustic reflexes can be used to confirm normal middle ear function, verifying that the air-bone gap does not result from an inefficient middle ear. Vestibular evoked myogenic potentials (VEMP) are used to test vestibular function. Acoustic or vibrational inputs stimulate vestibular hair cells, resulting in compensatory contraction of ipsilateral cervicofacial muscles as measured by

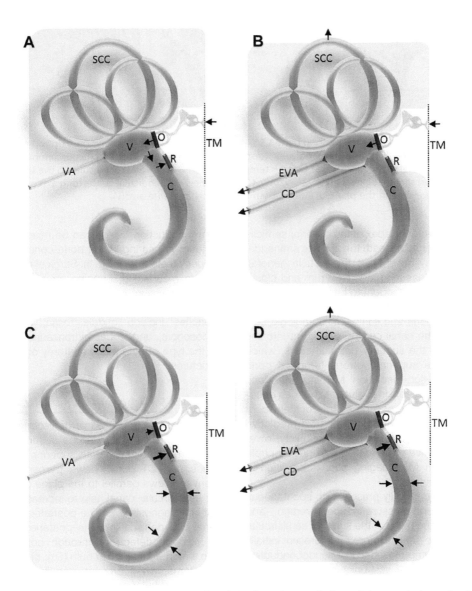

Fig. 2. Mechanisms of sound conduction in normal and third window pathology. (*A*) Normal air conduction (*arrows*). Vibrations are conducted from the tympanic membrane through auditory ossicles to the oval window. Acoustic energy from the oval window is then transmitted through incompressible perilymph, producing equal and outward motion of the round window. The differential pressure gradient between the oval and round windows is maintained across the basilar membrane and creates the perception of sound. (*B*) Abnormal air conduction (*arrows*). Third window lesions shunt acoustic energy inputted at the oval window, resulting in decreased motion of the round window. This decreases pressure across the basilar membrane and leads to reduced perception of air-conducted sounds. (*C*) Normal bone conduction (*arrows*). Vibrations are transmitted throughout the otic capsule. The oval and round windows are displaced outward to different extents, reflecting their unequal impedances. At low frequencies, the round window vibrates outward to a greater degree than the oval window. The resulting pressure difference across the basilar membrane enables sound perception. (*D*) Abnormal bone conduction (*arrows*). Third window lesions between the oval and round windows shunt acoustic energy away, especially from the less-vibrating oval window. There is minimal change in the vibration of the round window. However, the motion of the round window on the scala tympani side is unchanged. This artifactually elevates the pressure gradient across the basilar membrane, increasing the perception of bone-conducted sound. C, cochlea; CD, cochlear dehiscence; EVA, enlarged vestibular aqueduct; O, oval window; R, round window; SCC, semicircular canal; TM, tympanic membrane; V, vestibule; VA, vestibular aqueduct.

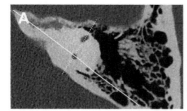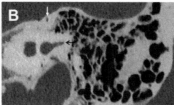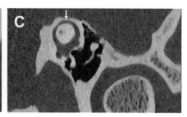

Fig. 3. Multiplanar reformats in temporal bone CT. (*A*) Axial temporal bone CT shows prescription of oblique reformats parallel (*solid line*) and perpendicular (*dotted line*) to the long axis of petrous temporal bone. (*B*) Stenvers view parallel to the long axis of petrous temporal bone. Images are perpendicular to the superior (*white arrow*) and lateral semicircular canals (*black arrow*). (*C*) Pöschl view perpendicular to the long axis of petrous temporal bone. Images are in the plane of superior semicircular canal (*white arrow*).

commonly affects the apex of the superior semicircular canal directly beneath the arcuate eminence, where the bony covering is thinnest. In general, dehiscences measuring at least 2 mm and closer to the vestibule are thought to be more significant, with variable correlations between linear/volumetric dimensions and clinical or audiologic outcomes.[34–44] The canal can be dehiscent into the dura mater or the superior petrosal sinus, which runs along the superior petrous temporal bone (**Fig. 4**).[45,46] High-resolution MR imaging does not play a primary role in evaluation, but can effectively exclude the presence of thin or dehiscent semicircular canals with high negative predictive value. However, because of the relatively lower positive predictive value, cases with questionable dehiscence on MR imaging should be referred for CT confirmation.[47–51]

Adult patients usually present with spontaneous dizziness, sound/pressure-induced vertigo, and nystagmus in the plane of the superior semicircular canal. Pediatric patients more often present initially with auditory symptoms, that is, pseudoconductive hearing loss. Severe vestibular dysfunction is an indication for surgery, because symptoms do not remit and tend to progress over the lifetime. Audiometry shows the characteristic low-frequency air-bone gap with decreased air and supranormal

bone conduction, which can be misdiagnosed as conductive hearing loss if bone conduction is not properly tested[13–17] (**Fig. 5**). Surgical repair options include resurfacing, capping, or plugging of the involved semicircular canal, versus reinforcement of the oval and/or round windows. Potential approaches include middle fossa, transmastoid, endoscopic, and endaural/transaural, depending on the type of defect and anatomy of surrounding structures.[31,52–56]

Posterior Semicircular Canal Dehiscence

Posterior semicircular canal dehiscence is a rare imaging finding, which can be observed in isolation or in combination with superior canal dehiscence. On CT, axial views perpendicular and Stenvers views parallel to the plane of the posterior semicircular canal help to increase the specificity of diagnosis.[57–67] The posterior semicircular canal can dehisce into the posterior fossa dura via a bony defect, or through communication with a high-riding jugular bulb (**Fig. 6**).[68–74] Clinical symptoms, when present, can include auditory and/or vestibular symptoms in the plane of the posterior semicircular canal. Audiometry is useful for confirming the characteristic low-frequency air-bone gap (**Fig. 7**).[61–63,75–80]

A   **B**

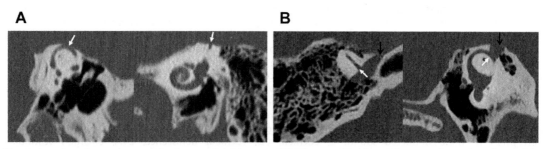

Fig. 4. Imaging of superior semicircular canal dehiscence. (*A*) CT scans, Pöschl and Stenvers views, show bony thinning of the roof of left superior semicircular canal, with focal dehiscence at the arcuate eminence (*white arrows*). (*B*) CT scans, axial and Pöschl views, show dehiscence of the right superior semicircular canal (*white arrows*) into the superior petrosal sinus (*black arrows*).

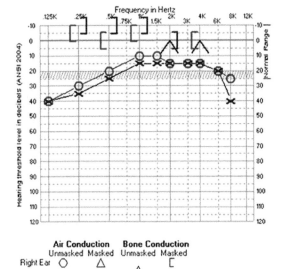

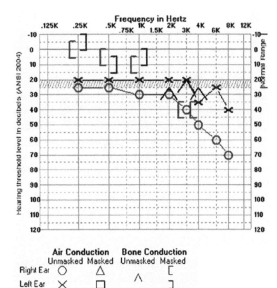

Fig. 5. Audiogram of bilateral superior semicircular canal dehiscence. Red cicle = right air conduction; red bracket = right bone conduction; blue cross = left air conduction; blue bracket = left masked bone conduction; caret = unmasked bone conduction; hatched line = normal range. Both ears demonstrate an air-bone gap with decreased air and increased bone conduction relative to the normal range, a phenomenon that is more apparent at low sound frequencies.

Lateral Semicircular Canal and Labyrinthine Fistula

The normal lateral semicircular canal is completely covered by otic capsule, which is the hardest and densest bone in the mammalian body. Therefore, isolated lateral semicircular canal dehiscence is extremely unusual and reported only in the presence of a dysplastic bony labyrinth. In such cases, patients can present with the characteristic auditory and vestibular symptoms in the plane of the lateral semicircular canal.[81,82] More commonly, destructive processes erode the otic capsule,

Fig. 7. Audiogram of bilateral posterior semicircular canal dehiscence. Both ears demonstrate an air-bone gap that is greater at low frequencies.

creating a third window into the lateral semicircular canal or other inner ear structures. This entity is known as a perilymphatic or labyrinthine fistula and is associated with chronic middle ear effusion and CSF leakage. The wide variety of potential causes includes infection, inflammation, neoplasia, CSF hypertension, trauma, and surgery.[79,80]

Infectious and inflammatory processes underlie most labyrinthine fistulae. Chronic otitis media refers to repeated middle ear infections with long-standing fluid opacification of the middle ear cavity, which can lead to demineralization and progressive erosions of the otic capsule (Figs. 8 and 9).[83–87] Rapid aggressive bone destruction can occur with direct extension of infection from soft tissue, promoting osteoclastic activity through localized hyperemia and acidosis. This process typically occurs in the setting of patient immunocompromise or fulminant pathogens, for example,

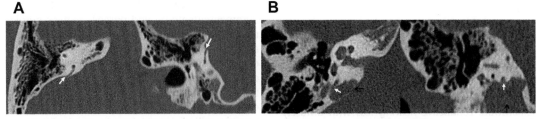

Fig. 6. Imaging of posterior semicircular canal dehiscence. (A) CT scans, axial and Pöschl views, show bony dehiscence of the superior limb of right posterior semicircular canal into the posterior fossa (white arrows). (B) CT scans, axial and Pöschl views, show bony dehiscence of the inferior limb of right posterior semicircular canal (white arrows) into a high-riding jugular bulb (black arrows).

A   **B**

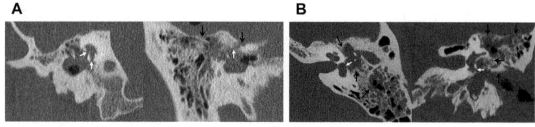

Fig. 8. Imaging of mastoiditis. (*A*) Chronic otitis media. CT scans, axial and coronal views, show fluid opacification of the right middle ear cavity with peripheral bony erosions involving the otic capsule and inner ear (*white arrows*), compatible with labyrinthine fistula. Dehiscence of the tegmen tympani and mastoideum (*black arrows*) predisposes to CSF leak. (*B*) Coalescent mastoiditis. CT scans, axial and coronal views, show diffuse fluid opacification of the left mastoid air cells and middle ear cavity with multifocal bone destruction (*black arrows*), including mastoid septae, epitympanic recess, tegmen tympani, and mastoideum resulting in CSF leakage. Bone erosions at the oval window (*white arrows*) are compatible with labyrinthine fistula.

Pseudomonas (necrotizing otitis); *Fusobacterium*, *Clostridium*, and beta-hemolytic *Streptococcus* (coalescent otomastoiditis); and *Mycobacterium* or invasive fungal infection.[88–97] More commonly, recurrent otitis media or otomastoid effusions produce granulation tissue with tympanic membrane perforations and/or retraction pockets, predisposing to acquired cholesteatoma formation.[98–103]

Cholesteatomas are epidermal inclusion cysts lined by stratified squamous epithelium that continually exfoliate keratin debris, analogous to epidermoid cysts in the skin and brain. When located in the temporal bone, these yield expansile

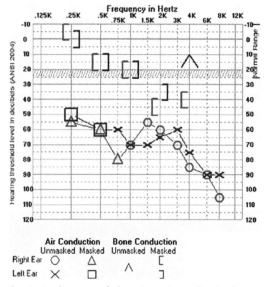

Fig. 9. Audiogram of chronic otitis media. Both ears demonstrate conductive hearing loss with diffusely decreased air conduction due to middle ear pathology. There is a superimposed air-bone gap with supranormal bone conduction at low frequencies, due to third window anatomy.

masses with progressive surrounding bone destruction. Proposed mechanisms of bone erosion include inflammatory osteoclastic activation with resorption osteitis, direct pressure by cholesteatoma growth, and/or secretion of osteolytic compounds by the cholesteatoma matrix. Reactive bone formation and protective "walling-off" mechanisms are uncommon.[104,105] Most acquired cholesteatomas originate in the middle ear cavity deep to the tympanic membrane. The most common location is the pars flaccida, or flaccid posterosuperior portion of tympanic membrane. Cholesteatomas arising in this location involve the epitympanic recess or Prussak space, initially eroding the scutum, tegmen tympani, lateral ossicles, and fallopian canal. A less common location is the pars tensa, or tense inferior two-thirds of the tympanic membrane. Cholesteatomas arising in this location involve the posterior mesotympanum medial to the ossicles, with erosions of aditus ad antrum, sinus tympani, facial recess, and otic capsule. In advanced stages, soft tissue and bone erosions can be present throughout the tympanic cavity, and the precise origin may be difficult to identify (**Fig. 10**).[106,107] Occasionally, with erosion through the tympanic membrane and/or external auditory canal, a cholesteatoma can decompress and completely drain its internal contents. This process is known as automastoidectomy and partially mimics surgical mastoidectomy at imaging, with a "hollowed-out" appearance of the middle ear and mastoid. Prior cholesteatoma is suggested by patient history, diffuse circumferential bone erosions, and a residual soft tissue rind.[108,109] In contrast, congenital cholesteatomas are thought to originate from embryonic epithelial rests deep to an intact tympanic membrane. Chronic otitis media is common in children; therefore, a superimposed inflammatory cause is likely. There is an association with

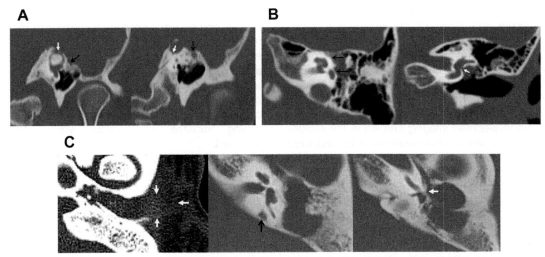

Fig. 10. Imaging of cholesteatoma. (A) CT scans, Pöschl views, show left pars flaccida acquired cholesteatoma. There is epitympanic soft tissue with multifocal bone erosion, including tegmen tympani (*black arrows*) and superior limb of superior semicircular canal (*white arrows*), compatible with labyrinthine fistula. (B) CT scans, axial and coronal views, show left congenital cholesteatoma. There is soft tissue centered at the cochlear promontory, with multifocal bone erosion of auditory ossicles, anterior tympanic wall, and otic capsule (*black arrows*). There is a labyrinthine fistula involving the oval window (*white arrow*). (C) CT scans, axial views, show left congenital external and middle ear anomaly. Soft tissue window shows microtia with bony stenosis and membranous atresia of the external auditory canal. A congenital cholesteatoma is present with soft tissue filling the rudimentary external auditory canal and middle ear cavity (*white arrows*). Bone windows show inner ear dysplasia with hypoplastic superior and lateral semicircular canals, underdeveloped vestibule, and enlarged vestibular aqueduct (*black arrow*). Extensive bone erosions are present involving the tympanic walls, auditory ossicles, tegmen tympani, and cochlear promontory with labyrinthine fistula, including round and oval windows (*white arrow*).

congenital external and middle ear anomalies, including microtia and syndromic dysplasias. Lesions most frequently originate in the anterosuperior tympanic cavity, near cochlear promontory and medial to the ossicles. Congenital cholesteatomas begin as well-circumscribed masses, but can grow to erode the ossicles, otic capsule, and tegmen tympani. At histopathology, these can present as enclosed epithelial cysts (closed type) of flat keratinizing epithelium with exposure of keratin (open type).[110–113]

Clinical symptoms of cholesteatoma vary according to the extent, location, and time course of disease. Some patients are asymptomatic, whereas others have varying degrees of auditory and/or vestibular systems. Patients can present with otorrhea, otalgia, conductive hearing loss, and vertiginous symptoms if a labyrinthine fistula is present. On audiometry, patients demonstrate a baseline conductive hearing loss with diffusely decreased air conduction. With isolated middle ear pathology, bone conduction remains normal and results in an air-bone gap across all sound frequencies. Superimposed third window effects produce supranormal bone conduction with exaggeration of the air-bone gap at low sound frequencies (**Fig. 11**).[114–120] Management options

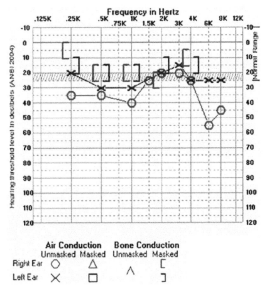

Fig. 11. Audiogram of right cholesteatoma with labyrinthine fistula. The right ear demonstrates conductive hearing loss due to middle ear pathology, with slightly decreased air conduction across multiple sound frequencies. There is a superimposed air-bone gap with supranormal bone conduction at low frequencies, due to third window anatomy.

include complete removal of cholesteatoma with exposure and repair of the labyrinthine fistula, versus near-total resection leaving a thin layer of cholesteatoma overlying the labyrinth. The former option can induce labyrinthitis and sensorineural hearing loss, whereas the latter option increases the likelihood of residual/recurrent disease.[121–124] In the postsurgical setting, MR imaging with diffusion-weighted imaging can aid in the evaluation of recurrent cholesteatoma with restricted diffusion and nonenhancement, as compared with postoperative granulation tissue, which enhances without diffusion abnormality.[125,126]

Langerhans cell histiocytosis (LCH) is characterized by aggressive proliferation of Langerhans cells. Originally considered a disorder of immune regulation, LCH has been reclassified as a dendritic cell neoplasm with strong inflammatory component, based on activating mutations in the BRAF-V600E proto-oncogene and dysregulation of the MAPK/ERK pathway.[127–129] Deposits can involve bone marrow, pituitary, brain, lung, liver, spleen, lymph nodes, thymus, and gastrointestinal tract. Within the temporal bone, lesions can be focal, multifocal, or diffuse with sharp geographic bone destruction. Common disease locations are the squamous and mastoid segments, with potential extension to the auditory ossicles and otic capsule. On MR imaging, T2 hypointensity can be seen due to hypercellular tissue as well as T1 hyperintensity, susceptibility, and fluid levels from spontaneous hemorrhage. Additional lesions within bone, dura, pituitary, and/or brain can support the diagnosis (**Fig. 12**).[130–134] Symptoms include otorrhea, otalgia, and conductive hearing loss. With inner ear fistula, vestibular and sensorineural hearing loss can also be present. LCH lesions can be confused for infection or neoplasia, and in the chronic setting, can be complicated by cholesteatoma.[135–141] Other histiocytic, granulomatous, and lymphocytic disorders can also yield destructive bone lesions and multisystem manifestations. These systemic inflammatory diseases are responsive to steroids and other immunosuppressive therapies, often resulting in complete radiographic and clinical resolution. Long-term follow-up is crucial, because multifocal and relapsing disease can occur years after treatment.[142–158]

Neoplastic processes can invade the temporal bone and fistulize to the inner ear. Rhabdomyosarcoma is the most common soft tissue sarcoma in children and is thought to arise from embryonic skeletal muscle precursor cells and/or pluripotent mesenchymal progenitor cells.[159,160] In the temporal bone, these present as rapidly growing soft tissue masses, commonly in the middle ear or petrous apex. Tumors can be complicated by inflammation or infection, leading to the misdiagnosis of primary otitis media or infectious mastoiditis. High clinical suspicion is crucial for curative surgery and/or adjuvant therapy. At-risk features include presumed infection refractory to antibiotics, discrete mass, regional lymphadenopathy, and cranial nerve signs. CT demonstrates aggressive bone destruction with variable periostitis and peri-inflammatory changes. On MR imaging, soft tissue may demonstrate T2-hypointense signal and restricted diffusion compatible with hypercellular tumor as well as heterogeneous avid enhancement. Because of the parameningeal location, intracranial invasion and metastases can occur early in the disease course (**Fig. 13**).[161–170]

Lymphoma, leukemia, myeloma, and neuroblastoma are other small round blue cell tumors with a capacity for diffuse marrow infiltration and cortical breakthrough.[171–180] Other metastatic tumors can infrequently involve the temporal bone and otic

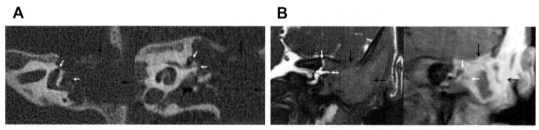

Fig. 12. Imaging of LCH. (*A*) CT scans, axial and coronal views, show invasive soft tissue with sharp bone destruction involving the left mastoid temporal bone (*black arrows*) and middle ear, resulting in erosions of auditory ossicles, tegmen mastoideum and tympani, and otic capsule. Labyrinthine fistula involves multiple inner ear structures, including oval window, superior and lateral semicircular canals (*white arrows*). (*B*) MR image, coronal fast imaging employing steady-state acquisition (FIESTA) and postcontrast T1 with fat saturation (FS), show a diffusely T2-hypointense and heterogeneously enhancing tissue through the left temporal bone (*black arrows*). There is extensive invasion of soft tissues and inner ear, with dehiscence of the superior and lateral semicircular canals (*white arrows*).

A   B

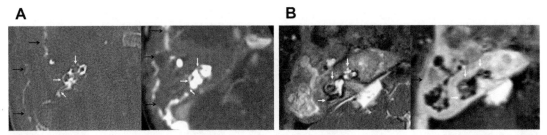

Fig. 13. Imaging of rhabdomyosarcoma. (*A*) CT scans, axial bone and soft tissue windows, show invasive right temporal bone mass with irregular bone erosions and multifocal breakthrough into soft tissues (*black arrows*), middle and inner ear, petrous apex, middle cranial fossa, and posterior fossa. Labyrinthine fistula involves multiple inner ear structures, including cochlear apex, oval window, and posterior semicircular canal (*white arrows*). (*B*) MR images, axial T2-weighted (T2W) and postcontrast T1-weighted (T1W) with FS, show abnormal T2-hypointense and avidly enhancing marrow throughout the right temporal bone (*black arrows*) with breakthrough into soft tissues and cranial cavity. Labyrinthine fistula involves multiple inner ear structures, including cochlear apex, lateral and posterior semicircular canals (*white arrows*).

capsule.[180–188] Vascular malformations and tumors can also permeate the temporal bone and produce vascular windows to the inner ear.[189–192] For example, glomus tumors or paragangliomas are smooth muscle tumors that arise from parasympathetic ganglia in the head and neck. Glomus jugulare tumors arise in the region of jugular foramen, with a characteristic superolateral vector of growth that can transgress the floor of middle ear and extend into the tympanic cavity (glomus jugulotympanicum). At CT, there is a characteristic "permeative" pattern of bone erosion. On MR imaging, a "salt and pepper" appearance results from hypervascularity with avid enhancement and flow voids (**Fig. 14**). Treatment options include surgery, radiation therapy, and/or selective embolization.[193–200] Malignant carcinomas can primarily or secondarily involve the temporal bone, with associated erosions. Occasionally, primary intracranial tumors such as gliosarcoma can extrude through the calvarium into extracranial soft tissues.[201,202]

Idiopathic intracranial hypertension or pseudotumor cerebri is a condition of elevated intracranial pressure without a primary inciting cause (tumor, infection, stroke). There is an association with obesity, because CSF opening pressures are positively associated with higher body mass index and cardiovascular risk factors. Patients can present with high-pressure headache, papilledema, progressive visual loss, and false localizing cranial nerve signs.[203–210] On CT, repeated CSF pulsations can result in effacement of the subarachnoid space with thinned diploe and prominent gyral convolutions along the inner table. Over time, these so-called arachnoid pits can progress to frank osteodural defects with labyrinthine fistulization, CSF leakage, and/or meningocele formation. Dehiscence is most likely to occur in areas where bone is already thin, including the middle cranial fossae, tegmen tympani, and arcuate eminences (**Fig. 15**). On MR imaging, additional features are reflective of the increased intracranial pressures: slit ventricles, empty sella, dural sinus

A   B

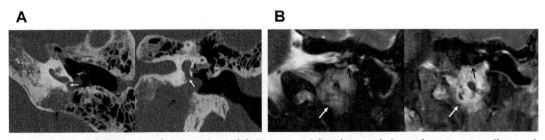

Fig. 14. Imaging of glomus jugulotympanicum. (*A*) CT scans, axial and coronal views, show an expansile mass in the left jugular foramen (*black arrows*) with superolateral growth into middle ear. There is a permeative pattern of surrounding bone destruction, including the cochlear promontory with dehiscence of oval and round windows (*white arrows*), jugular spine, and floor of middle ear cavity. (*B*) MR images, coronal T2W and postcontrast T1W with FS, show a T2-hyperintense and avidly enhancing left jugular foramen mass with internal vascular flow voids (*white arrows*). There is dehiscence into the inner ear, including round window of cochlea (*black arrows*).

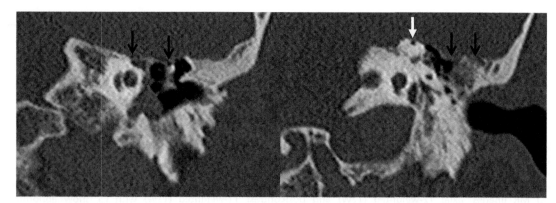

Fig. 15. Imaging of idiopathic intracranial hypertension. CT scans, coronal views, show diffuse osseous thinning with multiple arachnoid pits along the floor of left middle cranial fossa (*black arrows*), resulting in rarefaction of the tegmen tympani and predisposing to CSF leak. Superior semicircular canal dehiscence is also present (*white arrow*).

pseudostenosis, petrous apex cephaloceles, optic nerve sheath enlargement, superior ophthalmic vein dilation, posterior scleral flattening, and optic disc edema.[211–219] Accepted courses of treatment include weight loss, diuresis, and high-volume lumbar puncture. Severe cases may require surgery for CSF shunting, optic nerve sheath fenestration, and/or repair of skull defects.[220–224]

Traumatic fractures of the cranial vault and temporal bone can produce abnormal communications with the outside environment. Various complications can result, including CSF leakage with intracranial hypotension, meningocele formation, middle ear effusions, and otorrhea; and predisposition to infectious meningitis, labyrinthitis, and otitis. Longitudinal fractures parallel to the long axis of petrous temporal bone tend to involve the external and middle ear with conductive hearing loss. Transverse fractures perpendicular to the long axis of petrous temporal bone are more likely to violate the otic capsule with sensorineural

hearing loss. CT is important for delineating fracture planes and involvement of the otic capsule. The presence of pneumolabyrinth or pneumocochlea confirms that a labyrinthine fistula has occurred (**Fig. 16**).[225–232]

Iatrogenic labyrinthine fistulae can result from temporal bone surgery and posttherapy changes, either acutely or with a delayed time course. Patients can present with new-onset otorrhea, auditory, and/or vestibular symptoms. Complication rates are higher in the setting of more involved initial surgery, such as canal wall down tympanomastoidectomy. Causes are variable and include localized inflammation, infection, avascular necrosis, trauma, hardware migration, and recurrent disease (**Fig. 17**).[99,233–245]

Enlarged Vestibular Aqueduct

The bony vestibular aqueduct transmits the membranous endolymphatic duct, which drains fluid

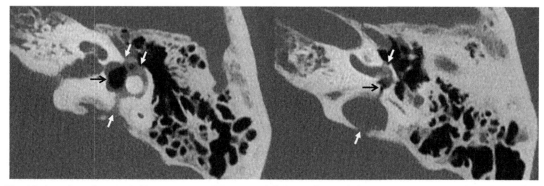

Fig. 16. Imaging of temporal bone trauma. CT scans, axial views, show a left transverse otic capsule-violating fracture (*white arrows*) extending through the cochlear promontory, round window, oval window, jugular bulb, and vestibular aqueduct. Free intralabyrinthine air in the vestibule (*black arrows*) is diagnostic of labyrinthine fistula.

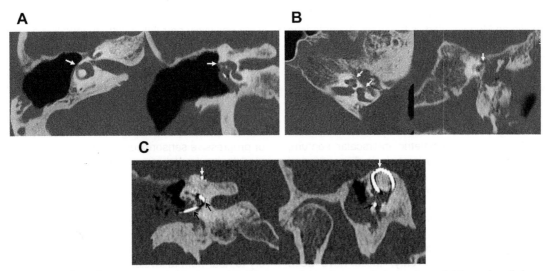

Fig. 17. Imaging of tympanomastoidectomy. (*A*) CT scans, axial and coronal views, show right canal wall down mastoidectomy and stapedectomy changes. There has been resection of otic capsule with exposure of the lateral semicircular canal (*white arrows*). (*B*) CT scans, axial and coronal views, show left canal wall down mastoidectomy complicated by chronic otitis media. The middle ear cavity is opacified with fluid, and there are surrounding bone erosions, including the cochlear apex and oval window (*white arrows*). (*C*) CT scans, coronal and Pöschl views, show malpositioned right cochlear implant traversing the oval window and vestibule (*black arrows*), coiling in a dehiscent superior semicircular canal (*white arrow*), and terminating near the common crus.

from the utricular and saccular ducts into the extraosseous endolymphatic sac, as well as the epithelium-lined perilymphatic duct, which communicates with the subarachnoid space. The overall morphology is that of an inverted J with multiple segments as described. The endolymphatic duct is a short single-lumen tubule that originates along the posteromedial vestibule (internal aperture), with a focal fusiform segment known as the sinus. Subsequent tapering leads into the proximal (ascending, horizontal, intermediate) segment, which curves superomedially with relatively constant size. Next is a sharp 70° angled constriction, known as the isthmus. The postisthmic segment corresponds roughly to the midpoint of the bony vestibular aqueduct and signifies the beginning of the intraosseous endolymphatic sac, which is conical in shape. The distal (descending, vertical) segment runs posteroinferiorly and progressively enlarges, more so in the axial than sagittal dimension. It opens to the external aperture on the posterior surface of the petrous pyramid, normally covered by a scale of bone known as the operculum. Beyond this is an extraosseous endolymphatic sac, a conical interconnecting network of tubules oriented posterolaterally. Distally, these tubules coalesce and terminate in a blind-ending pouch along the posterior wall of petrous temporal bone, enclosed between dural layers in close proximity to sigmoid sinus.[246]

The normal bony vestibular aqueduct is relatively long and proximally thinned, with a high effective impedance to sound transmission. When dilated, the vestibular aqueduct can serve as a third window with dissipation of acoustic energy from the inner ear into the posterior fossa dura or a high-riding jugular bulb.[1,2,72–74,247–250] Quantitative CT measurements have been established for diagnosis, most commonly the Cincinnati criteria: ≥1 mm at the midpoint (postisthmic segment) or ≥2 mm at the operculum (external aperture).[251,252] The older Valvassori criterion is more stringent, requiring a midpoint value of ≥1.5 mm.[253–255] Coronal reformats can better demonstrate the ovoid cross-sectional shape of the endolymphatic sac. Threshold values have been proposed as ≥2.4 mm at the midpoint and ≥4.34 mm at the operculum.[256,257] The oblique Pöschl projection allows for the most reliable depiction of the vestibular aqueduct throughout its length, and a threshold of ≥1.75 mm at the operculum has been proposed.[258–261] In practice, the adjacent inferior limb of posterior semicircular canal serves as an approximate reference to compare the size of the vestibular aqueduct. Dilation of the extraosseous endolymphatic sac can also be visualized on MR imaging.[262–264]

Enlarged vestibular aqueduct often occurs bilaterally and is seen with a spectrum of inner ear anomalies, which may be due to developmentally high inner ear pressures created by third window physiology. Incomplete partition type II, formerly known as Mondini triad, is the most characteristic malformation and includes the following: (1) "baseball cap" cochlea with bulbous nonseparation of the middle and apical turns; (2) enlarged vestibule with normal semicircular canals; (3) dilated vestibular aqueduct and endolymphatic sac. In practice, a spectrum of inner ear dysplasias can be seen, including cochleovestibular dysmorphism, deficient modiolus, asymmetric interscalar septum, and semicircular canal hypoplasia (Figs. 18 and 19). Genetic associations include Pendred (*SLC26A4, KCNJ10, FOXI1*), CHARGE (*CHD7*) (Figs. 20 and 21), and branchio-oto-renal (*EYA1, SIX1, SIX5*) (Figs. 22 and 23) syndromes.[264–276]

An often underrecognized imaging feature is the pattern of vestibular aqueductal enlargement. In order of increasing severity, these have been described as (1) mild focal dilation of aperture (borderline, filiform, wide notch); (2) similar moderate involvement of both aperture and midpoint (tubular, parallel); (3) severe involvement of aperture to a greater extent than the midpoint (funnel, flared). The latter morphologies have been significantly correlated with auditory and vestibular dysfunction, inner ear anomalies, and the presence of *SLC26A4* mutation. In a study performed at the author's institution, these morphologies were positively correlated with quantitative audiometric endpoints, including pure tone average, air-bone gap, and word recognition score. Imaging findings of dilated endolymphatic sac and inner ear malformations were additionally predictive of outcomes.[277–281]

Clinically, patients present with complex and variable patterns of hearing loss. Fluctuating and/or progressive sensorineural hearing loss is attributed to the underlying cochleovestibular malformations. At audiometry, this manifests with diffusely decreased air and bone conduction at both low and high frequencies. The presence of a third window can produce a superimposed air-bone gap at lower sound frequencies, which can artifactually increase bone conduction with recovery to near-normal levels.[12,18–20,282–288]

Cochlear Dehiscence

Cochlear dehiscence refers to deficiency of bone overlying the cochlea, permitting direct communication with the middle ear cavity or neurovascular structures. In order for third window mechanics to occur, the scala vestibuli side of the cochlea must be involved. Focal or diffuse thinning of the otic

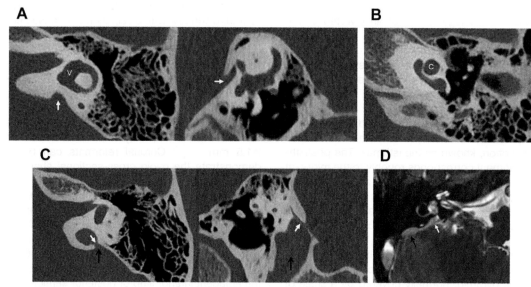

Fig. 18. Imaging of incomplete partition type II. Patient tested positive for *SLC26A4* mutation, diagnostic of Pendred syndrome. (*A*) CT scans, axial and Pöschl views, show dysplastic left vestibule (V) and enlarged vestibular aqueduct (*white arrows*), which has a "flared" morphology and is wider than the adjacent posterior semicircular canal. (*B*) CT scans, axial view, show a hypoplastic cochlea (C) with "baseball cap" morphology, including bulbous middle and apical turns with absent interscalar septum and deficient modiolus. (*C*) CT scans, axial and Pöschl views, show vestibular aqueduct dehiscence (*white arrows*) into a high-riding jugular bulb (*black arrows*). (*D*) MR images, axial FIESTA, show T2-intermediate signal within an enlarged right endolymphatic duct with flared morphology (*white arrow*) draining into a dilated endolymphatic sac (*black arrow*) along the posterior petrous face.

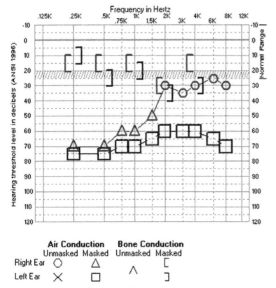

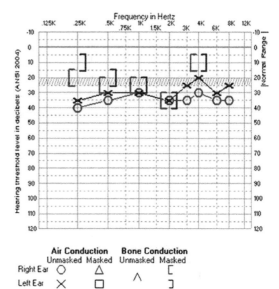

Fig. 19. Audiogram of bilateral incomplete partition type II. Both ears demonstrate sensorineural hearing loss with diffusely decreased air and bone conduction. There is a superimposed air-bone gap that artifactually increases bone conduction to near-normal levels, especially at lower sound frequencies.

Fig. 21. Audiogram of CHARGE syndrome. Both ears demonstrate mild sensorineural hearing loss with slightly decreased air and bone conduction. There is a superimposed air-bone gap that artifactually increases bone conduction to near-normal levels.

capsule can be congenital, postinflammatory, neoplastic, traumatic, or iatrogenic. Bone thinning enables fistulization to the carotid and fallopian canals, which can be hypomineralized as a normal variant. Defects can be minor (fissurelike) or major (gaping) and involve the nearest adjoining structure: petrous or lacerum segments of internal carotid artery; geniculate ganglion, labyrinthine, or tympanic segments of facial nerve; middle ear cavity or eustachian tube (Fig. 24).[289–299]

X-Linked Stapes Gusher

Stapes gusher syndrome is also known as X-linked deafness and incomplete partition type III.

It has been linked to mutations in the *POU3F4* gene on the X chromosome, which have been theorized to induce developmental otic placode ischemia with resulting abnormal bone development. Patients are usually boys and men and present with early-onset severe, progressive hearing loss. Female carriers can present with mild-moderate inner ear malformations and hearing loss, depending on the type of mutation.[300–306] The classic imaging appearance is a "corkscrew" cochlea with bulbous turns, absent modiolus, and patulous cochlear aperture. Images should be carefully scrutinized for deficiency of the bony lamina cribrosa, which normally separates the basal turn of cochlea from internal auditory canal fundus. Absence of the lamina cribrosa yields

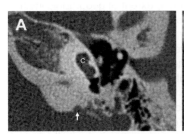

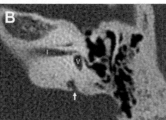

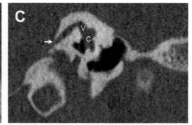

Fig. 20. Imaging of CHARGE syndrome. (A) CT scans, axial view, show a hypoplastic cochlea (C) with bulbous morphology, bulbous basal turn, undersegmented middle/apical turn, absent modiolus, and deficient interscalar septum. The vestibular aqueduct is slightly enlarged (*arrow*). (B) CT scans, axial view, show a hypoplastic vestibule (V) and stenotic internal auditory canal (I). The vestibular aqueduct is slightly enlarged (*arrow*). (C) CT scans, Pöschl view, show dysplasia of the cochlea (C) and vestibule (V). The vestibular aqueduct is slightly enlarged (*arrow*).

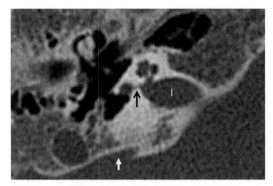

Fig. 22. Imaging of branchio-oto-renal syndrome. CT scans, axial view, show a dysplastic cochlea with "unwound" appearance consisting of a tapered basal turn (*black arrow*), hypoplastic and offset middle and apical turns, and flared internal auditory canal (I). The vestibular aqueduct is enlarged (*white arrow*).

direct communication between the perilymphatic and subarachnoid spaces, with variable transmission of intracranial pressures depending on the size of the bone defect. The vestibule, vestibular aqueduct, cochlear aqueduct, semicircular canals, internal auditory canal, and facial/vestibular nerve canals can also be enlarged and dysplastic, with diffuse thinning of the surrounding otic capsule (**Fig. 25**).[275,307–320] Clinical features include mixed hearing loss with severe

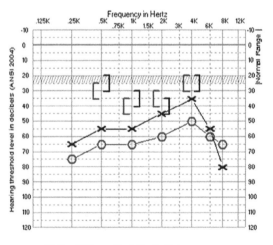

Fig. 23. Audiogram of branchio-oto-renal syndrome. Both ears demonstrate sensorineural hearing loss with diffusely decreased air and bone conduction. There is a superimposed air-bone gap that artifactually increases bone conduction to near-normal levels, especially at lower sound frequencies.

sensorineural component due to perilymphatic hydrops. A superimposed air-bone gap reflecting third window physiology may be detectable at low frequencies, mimicking conductive hearing loss (**Fig. 26**).[321–326] If patients have only conductive losses, they may benefit from external hearing aids. Stapes surgery should not be performed due to the high risk of CSF leak, meningitis, and labyrinthitis with further hearing loss. For patients with sensorineural hearing loss, cochlear implantation can be performed with control of fluid leakage. Outcomes remain poor compared with other inner ear malformations.[327–333]

Bone Dyscrasias

The otic capsule is the hardest and densest bone in the human body, forming from modified cartilaginous centers that ossify into a compact mineralized structure devoid of Haversian canals. Bone remodeling is inhibited later in life, due to antiresorptive chemicals secreted by the inner ear. High bone density enables intralabyrinthine fluid vibrations to be reflected rather than absorbed.[334,335] Bone dyscrasias can incite pathologic bone turnover with osteoclastic activation. The affected bone demonstrates decreased acoustic impedance and acts as a mechanically distributed third window, with dissipation of acoustic energy from the cochlea. This pathology results in a profound hearing loss with decreased air conduction (ossicular chain involvement) and/ or bone conduction (otic capsule involvement). Superimposed low-frequency air-bone gaps may be identified with partial recovery of bone thresholds.[336–340]

Otospongiosis or otosclerosis is the most common cause of hearing loss in young adults. The disease appears to be multifactorial with genetic, viral, inflammatory, and autoimmune associations. Abnormal bone remodeling is localized to the otic capsule endochondral bone.[341–344] Disease is graded according to extent of geographic involvement: 1 = fenestral, 2A = basal cochlear turn, 2B = cochlear middle/apical turn, 3 = diffuse cochlear involvement. Fenestral (stapedial) otospongiosis is the most common location and involves the fissula ante fenestram, a cartilaginous cleft anterior to the oval window, and progresses to stapes ankylosis with conductive hearing loss. Retrofenestral (cochlear) otospongiosis involves the pericochlear region and is typically seen in more advanced cases. The sensorineural component of hearing loss has been theorized to reflect microscopic impingement of the inner ear and/or regional inflammatory changes in the otic capsule.[345–350] Disease temporally progresses

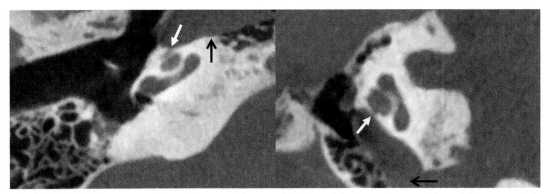

Fig. 24. Imaging of cochlear dehiscence. CT scans, axial and Pöschl views, show cochlear dehiscence of the cochlear apex (*white arrows*) into the carotid canal (*black arrows*).

through early, intermediate, and final phases. In the acute phase, there is deposition of unmineralized osteoid tissue within the otic capsule. With subacute disease, osteoclast activation induces focal bone resorption around preexisting blood vessels, yielding lucent woven bone (otospongiosis). In florid cases, frank cavitary plaques can develop within bone (cavitary otospongiosis) and communicate with inner ear structures, producing the appearance of diverticula (**Figs. 27** and **28**). Chronically, osteoblastic activity dominates and produces dense irregular cancellous bone (otosclerosis). MR imaging can demonstrate areas of marrow enhancement and edema reflective of inflammatory bone remodeling.[351–358] Bisphosphonates, which inhibit osteoclastic activity, and nutrient mineral supplements may help slow the progression of disease. Stapedectomy can be performed for isolated fenestral otospongiosis in the presence of an intact round window. For retrofenestral otospongiosis, cochlear implantation is

the operation of choice. Middle ear surgery in cavitary otosclerosis carries the risk of CSF gusher, due to macrocystic/microcystic spaces enabling communication between the perilymphatic and subarachnoid spaces.[359–363]

Osteogenesis imperfecta is the most common heritable connective tissue disorder. The disease is caused by various mutations in type I collagen synthesis (eg, *COL1A1*, *COL1A2*), yielding fragile connective tissue and brittle bones. Young patient age with diffuse skeletal abnormalities and fractures after minor trauma suggest the diagnosis.[339,364,365] The otic capsule is progressively undermineralized during life and can mimic lytic otospongiosis at CT. Osseous lucencies can be present at the fissula ante fenestram and bony labyrinth and can also affect auditory ossicles, oval window, round window, and fallopian canal (**Fig. 29**).[366–368] The pattern of disease involvement corresponds to the presence and type of hearing loss on audiometry (**Fig. 30**).[369–376]

A   **B**

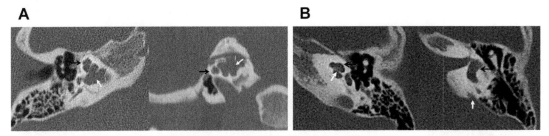

Fig. 25. Imaging of X-linked stapes gusher. (*A*) Male patient. CT scans, axial and Pöschl views, show dysplastic cochlea with "corkscrew" appearance demonstrating bulbous dilated turns (*black arrows*), absent interscalar septum and modiolus. There is absence of the lamina cribrosa (*white arrows*) that normally separates the cochlea from internal auditory canal (I), predisposing to CSF gusher with inner ear surgery. (*B*) Female *POU3F4* carrier. CT scans, axial views, show malformations similar to incomplete partition type II. There is an undersegmented "baseball cap" cochlea (*black arrow*) with hypoplastic lamina cribrosa between the basal turn of cochlea and internal auditory canal fundus. Vestibule (*black arrow*) and vestibular aqueduct (*white arrow*) are mildly dilated.

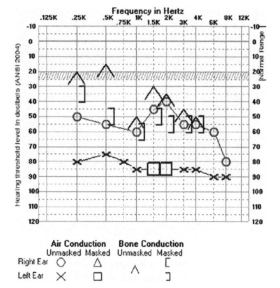

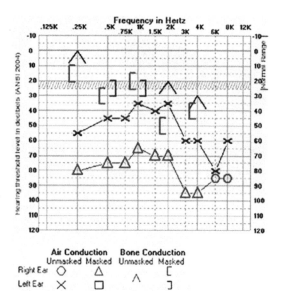

Fig. 26. Audiogram of X-linked stapes gusher. Both ears demonstrate sensorineural hearing loss with diffusely decreased air and bone conduction. There is a superimposed air-bone gap that artifactually increases bone conduction to near-normal levels, especially at lower sound frequencies.

Fig. 28. Audiogram of cavitary otospongiosis. Both ears demonstrate conductive hearing loss with diffusely decreased air conduction due to middle ear pathology. There is a superimposed low-frequency air-bone gap due to third window anatomy.

Bisphosphonates and dietary supplements can be used to promote otic capsule mineralization. Surgical options include stapes revision for fenestral disease and cochlear implantation for retrofenestral disease. Because of low bone stock, surgery is more technically difficult and associated with poorer patient outcomes.[377–383]

Fibrous dysplasia is a benign fibro-osseous condition of young adults. It is caused by sporadic mutations of the *GNAS* gene, with multiple associated syndromes including McCune-Albright (polyostotic fibrous dysplasia, café au lait spots, and hyperfunctional endocrinopathy). Defects in osteoblast maturation and differentiation yield immature woven (fibrous) bone, consisting of disorganized and structurally weak collagen fibers.[384–387] In early childhood and adolescence, there is active osteoclastic bone resorption with a lucent wispy or whorled

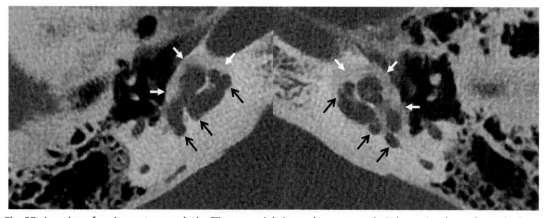

Fig. 27. Imaging of cavitary otospongiosis. CT scans, axial views, demonstrate lytic lucencies throughout the bony labyrinth (*white arrows*), including the fissula ante fenestram (fenestral) and pericochlear (retrofenestral) regions. Frank cavitary plaques create the appearance of cystic diverticula from the vestibule and cochlea (*black arrows*).

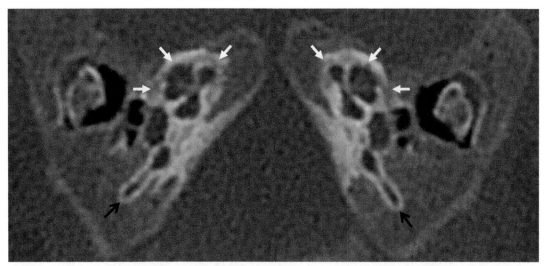

Fig. 29. Imaging of osteogenesis imperfecta. CT scans, axial views, demonstrate diffuse bone demineralization surrounding the semicircular canals (*black arrows*). There are lytic lucencies throughout the bony labyrinth (*white arrows*), including the fissula ante fenestram and pericochlear regions.

appearance on CT, and variable T2 hyperintensity and enhancement on MR imaging. The marrow space appears diffusely expanded but retains its overall morphology, blending smoothly into

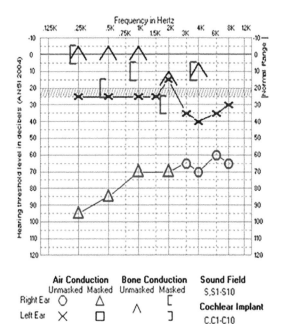

Fig. 30. Audiogram of osteogenesis imperfecta. Patient has history of trauma to the right side of the head with asymmetric hearing loss. The right ear demonstrates conductive hearing loss with diffusely decreased air conduction due to middle ear pathology. There is a superimposed low-frequency air-bone gap due to third window anatomy. The left ear demonstrates a mild air-bone gap without background conductive hearing loss.

overlying cortex. Following puberty, disease enters a static (quiescent) phase with greater osteoblastic activity. Bone becomes more sclerotic with a homogeneous (ground-glass) or heterogeneous (amorphous) appearance on CT, and progressive T2 hypointensity and hypoenhancement on MR imaging. Reactivation can rarely occur following trauma, surgery, or hormonal changes (**Fig. 31**).[387–391] Conductive hearing loss can result from external and middle ear involvement, particularly crowding of the ossicular chain. Sensorineural hearing loss has been linked to otic capsule and inner ear involvement, particularly stenosis and elongation of the internal auditory canal (**Fig. 32**).[392–404] Disease can be further complicated by infection, cholesteatoma, and rarely, malignant transformation into sarcoma. Management is conservative, with surgery reserved for functional preservation and prevention of complications.[405–410]

Paget disease or osteitis deformans is a multifactorial bone disease of older adults, in which there is excessive dystrophic remodeling as evidenced by elevated serum alkaline phosphatase. The initial osteolytic phase involves prominent bone resorption (osteoporosis circumscripta) by large osteoclasts. Hematopoietic marrow is replaced by fibrovascular connective tissue, which appears well defined and lucent on CT, with T2-hyperintense signal and enhancement on MR. As osteoblasts become activated, disease progresses to the mixed stage with disorganized bone formation. Bones show heterogeneous mosaic attenuation reflecting the combination of lytic and sclerotic activity.

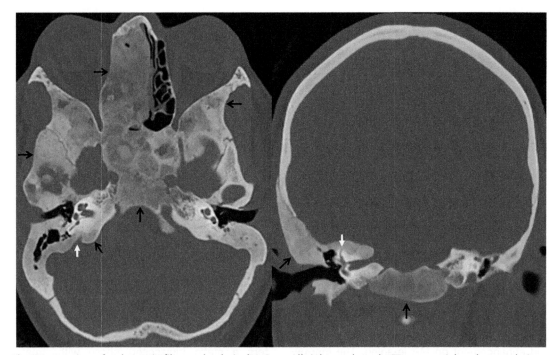

Fig. 31. Imaging of polyostotic fibrous dysplasia (McCune-Albright syndrome). CT scans, axial and coronal views, show multifocal expansion of right greater than left craniofacial bones and skull base (*black arrows*) with smooth cortical thinning, "ground-glass" marrow attenuation, and cystic degeneration. There is involvement of the right greater than left temporal bones, including right vestibular aqueduct and superior semicircular canal (*white arrows*).

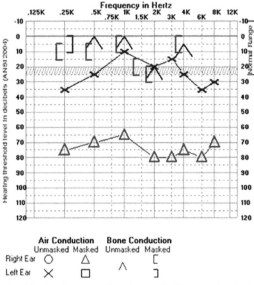

Fig. 32. Audiogram of polyostotic fibrous dysplasia (McCune-Albright syndrome). The right ear demonstrates conductive hearing loss with diffusely decreased air conduction due to middle ear pathology. There is a superimposed low-frequency air-bone gap due to third window anatomy. The left ear demonstrates a mild air-bone gap without background conductive hearing loss.

Expansion in all directions yields a coarsened morphology with irregular thickening of cortex and trabeculae. Over time, osteoblastic activity predominates, resulting in quiescent disease with dense "cotton-wool" sclerosis. In some cases, a final remodeling phase recruits osteoclasts to remodel inactive pagetic bone into more typically lamellar bone and restart the entire cycle (**Figs. 33** and **34**).[336,411–415] Patients present with progressive bilateral hearing loss due to diffuse multifocal involvement, including the temporal bone in advanced cases. Bone remodeling tracks from peripheral to central within the otic capsule, targeting the labyrinthine, endochondral, and tympanic layers. Sensorineural hearing loss can result from otic capsule erosions with cochlear dysfunction and internal auditory narrowing with compression of cranial nerve VIII. Conductive hearing loss can also be present when there is involvement of auditory ossicles and middle ear ligaments.[416–423] Bisphosphonate and calcitonin therapy help to limit bone remodeling. Cochlear implantation is advisable for patients with advanced hearing loss. Drug treatment before surgery helps reduce blood flow and decrease risks of disease hyperactivity at the instrumented area.[424–427]

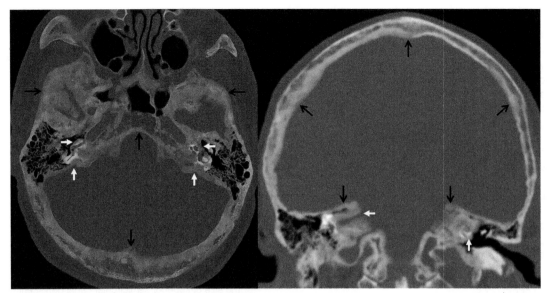

Fig. 33. Imaging of Paget disease. CT scans, axial and coronal views, show dystrophic craniofacial and skull base changes (*black arrows*) with irregular cortical expansion and mixed sclerosis/lysis. There is involvement of both bony labyrinths (*white arrows*) with narrowing of internal auditory canals.

Additional metabolic and inflammatory bone disorders can affect the temporal bone and generate diffuse third windows. Primary and secondary hyperparathyroidism (associated with renal osteodystrophy) involve disruptions in calcium and phosphate balance with subsequent inhibition of osteoclastogenesis. Metabolic disruption produces diffusely weakened bones (osteitis fibrosa cystica) with peritrabecular fibrosis and cystic collections of fibrovascular tissue and hemosiderin (brown tumors). Bone resorption occurs in various locations, including subperiosteal, subchondral, trabecular, endosteal, and subligamentous. In chronic disease, reactive periostitis can lead to narrowing and impingement of neurovascular structures.[428–432] Disseminated syphilis and tuberculosis infections can produce granulomatous otomastoiditis with aggressive bone destruction and fistulization.[428,433–436]

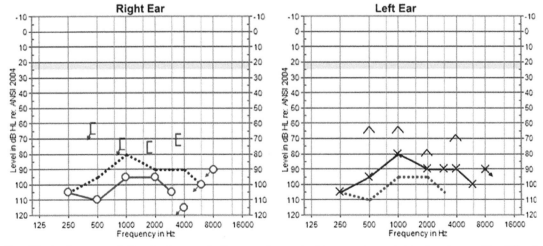

Fig. 34. Audiogram of Paget disease. Both ears demonstrate sensorineural hearing loss with diffusely decreased air and bone conduction. There is a superimposed low-frequency air-bone gap due to third window anatomy.

SUMMARY

Third window abnormalities are bony defects of the inner ear that enable abnormal communication with the middle ear and/or cranial cavity. Clinically, patients present clinically with vestibular (Tullio and Hennebert) signs as well as "pseudo-conductive" hearing loss with low-frequency air-bone gap. Third window lesions can occur at multiple anatomic locations, including the superior, posterior, and lateral semicircular canals; vestibule and vestibular aqueduct; and scala vestibuli of the cochlea. Causes include idiopathic dehiscence, infection, inflammation, neoplasia, CSF hypertension, trauma, surgery, congenital malformations, and bone dyscrasias. High-resolution temporal bone CT is critical for accurate diagnosis and management of third window pathologies.

REFERENCES

1. Merchant SN, Rosowski JJ. Conductive hearing loss caused by third-window lesions of the inner ear. Otol Neurotol 2008;29:282–9.

2. Ho ML, Moonis G, Halpin CF, et al. Spectrum of third window abnormalities: semicircular canal dehiscence and beyond. AJNR Am J Neuroradiol 2017;38(1):2–9.

3. Kaski D, Davies R, Luxon L, et al. The Tullio phenomenon: a neurologically neglected presentation. J Neurol 2012;259(1):4–21.

4. Shuman AG, Rizvi SS, Pirouet CW, et al. Hennebert's sign in superior semicircular canal dehiscence syndrome: a video case report. Laryngoscope 2012;122(2):412–4.

5. Branstetter BF 4th, Harrigal C, Escott EJ, et al. Superior semicircular canal dehiscence: oblique reformatted CT images for diagnosis. Radiology 2006;238:938–42.

6. Lee YH, Rivas-Rodriguez F, Song JJ, et al. The prevalence of superior semicircular canal dehiscence in conductive and mixed hearing loss in the absence of other pathology using submillimetric temporal bone computed tomography. J Comput Assist Tomogr 2014;38(2):190–5.

7. Ekdale EG. Form and function of the mammalian inner ear. J Anat 2016;228(2):324–37.

8. Thomson S1, Madani G2. The windows of the inner ear. Clin Radiol 2014;69(3):e146–52.

9. Stenfelt S, Hato N, Goode RL. Fluid volume displacement at the oval and round windows with air and bone conduction stimulation. J Acoust Soc Am 2004;115(2):797–812.

10. Chhana D, Thompson C, Ahob K. Two-dimensional analysis of fluid motion in the cochlea resulting from compressional bone conduction. J Sound Vib 2014;333(3):1067–78.

11. Tonndorf J, Tabor JR. Closure of the cochlear windows: its effect upon air- and bone-conduction. Ann Otol Rhinol Laryngol 1962;71:5–29.

12. Bance M. When is a conductive hearing loss not a conductive hearing loss? Causes of a mismatch in air-bone threshold measurements or a "pseudoconductive" hearing loss. J Otolaryngol 2004;33:135–8.

13. Minor LB. Superior canal dehiscence syndrome. Am J Otol 2000;21:9–19.

14. Minor LB, Solomon D, Zinreich JS, et al. Sound- and/or pressure-induced vertigo due to bone dehiscence of the superior semicircular canal. Arch Otolaryngol Head Neck Surg 1998;124:249–58.

15. Belden CJ, Weg N, Minor LB, et al. CT evaluation of bone dehiscence of the superior semi-circular canal as a cause of sound- and/or pressure-induced vertigo. Radiology 2003;226:337–43.

16. Yuen HW, Boeddinghaus R, Eikelboom RH, et al. The relationship between the air-bone gap and the size of superior semicircular canal dehiscence. Otolaryngol Head Neck Surg 2009;141(6):689–94.

17. Noij KS, Duarte MJ, Wong K, et al. Toward optimizing cervical vestibular evoked myogenic potentials (cvemp): combining air-bone gap and cVEMP thresholds to improve diagnosis of superior canal dehiscence. Otol Neurotol 2018;39(2):212–20.

18. Merchant SN, Nakajima HH, Halpin C, et al. Clinical investigation and mechanism of air-bone gaps in large vestibular aqueduct syndrome. Ann Otol Rhinol Laryngol 2007;116(7):532–41.

19. Seo YJ, Kim J, Choi JY. Correlation of vestibular aqueduct size with air-bone gap in enlarged vestibular aqueduct syndrome. Laryngoscope 2016;126(7):1633–8.

20. Sheykholeslami K, Schmerber S, Habiby Kermany M, et al. Vestibular-evoked myogenic potentials in three patients with large vestibular aqueduct. Hear Res 2004;190(1–2):161–8.

21. Fatterpekar GM, Doshi AH, Dugar M, et al. Role of 3D CT in the evaluation of the temporal bone. Radiographics 2006;26(Suppl 1):S117–32.

22. Veillon F, Riehm S, Emachescu B, et al. Imaging of the windows of the temporal bone. Semin Ultrasound CT MR 2001;22(3):271–80.

23. Giesemann A, Hofmann E. Some remarks on imaging of the inner ear: options and limitations. Clin Neuroradiol 2015;25(Suppl 2):197–203.

24. Ward BK, Carey JP, Minor LB. Superior canal dehiscence syndrome: lessons from the first 20 years. Front Neurol 2017;8:177.

25. Nadgir RN, Ozonoff A, Devaiah AK, et al. Superior semicircular canal dehiscence: congenital or acquired condition? AJNR Am J Neuroradiol 2011;32(5):947–9.

26. Minor LB, Cremer PD, Carey JP, et al. Symptoms and signs in superior canal dehiscence syndrome. Ann N Y Acad Sci 2001;942:259–73.

27. Naert L, Van de Berg R, Van de Heyning P, et al. Aggregating the symptoms of superior semicircular canal dehiscence syndrome. Laryngoscope 2018;128(8):1932–8.

28. Curtin HD. Superior semicircular canal dehiscence syndrome and multi-detector row CT. Radiology 2003;226:312–4.

29. Hagiwara M, Shaikh JA, Fang Y, et al. Prevalence of radiographic semicircular canal dehiscence in very young children: an evaluation using high-resolution computed tomography of the temporal bones. Pediatr Radiol 2012;42(12):1456–64.

30. Sequeira SM, Whiting BR, Shimony JS, et al. Accuracy of computed tomography detection of superior canal dehiscence. Otol Neurotol 2011;32(9): 1500–5.

31. Stimmer H, Hamann KF, Zeiter S, et al. Semicircular canal dehiscence in HR multislice computed tomography: distribution, frequency, and clinical relevance. Eur Arch Otorhinolaryngol 2012;269(2): 475–80.

32. Cloutier JF, Bélair M, Saliba I. Superior semicircular canal dehiscence: positive predictive value of high-resolution CT scanning. Eur Arch Otorhinolaryngol 2008;265(12):1455–60.

33. Tavassolie TS, Penninger RT, Zuñiga MG, et al. Multislice computed tomography in the diagnosis of superior canal dehiscence: how much error, and how to minimize it? Otol Neurotol 2012;33(2):215–22.

34. Mikulec AA, McKenna MJ, Ramsey MJ, et al. Superior semicircular canal dehiscence presenting as conductive hearing loss without vertigo. Otol Neurotol 2004;25:121–9.

35. Beutner D. The relationship between the air-bone gap and the size of superior semicircular canal dehiscence. Otolaryngol Head Neck Surg 2010; 142(4):634 [author reply: 634–6].

36. Pfammatter A, Darrouzet V, Gärtner M, et al. A superior semicircular canal dehiscence syndrome multicenter study: is there an association between size and symptoms? Otol Neurotol 2010; 31(3):447–54.

37. Chien WW, Janky K, Minor LB, et al. Superior canal dehiscence size: multivariate assessment of clinical impact. Otol Neurotol 2012;33(5):810–5.

38. Sood D, Rana L, Chauhan R, et al. Superior semicircular canal dehiscence: a new perspective. Eur J Radiol Open 2017;4:144–6.

39. Niesten ME, Stieger C, Lee DJ, et al. Assessment of the effects of superior canal dehiscence location and size on intracochlear sound pressures. Audiol Neurootol 2015;20(1):62–71.

40. Hunter JB, O'Connell BP, Wang J, et al. Correlation of superior canal dehiscence surface area with vestibular evoked myogenic potentials, audiometric thresholds, and dizziness handicap. Otol Neurotol 2016;37(8):1104–10.

41. Saliba I, Maniakas A, Benamira LZ, et al. Superior canal dehiscence syndrome: clinical manifestations and radiologic correlations. Eur Arch Otorhinolaryngol 2014;271(11):2905–14.

42. Kim N, Steele CR, Puria S. Superior-semicircular-canal dehiscence: effects of location, shape, and size on sound conduction. Hear Res 2013;301:72–84.

43. Rajan GP, Leaper MR, Goggin L, et al. The effects of superior semicircular canal dehiscence on the labyrinth: does size matter? Otol Neurotol 2008; 29(7):972–5.

44. Lagman C, Beckett JS, Chung LK, et al. Novel method of measuring canal dehiscence and evaluation of its potential as a predictor of symptom outcomes after middle fossa craniotomy. Neurosurgery 2018;83(3):459–64.

45. McCall AA, McKenna MJ, Merchant SN, et al. Superior canal dehiscence syndrome associated with the superior petrosal sinus in pediatric and adult patients. Otol Neurotol 2011;32:1312–9.

46. Koo JW, Hong SK, Kim DK, et al. Superior semicircular canal dehiscence syndrome by the superior petrosal sinus. J Neurol Neurosurg Psychiatry 2010;81(4):465–7.

47. Browaeys P, Larson TL, Wong ML, et al. Can MRI replace CT in evaluating semicircular canal dehiscence? AJNR Am J Neuroradiol 2013;34(7):1421–7.

48. Inal M, Burulday V, Bayar Muluk N, et al. Magnetic resonance imaging and computed tomography for diagnosing semicircular canal dehiscence. J Craniomaxillofac Surg 2016;44(8):998–1002.

49. Spear SA, Jackson NM, Mehta R, et al. Is MRI equal to CT in the evaluation of thin and dehiscent superior semicircular canals? Otol Neurotol 2016; 37(2):167–70.

50. Beyazal Çeliker F, Özgür A, Çeliker M, et al. The efficacy of magnetic resonance imaging for the diagnosis of superior semicircular canal dehiscence. J Int Adv Otol 2018;14(1):68–71.

51. Benamira LZ, Maniakas A, Alzahrani M, et al. Common features in patients with superior canal dehiscence declining surgical treatment. J Clin Med Res 2015;7(5):308–14.

52. Chilvers G, McKay-Davies I. Recent advances in superior semicircular canal dehiscence syndrome. J Laryngol Otol 2015;129(3):217–25.

53. Lookabaugh S, Kelly HR, Carter MS, et al. Radiologic classification of superior canal dehiscence: implications for surgical repair. Otol Neurotol 2015;36(1):118–25.

54. Palma Diaz M, Cisneros Lesser JC, Vega Alarcón A. Superior semicircular canal dehiscence syndrome - diagnosis and surgical management. Int Arch Otorhinolaryngol 2017;21(2):195–8.

55. Mau C, Kamal N, Badeti S, et al. Superior semicircular canal dehiscence: diagnosis and management. J Clin Neurosci 2018;48:58–65.

56. Lee GS, Zhou G, Poe D, et al. Clinical experience in diagnosis and management of superior semicircular canal dehiscence in children. Laryngoscope 2011;121(10):2256–61.

57. Crovetto M, Whyte J, Rodriguez OM, et al. Anatomo-radiological study of the superior semicircular canal dehiscence: radiological considerations of superior and posterior semicircular canals. Eur J Radiol 2010;76:167–72.

58. Saxby AJ, Gowdy C, Fandiño M, et al. Radiological prevalence of superior and posterior semicircular canal dehiscence in children. Int J Pediatr Otorhinolaryngol 2015;79(3):411–8.

59. Dang PT, Kennedy TA, Gubbels SP. Simultaneous, unilateral plugging of superior and posterior semicircular canal dehiscences to treat debilitating hyperacusis. J Laryngol Otol 2014; 128(2):174–8.

60. Elmali M, Polat AV, Kucuk H, et al. Semicircular canal dehiscence: frequency and distribution on temporal bone CT and its relationship with the clinical outcomes. Eur J Radiol 2013;82(10):e606–9.

61. Russo JE, Crowson MG, DeAngelo EJ, et al. Posterior semicircular canal dehiscence: CT prevalence and clinical symptoms. Otol Neurotol 2014;35(2):310–4.

62. Meiklejohn DA, Corrales CE, Boldt BM, et al. Pediatric semicircular canal dehiscence: radiographic and histologic prevalence, with clinical correlation. Otol Neurotol 2015;36(8):1383–9.

63. Nomiya S, Cureoglu S, Kariya S, et al. Posterior semicircular canal dehiscence: a histopathologic human temporal bone study. Otol Neurotol 2010; 31:1122–7.

64. Whyte J, Cisneros AI, Martínez C, et al. Congenital dehiscence in the posterior semicircular canal. Otol Neurotol 2013;34(6):1134–7.

65. Peress L, Telian SA, Srinivasan A. Dehiscence of the posterior semicircular canal. Am J Otolaryngol 2015;36(1):77–9.

66. Gopen Q, Zhou G, Poe D, et al. Posterior semicircular canal dehiscence: first reported case series. Otol Neurotol 2010;31(2):339–44.

67. Schutt CA, Kveton JF. Posterior semicircular canal dehiscence secondary to jugular enlargement. Am J Otolaryngol 2016;37(3):173–4.

68. Kundaragi NG, Mudali S, Karpagam B, et al. Intracranially protruded bilateral posterior and superior SCCs with multiple dehiscences in a patient with positional vertigo: CT and MR imaging findings and review of literature. Indian J Radiol Imaging 2014;24(4):406–9.

69. Gubbels SP, Zhang Q, Lenkowski PW, et al. Repair of posterior semicircular canal dehiscence from a high jugular bulb. Ann Otol Rhinol Laryngol 2013; 122(4):269–72.

70. Lim HW, Park HJ, Jung JH, et al. Surgical treatment of posterior semicircular canal dehiscence syndrome caused by jugular diverticulum. J Laryngol Otol 2012;126(9):928–31.

71. Park JJ, Shen A, Loberg C, et al. The relationship between jugular bulb position and jugular bulb related inner ear dehiscence: a retrospective analysis. Am J Otolaryngol 2015;36(3): 347–51.

72. Friedmann DR, Eubig J, Winata LS, et al. Prevalence of jugular bulb abnormalities and resultant inner ear dehiscence: a histopathologic and radiologic study. Otolaryngol Head Neck Surg 2012; 147(4):750–6.

73. Sone M, Katayama N, Naganawa S, et al. Audiological signs in pediatric cases with dehiscence of the bony labyrinth caused by a high jugular bulb. Int J Pediatr Otorhinolaryngol 2012;76(3):447–51.

74. Erdogan N, Songu M, Akay E, et al. Posterior semicircular canal dehiscence in asymptomatic ears. Acta Otolaryngol 2011;131(1):4–8.

75. Kubota M, Kubo K, Yasui T, et al. Development of conductive hearing loss due to posterior semicircular canal dehiscence. Auris Nasus Larynx 2015;42(3):245–8.

76. Bear ZW, McEvoy TP, Mikulec AA. Quantification of hearing loss in patients with posterior semicircular canal dehiscence. Acta Otolaryngol 2015; 135(10):974–7.

77. Krombach GA, DiMartino E, Schmitz-Rode T, et al. Posterior semicircular canal dehiscence: a morphologic cause of vertigo similar to superior semicircular canal dehiscence. Eur Radiol 2003; 13:1444–50.

78. Spasic M, Trang A, Chung LK, et al. Clinical characteristics of posterior and lateral semicircular canal dehiscence. J Neurol Surg B Skull Base 2015; 76(6):421–5.

79. Chien WW, Carey JP, Minor LB. Canal dehiscence. Curr Opin Neurol 2011;24:25–31.

80. Zhang LC, Sha Y, Dai CF. Another etiology for vertigo due to idiopathic lateral semicircular canal bony defect. Auris Nasus Larynx 2011;38(3): 402–5.

81. Zhang YB, Dai CF, Sha Y. Sound-induced vertigo due to bone dehiscence of the lateral semicircular canal. Eur Arch Otorhinolaryngol 2010;267(8): 1319–21.

82. Bhalla AS, Singh A, Jana M. Chronically discharging ears: evelution with high resolution computed tomography. Pol J Radiol 2017;82:478–89.

83. Payal G, Pranjal K, Gul M, et al. Computed tomography in chronic suppurative otitis media: value in surgical planning. Indian J Otolaryngol Head Neck Surg 2012;64(3):225–9.

84. Faramarzi AH, Heydari ST, Rusta M. The prevalence of labyrinthine fistula in chronic otitis media surgery in shiraz, southern iran. Iran Red Crescent Med J 2011;13(8):582–5.

85. Busaba NY. Clinical presentation and management of labyrinthine fistula caused by chronic otitis media. Ann Otol Rhinol Laryngol 1999; 108(5):435–9.

86. Jang CH, Merchant SN. Histopathology of labyrinthine fistulae in chronic otitis media with clinical implications. Am J Otol 1997;18(1):15–25.

87. Matsubara K, Omori K, Baba K. Acute coalescent mastoiditis and acoustic sequelae in an infant with severe congenital neutropenia. Int J Pediatr Otorhinolaryngol 2002;62(1):63–7.

88. Arcand P, Cérat J, Spénard JR. Acute otomastoiditis in the leukemic child. J Otolaryngol 1989;18(7): 380–3.

89. Yunus TM, Molina RM, Prevatt AR, et al. Hearing loss with semicircular canal fistula in exotoxin A-deficient Pseudomonas otitis media. Otolaryngol Head Neck Surg 2004;130(4):430–6.

90. Stiernberg CM, Stiernberg C, Bailey BJ, et al. Acute necrotizing otitis media. Otolaryngol Head Neck Surg 1986;94(5):648–51.

91. Shen KH, Shiao AS. Acute necrotizing otitis media in an infant: a case report. Zhonghua Yi Xue Za Zhi (Taipei) 1999;62(3):175–8.

92. Gebhardt B, Giers A, Arens C, et al. Fusobacterium necrophorum–cause of a mastoiditis with skull- and mandibular joint osteomyelitis. Laryngorhinootologie 2011;90(7):403–8 [in German].

93. Aldana-Aguirre JC, El-Hakim H, Phillipos E, et al. Congenital tuberculosis presenting as otorrhoea in a preterm infant. BMJ Case Rep 2018.

94. Viswanatha B, Naseeruddin K. Fungal infections of the ear in immunocompromised host: a review. Mediterr J Hematol Infect Dis 2011;3(1): e2011003.

95. Rutt AL, Sataloff RT. Aspergillus otomycosis in an immunocompromised patient. Ear Nose Throat J 2008;87(11):622–3.

96. Bryce GE, Phillips P, Lepawsky M, et al. Invasive Aspergillus tympanomastoiditis in an immunocompetent patient. J Otolaryngol 1997;26(4):266–9.

97. Marzo SJ, Leonetti JP. Invasive fungal and bacterial infections of the temporal bone. Laryngoscope 2003;113(9):1503–7.

98. Ghiasi S. Labyrinthine fistula in chronic otitis media with cholesteatoma. J Pak Med Assoc 2011;61(4): 352–5.

99. Kitahara T, Kamakura T, Ohta Y, et al. Chronic otitis media with cholesteatoma with canal fistula and bone conduction threshold after tympanoplasty with mastoidectomy. Otol Neurotol 2014;35(6): 981–8.

100. Shinnabe A, Hara M, Hasegawa M, et al. Clinical characteristics and surgical benefits and problems of chronic otitis media and middle ear cholesteatoma in elderly patients older than 70 years. Otol Neurotol 2012;33(7):1213–7.

101. Blom EF, Gunning MN, Kleinrensink NJ, et al. Influence of ossicular chain damage on hearing after chronic otitis media and cholesteatoma surgery: a systematic review and meta-analysis. JAMA Otolaryngol Head Neck Surg 2015;141(11):974–82.

102. Bulğurcu S, Arslan İB, Dikilitaş B, et al. Relation between ossicular erosion and destruction of facial and lateral semicircular canals in chronic otitis media. Int Arch Otorhinolaryngol 2017; 21(3):239–42.

103. Jang CH, Choi YH, Jeon ES, et al. Extradural granulation complicated by chronic suppurative otitis media with cholesteatoma. In Vivo 2014;28(4): 651–5.

104. Maniu A, Harabagiu O, Perde Schrepler M, et al. Molecular biology of cholesteatoma. Rom J Morphol Embryol 2014;55(1):7–13.

105. Kuo CL, Shiao AS, Yung M, et al. Updates and knowledge gaps in cholesteatoma research. Biomed Res Int 2015;2015:854024.

106. Corrales CE, Blevins NH. Imaging for evaluation of cholesteatoma: current concepts and future directions. Curr Opin Otolaryngol Head Neck Surg 2013;21(5):461–7.

107. Rosito LS, Netto LF, Teixeira AR, et al. Classification of cholesteatoma according to growth patterns. JAMA Otolaryngol Head Neck Surg 2016;142(2): 168–72.

108. Blake DM, Vazquez A, Tomovic S, et al. Automastoidectomy. Ear Nose Throat J 2014;93(6):E53–4.

109. Miranda JA, Suzuki FA, de Carvalho Borges MH, et al. Automastoidectomy. Braz J Otorhinolaryngol 2006;72(3):429.

110. Jang CH, Cho YB. Congenital cholesteatoma extending into the internal auditory canal and cochlea: a case report. In Vivo 2008;22(5): 651–4.

111. Tos M. A new pathogenesis of mesotympanic (congenital) cholesteatoma. Laryngoscope 2000; 110(11):1890–7.

112. Bacciu A, Di Lella F, Pasanisi E, et al. Open vs closed type congenital cholesteatoma of the middle ear: two distinct entities or two aspects of the same phenomenon? Int J Pediatr Otorhinolaryngol 2014;78(12):2205–9.

113. McGill TJ, Merchant S, Healy GB, et al. Congenital cholesteatoma of the middle ear in children: a clinical and histopathological report. Laryngoscope 1991;101(6 Pt 1):606–13.

114. Kim SH, Cho YS, Chu HS, et al. Open-type congenital cholesteatoma: differential diagnosis for conductive hearing loss with a normal tympanic membrane. Acta Otolaryngol 2012;132:618–23.

115. Fiorino F, Pizzini FB, Mattellini B, et al. Vestibular dehiscence syndrome caused by a labyrinthine congenital cholesteatoma. Ear Nose Throat J 2015;94(2):E1–5.

116. Ikeda R, Kobayashi T, Kawase T, et al. Risk factors for deterioration of bone conduction hearing in cases of labyrinthine fistula caused by middle ear cholesteatoma. Ann Otol Rhinol Laryngol 2012; 121(3):162–7.

117. Katsura H, Mishiro Y, Adachi O, et al. Long-term deterioration of bone-conduction hearing level in patients with labyrinthine fistula. Auris Nasus Larynx 2014;41(1):6–9.

118. Rosito LPS, Canali I, Teixeira A, et al. Cholesteatoma labyrinthine fistula: prevalence and impact. Braz J Otorhinolaryngol 2018. https://doi.org/10.1016/j.bjorl.2018.01.005 [pii:S1808-8694(18)30059-4].

119. Shim DB, Ko KM, Song MH, et al. A case of labyrinthine fistula by cholesteatoma mimicking lateral canal benign paroxysmal positional vertigo. Korean J Audiol 2014;18(3):153–7.

120. Casale M, Errante Y, Sabatino L, et al. Perilymphatic fistula test: a video clip demonstration. Eur Rev Med Pharmacol Sci 2014;18(23):3549–50.

121. Eliades SJ, Limb CJ. The role of mastoidectomy in outcomes following tympanic membrane repair: a review. Laryngoscope 2013;123(7): 1787–802.

122. Meyer A, Bouchetemblé P, Costentin B, et al. Lateral semicircular canal fistula in cholesteatoma: diagnosis and management. Eur Arch Otorhinolaryngol 2016;273(8):2055–63.

123. Kobayashi T, Sato T, Toshima M, et al. Treatment of labyrinthine fistula with interruption of the semicircular canals. Arch Otolaryngol Head Neck Surg 1995;121(4):469–75.

124. Debruyne F, Vantrappen G, Feenstra L, et al. Computed tomographic imaging of repaired fistulas of the lateral semicircular canal. Am J Otol 1994;15(4):549–50.

125. Muzaffar J, Metcalfe C, Colley S, et al. Diffusion-weighted magnetic resonance imaging for residual and recurrent cholesteatoma: a systematic review and meta-analysis. Clin Otolaryngol 2017;42(3): 536–43.

126. van Egmond SL, Stegeman I, Grolman W, et al. A systematic review of non-echo planar diffusion-weighted magnetic resonance imaging for detection of primary and postoperative cholesteatoma. Otolaryngol Head Neck Surg 2016;154(2):233–40.

127. Tran G, Huynh TN, Paller AS. Langerhans cell histiocytosis: a neoplastic disorder driven by Ras-ERK pathway mutations. J Am Acad Dermatol 2018;78(3):579–90.e4.

128. Abla O, Weitzman S. Treatment of Langerhans cell histiocytosis: role of BRAF/MAPK inhibition. Hematology Am Soc Hematol Educ Program 2015;2015: 565–70.

129. Roden AC, Hu X, Kip S, et al. BRAF V600E expression in Langerhans cell histiocytosis: clinical and immunohistochemical study on 25 pulmonary and 54 extrapulmonary cases. Am J Surg Pathol 2014;38(4):548–51.

130. Zheng H, Xia Z, Cao W, et al. Pediatric Langerhans cell histiocytosis of the temporal bone: clinical and imaging studies of 27 cases. World J Surg Oncol 2018;16(1):72.

131. Ginat DT, Johnson DN, Cipriani NA. Langerhans cell histiocytosis of the temporal bone. Head Neck Pathol 2016;10(2):209–12.

132. Neilan RE, Kutz JW Jr. Langerhans cell histiocytosis of the temporal bone. Otol Neurotol 2012; 33(4):e31–2.

133. Yildirim-Baylan M, Cureoglu S, Paparella MM. Langerhans' cell histiocytosis of the temporal bone. Otol Neurotol 2012;33(2):e15–6.

134. Nicollas R, Rome A, Belaïch H, et al. Head and neck manifestation and prognosis of Langerhans' cell histiocytosis in children. Int J Pediatr Otorhinolaryngol 2010;74(6):669–73.

135. Ong HY, Goh LC, Santhi K, et al. Concurrent mastoid cellulitis and langerhans cells histiocytosis: a challenging diagnosis. Oman Med J 2018;33(2): 167–70.

136. Simmonds JC, Vecchiotti M. Cholesteatoma as a complication of Langerhans Cell Histiocytosis of the temporal bone: a nationwide cross-sectional analysis. Int J Pediatr Otorhinolaryngol 2017;100:66–70.

137. Losie JA, Yong M, Kozak FK, et al. Unique case of hearing recovery after otic capsule destruction and complete sensorineural hearing loss caused by langerhans cell histiocytosis. Otol Neurotol 2017; 38(8):1129–32.

138. Blumberg JM, Malhotra A, Wu X, et al. Langerhans cell histiocytosis of the temporal bone with otic capsule involvement. Clin Neuroradiol 2017;27(2): 163–8.

139. Modest MC, Garcia JJ, Arndt CS, et al. Langerhans cell histiocytosis of the temporal bone: a review of 29 cases at a single center. Laryngoscope 2016; 126(8):1899–904.

140. Giovannetti F, Aboh IV, Chisci G, et al. Langerhans cell histiocytosis: treatment strategies. J Craniofac Surg 2014;25(3):1134–6.

141. Nakamaru Y, Takagi D, Oridate N, et al. Otolaryngologic manifestations of antineutrophil cytoplasmic antibody-associated vasculitis. Otolaryngol Head Neck Surg 2012;146(1):119–21.

142. Uppal P, Taitz J, Wainstein B, et al. Refractory otitis media: an unusual presentation of childhood granulomatosis with polyangiitis. Pediatr Pulmonol 2014;49(3):E21–4.

143. Mercan GC, Mercan B, Cukurova I. Wegener granulomatosis presenting as refractory otitis media: a case report. Kulak Burun Bogaz Ihtis Derg 2012; 22(5):293–6.

144. Goderis J, De Schepper S, Vannieuwenhuyze P, et al. Wegener granulomatosis as possible cause

of vertigo: case report and review. B-ENT 2015; 11(1):67–72.

145. Elmas F, Shrestha BL, Linder TE. Subtotal petrosectomy and cochlear implant placement in otologic presentation of "Wegener's Granulomatosis". Kathmandu Univ Med J (KUMJ) 2017;15(57):94–8.

146. Ovadia S, Dror I, Zubkov T, et al. Churg-Strauss syndrome: a rare presentation with otological and pericardial manifestations: case report and review of the literature. Clin Rheumatol 2009;28(Suppl 1): S35–8.

147. Gross M, Maly B, Arevalo C, et al. Acute otitis media and subdural abscess as primary manifestations of Kikuchi's disease. Otolaryngol Head Neck Surg 2004;130(3):391–4.

148. Tian XF, Li TJ, Yu SF. Giant cell granuloma of the temporal bone: a case report with immunohistochemical, enzyme histochemical, and in vitro studies. Arch Pathol Lab Med 2003;127(9): 1217–20.

149. Lee TK, Jung TY, Baek HJ, et al. Disseminated juvenile xanthogranuloma occurring after treatment of Langerhans cell histiocytosis: a case report. Childs Nerv Syst 2018;34(4):765–70.

150. Wenig BM, Abbondanzo SL, Childers EL, et al. Extranodal sinus histiocytosis with massive lymphadenopathy (Rosai-Dorfman disease) of the head and neck. Hum Pathol 1993;24(5):483–92.

151. Calandra CR, Bustos A, Falcon F, et al. Erdheim-Chester disease: atypical presentation of a rare disease. BMJ Case Rep 2017;2017 [pii:bcr-2017-220827].

152. Pollack IF, Hamilton RL, Fitz C, et al. Congenital reactive myofibroblastic tumor of the petrous bone: case report. Neurosurgery 2001;48(2): 430–5.

153. Lovisari F, Terzi V, Lippi MG, et al. Hemophagocytic lymphohistiocytosis complicated by multiorgan failure: a case report. Medicine (Baltimore) 2017; 96(50):e9198.

154. Ortlip TE, Drake VE, Raghavan P, et al. Inflammatory pseudotumor of the temporal bone: a case series. Otol Neurotol 2017;38(7):1024–31.

155. Rodgers B, Bhalla V, Zhang D, et al. Bilateral inflammatory myofibroblastic tumor mastoiditis. Head Neck 2015;37(11):E142–5.

156. Zhou X, Liu T, Chen Z, et al. Inflammatory myofibroblastic tumor of the temporal bone presenting with pulsatile tinnitus: a case report. J Med Case Rep 2013;7:157.

157. Maniu AA, Harabagiu O, Damian LO, et al. Mastoiditis and facial paralysis as initial manifestations of temporal bone systemic diseases - the significance of the histopathological examination. Rom J Morphol Embryol 2016;57(1):243–8.

158. Nwawka OK, Nadgir R, Fujita A, et al. Granulomatous disease in the head and neck: developing a differential diagnosis. Radiographics 2014;34(5): 1240–56.

159. Péault B, Rudnicki M, Torrente Y, et al. Stem and progenitor cells in skeletal muscle development, maintenance, and therapy. Mol Ther 2007;15(5):867–77.

160. Chal J, Pourquié O. Making muscle: skeletal myogenesis in vivo and in vitro. Development 2017; 144(12):2104–22.

161. Goldberg MJ. Pediatric temporal bone rhabdomyosarcoma. JAAPA 2016;29(8):1–3.

162. Gluth MB. Rhabdomyosarcoma and other pediatric temporal bone malignancies. Otolaryngol Clin North Am 2015;48(2):375–90.

163. Freling NJ, Merks JH, Saeed P, et al. Imaging findings in craniofacial childhood rhabdomyosarcoma. Pediatr Radiol 2010;40(11):1723–38 [quiz: 1855].

164. Kariya S, Cureoglu S, Schachern PA, et al. Histopathological temporal bone study of the metastatic rhabdomyosarcoma. Auris Nasus Larynx 2009; 36(2):221–3.

165. Sbeity S, Abella A, Arcand P, et al. Temporal bone rhabdomyosarcoma in children. Int J Pediatr Otorhinolaryngol 2007;71(5):807–14.

166. Abbas A, Awan S. Rhabdomyosarcoma of the middle ear and mastoid: a case report and review of the literature. Ear Nose Throat J 2005;84(12):780, 782, 784.

167. Durve DV, Kanegaonkar RG, Albert D, et al. 1. Paediatric rhabdomyosarcoma of the ear and temporal bone. Clin Otolaryngol Allied Sci 2004;29(1):32–7.

168. Lee CA, Aga L, Lie QY, et al. Rhabdomyosarcoma presenting as an acute suppurative mastoiditis. Otolaryngol Head Neck Surg 2004;131(5):791–2.

169. Chevallier KM, Wiggins RH, Quinn NA, et al. Differentiating pediatric rhabdomyosarcoma and Langerhans cell histiocytosis of the temporal bone by imaging appearance. AJNR Am J Neuroradiol 2016;37(6):1185–9.

170. Zhang X, Ma K, Wang J, et al. A prospective evaluation of the combined helical tomotherapy and chemotherapy in pediatric patients with unresectable rhabdomyosarcoma of the temporal bone. Cell Biochem Biophys 2014;70(1):103–8.

171. Sung L, Dix D, Allen U, et al. Epstein-Barr virus-associated lymphoproliferative disorder in a child undergoing therapy for localized rhabdomyosarcoma. Med Pediatr Oncol 2000;34(5):358–60.

172. Alvi SA, Flynn JP, Gener M, et al. Burkitt lymphoma of the temporal bone. Otol Neurotol 2018;39(5): e410–2.

173. Vaid S, Jadhav J, Chandorkar A, et al. Bilateral non-hodgkin's lymphoma of the temporal bone: a rare and unusual presentation. Case Rep Otolaryngol 2016;2016:2641876.

174. Liu Y, Chen Q, Si Y, et al. Hodgkin's lymphoma of the temporal bone accompanied by intracranial abscess. Otol Neurotol 2014;35(2):e95–6.

175. Aljafar HM, Alsuhibani SS, Alahmari MS, et al. Temporal bone metastasis as a sign of relapsing chronic lymphocytic leukemia. Saudi Med J 2015; 36(10):1233–5.

176. Kumar R, Kumar N, Mohindro S, et al. Solitary plasmacytoma of temporal bone: a rare case report. Asian J Neurosurg 2017;12(1):95–7.

177. Sweeney AD, Hunter JB, Rajkumar SV, et al. Plasmacytoma of the temporal bone, a great imitator: report of seven cases and comprehensive review of the literature. Otol Neurotol 2017;38(3):400–7.

178. Silva C, Silvestre N, Amorim AM, et al. Temporal bone myeloid sarcoma. Acta Otorrinolaringol Esp 2015;66(3):175–7.

179. Almofada HS, Timms MS, Dababo MA. Ganglioneuroma of the external auditory canal and middle ear. Case Rep Otolaryngol 2017;2017:4736895.

180. Hensley MF. Metastatic neuroblastoma in a 16-month-old child. J Am Osteopath Assoc 1985; 85(8):534–6.

181. Bellarbi S, Harmouch A, El Ochi MR, et al. Melanotic progonoma of temporal and occipital bones: a case report. Neurochirurgie 2013;59(3):138–40.

182. Hızlı Ö, Salduz A, Kaya S, et al. A rare location for sarcoma metastasis: the temporal bone. Am J Otolaryngol 2015;36(6):772–7.

183. Clamp PJ, Jardine AH. Mastoiditis secondary to metastatic lung carcinoma: case report and literature review. J Laryngol Otol 2011;125(11): 1173–5.

184. Choi SH, Park IS, Kim YB, et al. Unusual presentation of a metastatic tumor to the temporal bone: severe otalgia and facial paralysis. Korean J Audiol 2014;18(1):34–7.

185. Su P, Kuan CC, Kondo K, et al. Temporal bone pathological study on maxillary sinus carcinoma with bilateral temporal bone metastasis. Acta Otolaryngol 2007;127(12):1338–44.

186. Nagai M, Yamada H, Kitamoto M, et al. J Facial nerve palsy due to temporal bone metastasis from hepatocellular carcinoma. Gastroenterol Hepatol 2005;20(7):1131–2.

187. Wu Ch, Kaga K, Ohira Y, et al. Histopathology of multiple temporal bone metastasis from pancreatic adenocarcinoma: a case showing bilateral hearing loss and Bechterew's phenomenon. Otolaryngol Head Neck Surg 2000;122(4):613–5.

188. Ohira Y, Kaga K, Kodama A. A case of bilateral sudden hearing loss and vertigo caused by bilateral temporal bone metastasis from pancreatic carcinoma–comparison of clinical findings and temporal bone pathological findings. Nihon Jibiinkoka Gakkai Kaiho 1991;94(1):9–15 [in Japanese].

189. Yue Y, Jin Y, Yang B, et al. Retrospective case series of the imaging findings of facial nerve hemangioma. Eur Arch Otorhinolaryngol 2015;272(9): 2497–503.

190. Dai YY, Sha Y, Zhang F, et al. Imaging diagnosis of masses in temporal bone associated with pulsatile tinnitus. Zhonghua Yi Xue Za Zhi 2013;93(33): 2617–21 [in Chinese].

191. Benoit MM, North PE, McKenna MJ, et al. Facial nerve hemangiomas: vascular tumors or malformations? Otolaryngol Head Neck Surg 2010;142(1): 108–14.

192. Lalaji TA, Haller JO, Burgess RJ. A case of head and neck kaposiform hemangioendothelioma simulating a malignancy on imaging. Pediatr Radiol 2001;31(12):876–8.

193. Gosepath J, Welkoborsky HJ, Mann W. [Biology and growth velocity of tumors of the globus jugulotympanicum and glomus caroticum]. Laryngorhinootologie 1998;77(8):429–33 [in German].

194. Steiner MA, Khan M, May BB, et al. Giant recurrent glomus jugulotympanicum with intracranial, extracranial, and nasophayngeal extension: the imaging role in clinical management. Radiol Case Rep 2015;4(4):314.

195. Tasar M, Yetiser S. Glomus tumors: therapeutic role of selective embolization. J Craniofac Surg 2004; 15(3):497–505.

196. Sur RK, Levin CV, Donde B, et al. Jugulotympanic paragangliomas. S Afr J Surg 1995;33(3):112–4.

197. Goebel JA, Smith PG, Kemink JL, et al. Primary adenocarcinoma of the temporal bone mimicking paragangliomas: radiographic and clinical recognition. Otolaryngol Head Neck Surg 1987;96(3): 231–8.

198. Devaney KO, Ferlito A, Rinaldo A. Endolymphatic sac tumor (low-grade papillary adenocarcinoma) of the temporal bone. Acta Otolaryngol 2003; 123(9):1022–6.

199. Mukherji SK, Castillo M. Adenocarcinoma of the endolymphatic sac: imaging features and preoperative embolization. Neuroradiology 1996;38(2): 179–80.

200. Devaney KO, Boschman CR, Willard SC, et al. Tumours of the external ear and temporal bone. Lancet Oncol 2005;6(6):411–20.

201. Borota OC, Scheie D, Bjerkhagen B, et al. Gliosarcoma with liposarcomatous component, bone infiltration and extracranial growth. Clin Neuropathol 2006;25(4):200–3.

202. Schuss P, Ulrich CT, Harter PN, et al. Gliosarcoma with bone infiltration and extracranial growth: case report and review of literature. J Neurooncol 2011; 103(3):765–70.

203. Friedman DI. The pseudotumor cerebri syndrome. Neurol Clin 2014;32(2):363–96.

204. McGeeney BE, Friedman DI. Pseudotumor cerebri pathophysiology. Headache 2014;54(3):445–58.

205. Bezerra MLS, Ferreira ACAF, de Oliveira-Souza R. Pseudotumor cerebri and glymphatic dysfunction. Front Neurol 2018;8:734.

206. Gilland O, Tourtellotte WW, O'Tauma L, et al. Normal cerebrospinal fluid pressure. J Neurosurg 1974;40:587–93.

207. Corbett JJ, Mehta MP. Cerebrospinal fluid pressure in normal obese subjects and patients with pseudotumor cerebri. Neurology 1983;33:1386–8.

208. Whiteley W, Al-Shahi R, Warlow CP, et al. CSF opening pressure: reference interval and the effect of body mass index. Neurology 2006;67:1690–1.

209. Avery RA, Shah SS, Licht DJ, et al. Reference range for cerebrospinal fluid opening pressure in children. N Engl J Med 2010;363:891–3.

210. Contreras-Martin Y, Bueno-Perdomo JH. Idiopathic intracranial hypertension: descriptive analysis in our setting. Neurologia 2015;30(2):106–10.

211. Tuncel SA, Yılmaz E, Çağlı B, et al. Lumbar opening pressure and radiologic scoring in idiopathic intracranial hypertension: is there any correlation? Pol J Radiol 2017;82:701–5.

212. Rizk HG, Hatch JL, Stevens SM, et al. Lateral skull base attenuation in superior semicircular canal dehiscence and spontaneous cerebrospinal fluid otorrhea. Otolaryngol Head Neck Surg 2016;155(4):641–8.

213. Jan TA, Cheng YS, Landegger LD, et al. Relationship between surgically treated superior canal dehiscence syndrome and body mass index. Otolaryngol Head Neck Surg 2017;156(4):722–7.

214. Schutt CA, Neubauer P, Samy RN, et al. The correlation between obesity, obstructive sleep apnea, and superior semicircular canal dehiscence: a new explanation for an increasingly common problem. Otol Neurotol 2015;36(3):551–4.

215. Bialer OY, Rueda MP, Bruce BB, et al. Meningoceles in idiopathic intracranial hypertension. AJR Am J Roentgenol 2014;202(3):608–13.

216. Jamjoom DZ, Alorainy IA. The association between petrous apex cephalocele and empty sella. Surg Radiol Anat 2015;37(10):1179–82.

217. Brainard L, Chen DA, Aziz KM, et al. Association of benign intracranial hypertension and spontaneous encephalocele with cerebrospinal fluid leak. Otol Neurotol 2012;33(9):1621–4.

218. Silver RI, Moonis G, Schlosser RJ, et al. Radiographic signs of elevated intracranial pressure in idiopathic cerebrospinal fluid leaks: a possible presentation of idiopathic intracranial hypertension. Am J Rhinol 2007;21(3):257–61.

219. Wang YX, Jonas JB, Wang N, et al. Intraocular pressure and estimated cerebrospinal fluid pressure. The Beijing Eye Study 2011. PLoS One 2014;9(8):e104267.

220. Burkett JG, Ailani J. An up to date review of pseudotumor cerebri syndrome. Curr Neurol Neurosci Rep 2018;18(6):33.

221. Aylward SC, Way AL. Pediatric intracranial hypertension: a current literature review. Curr Pain Headache Rep 2018;22(2):14.

222. Cleves-Bayon C. Idiopathic intracranial hypertension in children and adolescents: an update. Headache 2018;58(3):485–93.

223. Galgano MA, Deshaies EM. An update on the management of pseudotumor cerebri. Clin Neurol Neurosurg 2013;115(3):252–9.

224. Gilbert AL, Chwalisz B, Mallery R. Complications of optic nerve sheath fenestration as a treatment for idiopathic intracranial hypertension. Semin Ophthalmol 2018;33(1):36–41.

225. Swartz JD. Temporal bone trauma. Semin Ultrasound CT MR 2001;22(3):219–28.

226. Exadaktylos AK, Sclabas GM, Nuyens M, et al. The clinical correlation of temporal bone fractures and spiral computed tomographic scan: a prospective and consecutive study at a level I trauma center. J Trauma 2003;55(4):704–6.

227. Yetiser S, Hidir Y, Gonul E. Facial nerve problems and hearing loss in patients with temporal bone fractures: demographic data. J Trauma 2008; 65(6):1314–20.

228. Ishman SL, Friedland DR. Temporal bone fractures: traditional classification and clinical relevance. Laryngoscope 2004;114(10):1734–41.

229. Rafferty MA, Mc Conn Walsh R, Walsh MA. A comparison of temporal bone fracture classification systems. Clin Otolaryngol 2006;31(4): 287–91.

230. Dahiya R, Keller JD, Litofsky NS, et al. Temporal bone fractures: otic capsule sparing versus otic capsule violating clinical and radiographic considerations. J Trauma 1999;47(6):1079–83.

231. Gross M, Ben-Yaakov A, Goldfarb A, et al. Pneumolabyrinth: an unusual finding in a temporal bone fracture. Int J Pediatr Otorhinolaryngol 2003; 67(5):553–5.

232. Johnson F, Semaan MT, Megerian CA. Temporal bone fracture: evaluation and management in the modern era. Otolaryngol Clin North Am 2008; 41(3):597–618, x.

233. Kao R, Wannemuehler T, Yates CW, et al. Outpatient management of cholesteatoma with canal wall reconstruction tympanomastoidectomy. Laryngoscope Investig Otolaryngol 2017;2(6): 351–7.

234. Kuhweide R, Van de Steene V, Vlaminck S, et al. Reparative granuloma related to perilymphatic fistula. Adv Otorhinolaryngol 2007;65:296–9.

235. Hakuba N, Hato N, Shinomori Y, et al. Labyrinthine fistula as a late complication of middle ear surgery using the canal wall down technique. Otol Neurotol 2002;23(6):832–5.

236. Cox MD, Page JC, Trinidade A, et al. Long-term complications and surgical failures after ossiculoplasty. Otol Neurotol 2017;38(10):1450–5.

237. Lesinski SG. Causes of conductive hearing loss after stapedectomy or stapedotomy: a prospective

study of 279 consecutive surgical revisions. Otol Neurotol 2002;23(3):281–8.

238. Incesulu A, Häusler R. Advantages and risks of various sealing procedures of the oval window: vein graft, adipose tissue, gelfoam, merogel. Adv Otorhinolaryngol 2007;65:206–9.

239. Kusuma S, Liou S, Haynes DS. Disequilibrium after cochlear implantation caused by a perilymph fistula. Laryngoscope 2005;115(1):25–6.

240. Chiesa Estomba CM, Rivera Schmitz T, Betances Reinoso FA, et al. Complications after cochlear implantation in adult patients. 10-Year retrospective analysis of a tertiary academic centre. Auris Nasus Larynx 2017;44(1):40–5.

241. Gadre AK, Hammerschlag PE. Labyrinthine fistula: an unreported complication of the Grote prosthesis. Laryngoscope 2001;111(5):796–800.

242. Ayache D, Lejeune D, Williams MT. Imaging of postoperative sensorineural complications of stapes surgery: a pictorial essay. Adv Otorhinolaryngol 2007;65:308–13.

243. Portmann D, Rezende Ferreira D. Delayed labyrinthine fistula in canal wall down mastoidectomy. Rev Laryngol Otol Rhinol (Bord) 2003;124(4):265–8.

244. Phillips DJ, Njoku IU, Brown KD, et al. Radiation-induced necrosis of the temporal bone: diagnosis and management. Otol Neurotol 2015;36(8): 1374–7.

245. Roberts SA, Kamdar DJ, Mehta H, et al. Post-radiotherapy radionecrosis of the temporal bone resulting in delayed CSF otorrhoea: a case report. Br J Neurosurg 2013;27(1):125–7.

246. Lo WW, Daniels DL, Chakeres DW, et al. The endolymphatic duct and sac. AJNR Am J Neuroradiol 1997;18(5):881–7.

247. Hourani R, Carey J, Yousem DM. Dehiscence of the jugular bulb and vestibular aqueduct: findings on 200 consecutive temporal bone computed tomography scans. J Comput Assist Tomogr 2005; 29(5):657–62.

248. Friedmann DR, Eubig J, Winata LS, et al. A clinical and histopathologic study of jugular bulb abnormalities. Arch Otolaryngol Head Neck Surg 2012; 138(1):66–71.

249. Friedmann DR, Le BT, Pramanik BK, et al. Clinical spectrum of patients with erosion of the inner ear by jugular bulb abnormalities. Laryngoscope 2010;120(2):365–72.

250. Kupfer RA, Hoesli RC, Green GE, et al. The relationship between jugular bulb-vestibular aqueduct dehiscence and hearing loss in pediatric patients. Otolaryngol Head Neck Surg 2012;146(3):473–7.

251. Boston M, Halsted M, Meinzen-Derr J, et al. The large vestibular aqueduct: a new definition based on audiologic and computed tomography correlation. Otolaryngol Head Neck Surg 2007;136(6): 972–7.

252. Vijayasekaran S, Halsted MJ, Boston M, et al. When is the vestibular aqueduct enlarged? A statistical analysis of the normative distribution of vestibular aqueduct size. AJNR Am J Neuroradiol 2007;28(6):1133–8.

253. Valvassori G, Clemis J. The large vestibular aqueduct syndrome. Laryngoscope 1978;88:273–8.

254. El-Badry MM, Osman NM, Mohamed HM, et al. Evaluation of the radiological criteria to diagnose large vestibular aqueduct syndrome. Int J Pediatr Otorhinolaryngol 2016;81:84–91.

255. Dewan K, Wippold FJ 2nd, Lieu JE. Enlarged vestibular aqueduct in pediatric sensorineural hearing loss. Otolaryngol Head Neck Surg 2009; 140(4):552–8.

256. Murray LN, Tanaka GJ, Cameron DS, et al. Coronal computed tomography of the normal vestibular aqueduct in children and young adults. Arch Otolaryngol Head Neck Surg 2000;126(11): 1351–7.

257. Saliba I, Gingras-Charland ME, St-Cyr K, et al. Coronal CT scan measurements and hearing evolution in enlarged vestibular aqueduct syndrome. Int J Pediatr Otorhinolaryngol 2012;76(4):492–9.

258. Lane JI, Lindell EP, Witte RJ, et al. Middle and inner ear: improved depiction with multiplanar reconstruction of volumetric CT data. Radiographics 2006;26(1):115–24.

259. Ozgen B, Cunnane ME, Caruso PA, et al. Comparison of 45 degrees oblique reformats with axial reformats in CT evaluation of the vestibular aqueduct. AJNR Am J Neuroradiol 2008;29(1):30–4.

260. Juliano AF, Ting EY, Mingkwansook V, et al. Vestibular aqueduct measurements in the 45° oblique (Pöschl) plane. AJNR Am J Neuroradiol 2016; 37(7):1331–7.

261. Hwang M, Marovich R, Shinc SS, et al. Optimizing CT for the evaluation of vestibular aqueduct enlargement: inter-rater reproducibility and predictive value of reformatted CT measurements. J Otology 2015; 10(1):13–7.

262. Naganawa S1, Koshikawa T, Iwayama E, et al. MR imaging of the enlarged endolymphatic duct and sac syndrome by use of a 3D fast asymmetric spin-echo sequence: volume and signal-intensity measurement of the endolymphatic duct and sac and area measurement of the cochlear modiolus. AJNR Am J Neuroradiol 2000;21(9): 1664–9.

263. Thylur DS, Jacobs RE, Go JL, et al. Ultra-high-field magnetic resonance imaging of the human inner ear at 11.7 tesla. Otol Neurotol 2017;38(1): 133–8.

264. Joshi VM, Navlekar SK, Kishore GR, et al. CT and MR imaging of the inner ear and brain in children with congenital sensorineural hearing loss. Radiographics 2012;32(3):683–98.

265. Lo WW. What is a 'Mondini' and what difference does a name make? AJNR Am J Neuroradiol 1999;20(8):1442–4.

266. Sennaroglu L, Saatci I. A new classification for cochleovestibular malformations. Laryngoscope 2002;112:2230–41.

267. Liu YK, Qi CL, Tang J, et al. The diagnostic value of measurement of cochlear length and height in temporal bone CT multiplanar reconstruction of inner ear malformation. Acta Otolaryngol 2017;137(2):119–26.

268. D'Arco F, Talenti G, Lakshmanan R, et al. Do measurements of inner ear structures help in the diagnosis of inner ear malformations? a review of literature. Otol Neurotol 2017;38(10):e384–92.

269. Talenti G, Manara R, Brotto D, et al. High-resolution 3T magnetic resonance findings in cochlear hypoplasias and incomplete partition anomalies: a pictorial review. Br J Radiol 2018;91:2018120.

270. Reinshagen KL, Curtin HD, Quesnel AM, et al. Measurement for detection of incomplete partition type II anomalies on MR imaging. AJNR Am J Neuroradiol 2017;38(10):2003–7.

271. Ahadizadeh E, Ascha M, Manzoor N, et al. Hearing loss in enlarged vestibular aqueduct and incomplete partition type II. Am J Otolaryngol 2017;38(6):692–7.

272. Leung KJ, Quesnel AM, Juliano AF, et al. Correlation of CT, MR, and histopathology in incomplete partition-II cochlear anomaly. Otol Neurotol 2016;37(5):434–7.

273. Sennaroglu L. Histopathology of inner ear malformations: do we have enough evidence to explain pathophysiology? Cochlear Implants Int 2016;17(1):3–20.

274. Aimoni C, Ciorba A, Cerritelli L, et al. Enlarged vestibular aqueduct: audiological and genetical features in children and adolescents. Int J Pediatr Otorhinolaryngol 2017;101:254–8.

275. Mey K, Bille M, Cayé-Thomasen P. Cochlear implantation in Pendred syndrome and non-syndromic enlarged vestibular aqueduct - clinical challenges, surgical results, and complications. Acta Otolaryngol 2016;136(10):1064–8.

276. Huang BY, Zdanski C, Castillo M. Pediatric sensorineural hearing loss, part 2: syndromic and acquired causes. AJNR Am J Neuroradiol 2012;33(3):399–406.

277. Papsin BC. Cochlear implantation in children with anomalous cochleovestibular anatomy. Laryngoscope 2005;115(1 Pt 2 Suppl 106):1–26.

278. Marques SR, Smith RL, Isotani S, et al. Morphological analysis of the vestibular aqueduct by computerized tomography images. Eur J Radiol 2007;61(1):79–83.

279. Okamoto Y, Mutai H, Nakano A, et al. Subgroups of enlarged vestibular aqueduct in relation to SLC26A4 mutations and hearing loss. Laryngoscope 2014;124(4):E134–40.

280. Maiolo V, Savastio G, Modugno GC, et al. Relationship between multidetector CT imaging of the vestibular aqueduct and inner ear pathologies. Neuroradiol J 2013;26(6):683–92.

281. Ho ML, Deep NL, Carlson ML, et al. Paper SPS1_107, Classifying the Large Vestibular Aqueduct: Morphometry to Audiometry, September 09, 2016. American Society of Head and Neck Radiology, Washington, DC.

282. Berrettini S, Forli F, Bogazzi F, et al. Large vestibular aqueduct syndrome: audiological, radiological, clinical, and genetic features. Am J Otolaryngol 2005;26(6):363–71.

283. Madden C, Halsted M, Benton C, et al. Enlarged vestibular aqueduct syndrome in the pediatric population. Otol Neurotol 2003;24(4):625–32.

284. Mimura T, Sato E, Sugiura M, et al. Hearing loss in patients with enlarged vestibular aqueduct: air-bone gap and audiological Bing test. Int J Audiol 2005;44(8):466–9.

285. Arjmand EM, Webber A. Audiometric findings in children with a large vestibular aqueduct. Arch Otolaryngol Head Neck Surg 2004;130(10):1169–74.

286. Zhou G, Gopen Q, Kenna MA. Delineating the hearing loss in children with enlarged vestibular aqueduct. Laryngoscope 2008;118:2062–6.

287. Zhou G, Gopen Q. Characteristics of vestibular evoked myogenic potentials in children with enlarged vestibular aqueduct. Laryngoscope 2011;121(1):220–5.

288. Yang CJ, Lavender V, Meinzen-Derr JK, et al. Vestibular pathology in children with enlarged vestibular aqueduct. Laryngoscope 2016;126(10):2344–50.

289. Young RJ, Shatzkes DR, Babb JS, et al. The cochlear-carotid interval: anatomic variation and potential clinical implications. AJNR Am J Neuroradiol 2006;27(7):1486–90.

290. Shoman NM, Samy RN, Pensak ML, et al. Contemporary neuroradiographic assessment of the cochleo-carotid partition. ORL J Otorhinolaryngol Relat Spec 2016;78(4):193–8.

291. Penido Nde O, Borin A, Fukuda Y, et al. Microscopic anatomy of the carotid canal and its relations with cochlea and middle ear. Braz J Otorhinolaryngol 2005;71(4):410–4.

292. Hearst MJ, Kadar A, Keller JT, et al. Petrous carotid canal dehiscence: an anatomic and radiographic study. Otol Neurotol 2008;29(7):1001–4.

293. Spiessberger A, Baumann F, Kothbauer KF, et al. Bony dehiscence of the horizontal petrous internal carotid artery canal: an anatomic study with surgical implications. World Neurosurg 2018. https://doi.org/10.1016/j.wneu.2018.03.172 [pii:S1878-8750(18)30654-30655].

294. Lund AD, Palacios SD. Carotid artery-cochlear dehiscence: a review. Laryngoscope 2011; 121(12):2658–60.

295. Neyt P, Govaere F, Forton GE. Simultaneous true stapes fixation and bilateral bony dehiscence between the internal carotid artery and the apex of the cochlea: the ultimate pitfall. Otol Neurotol 2011;32:909–13.

296. Kim HH, Wilson DF. A third mobile window at the cochlear apex. Otolaryngol Head Neck Surg 2006;135(6):965–6.

297. Schart-Morén N, Larsson S, Rask-Andersen H, et al. Anatomical characteristics of facial nerve and cochlea interaction. Audiol Neurootol 2017; 22(1):41–9.

298. Fang CH, Chung SY, Blake DM, et al. Prevalence of cochlear-facial dehiscence in a study of 1,020 temporal bone specimens. Otol Neurotol 2016;37(7): 967–72.

299. Pauna HF, Monsanto RC, Schachern PA, et al. The surgical challenge of carotid artery and Fallopian canal dehiscence in chronic ear disease: a pitfall for endoscopic approach. Clin Otolaryngol 2017; 42(2):268–74.

300. Friedman RA, Bykhovskaya Y, Tu G, et al. Molecular analysis of the POU3F4 gene in patients with clinical and radiographic evidence of X-linked mixed deafness with perilymphatic gusher. Ann Otol Rhinol Laryngol 1997;106(4): 320–5.

301. Schild C, Prera E, Lüblinghoff N, et al. Novel mutation in the homeobox domain of transcription factor POU3F4 associated with profound sensorineural hearing loss. Otol Neurotol 2011;32(4): 690–4.

302. Anger GJ, Crocker S, McKenzie K, et al. X-linked deafness-2 (DFNX2) phenotype associated with a paracentric inversion upstream of POU3F4. Am J Audiol 2014;23(1):1–6.

303. Wester JL, Merna C, Peng KA, et al. Facial nerve stimulation following cochlear implantation for X-linked stapes gusher syndrome leading to identification of a novel POU3F4 mutation. Int J Pediatr Otorhinolaryngol 2016;91:121–3.

304. Marlin S, Moizard MP, David A, et al. Phenotype and genotype in females with POU3F4 mutations. Clin Genet 2009;76(6):558–63.

305. Papadaki E, Prassopoulos P, Bizakis J, et al. X-linked deafness with stapes gusher in females. Eur J Radiol 1998;29(1):71–5.

306. Choi JW, Min B, Kim A, et al. De novo large genomic deletions involving POU3F4 in incomplete partition type III inner ear anomaly in East Asian populations and implications for genetic counseling. Otol Neurotol 2015;36(1):184–90.

307. Saylisoy S, Incesulu A, Gurbuz MK, et al. Computed tomographic findings of X-linked

deafness: a spectrum from child to mother, from young to old, from boy to girl, from mixed to sudden hearing loss. J Comput Assist Tomogr 2014; 38(1):20–4.

308. Alizadeh H, Nasri F, Mehdizadeh M, et al. Computed tomography findings of a patient with severe dysplasia of the inner ear and recurrent meningitis: a case report of gusher ear in a five-year old boy. Iran J Radiol 2014;11(3):e4168.

309. Talbot JM, Wilson DF. Computed tomographic diagnosis of X-linked congenital mixed deafness, fixation of the stapedial footplate, and perilymphatic gusher. Am J Otol 1994;15:177–82.

310. Kumar G, Castillo M, Buchman CA. X-linked stapes gusher: CT findings in one patient. AJNR Am J Neuroradiol 2003;24(6):1130–2.

311. Phelps PD, Reardon W, Pembrey M, et al. X-linked deafness, stapes gushers and a distinctive defect of the inner ear. Neuroradiology 1991;33(4):326–30.

312. Eluvathingal Muttikkal TJ, Nicolasjilwan M. Congenital X-linked Stapes Gusher Syndrome in an Infant. A Case Report. Neuroradiol J 2012;25(1):76–80.

313. El Beltagi AH, Elsherbiny MM, El-Nil H. Letter to the editor. Congenital X-linked stapes gusher syndrome. Neuroradiol J 2012;25(4):486–8.

314. Cabbarzade C, Sennaroglu L, Süslü N. CSF gusher in cochlear implantation: the risk of missing CT evidence of a cochlear base defect in the presence of otherwise normal cochlear anatomy. Cochlear Implants Int 2015;16(4):233–6.

315. Jackler RK, Hwang PH. Enlargement of the cochlear aqueduct: fact or fiction? Otolaryngol Head Neck Surg 1993;109(1):14–25.

316. Gong WX, Gong RZ, Zhao B. HRCT and MRI findings in X-linked non-syndromic deafness patients with a POU3F4 mutation. Int J Pediatr Otorhinolaryngol 2014;78(10):1756–62.

317. Kamogashira T, Iwasaki S, Kashio A, et al. Prediction of intraoperative CSF gusher and postoperative facial nerve stimulation in patients with cochleovestibular malformations undergoing cochlear implantation surgery. Otol Neurotol 2017;38(6):e114–9.

318. Cremers CW, Snik AF, Huygen PL, et al. X-linked mixed deafness syndrome with congenital fixation of the stapedial footplate and perilymphatic gusher (DFN3). Adv Otorhinolaryngol 2002;61:161–7.

319. McFadden MD, Wilmoth JG, Mancuso AA, et al. Preoperative computed tomography may fail to detect patients at risk for perilymph gusher. Ear Nose Throat J 2005;84(12):770, 772–4.

320. Choi BY, An YH, Song JJ, et al. Clinical observations and molecular variables of patients with hearing loss and incomplete partition type III. Laryngoscope 2016;126(3):E123–8.

321. Wahba H, Youssef T. Stapedectomy gusher: a clinical experience. Int Adv Otol 2010;6(2): 149–54.

322. Kanno A, Mutai H, Namba K, et al. Frequency and specific characteristics of the incomplete partition type III anomaly in children. Laryngoscope 2017; 127(7):1663–9.

323. Glasscock ME. The stapes gusher. Arch Otolaryngol 1973;98(2):82–91.

324. Choi BY, An YH, Park JH, et al. Audiological and surgical evidence for the presence of a third window effect for the conductive hearing loss in DFNX2 deafness irrespective of types of mutations. Eur Arch Otorhinolaryngol 2013;270(12): 3057–62.

325. Snik AF, Hombergen GC, Mylanus EA, et al. Air-bone gap in patients with X-linked stapes gusher syndrome. Am J Otol 1995;16(2):241–6.

326. Özbal Batuk M, Çınar BÇ, Özgen B, et al. Audiological and radiological characteristics in incomplete partition malformations. J Int Adv Otol 2017; 13(2):233–8.

327. Smeds H, Wales J, Asp F, et al. X-linked malformation and cochlear implantation. Otol Neurotol 2017; 38(1):38–46.

328. Kim CS, Maxfield AZ, Foyt D, et al. Utility of intraoperative computed tomography for cochlear implantation in patients with difficult anatomy. Cochlear Implants Int 2018;19(3):170–9.

329. Vashist S, Singh S. CSF Gusher in Cochlear Implant Surgery-does it affect surgical outcomes? Eur Ann Otorhinolaryngol Head Neck Dis 2016; 133(Suppl 1):S21–4.

330. Incesulu A, Adapinar B, Kecik C. Cochlear implantation in cases with incomplete partition type III (X-linked anomaly). Eur Arch Otorhinolaryngol 2008; 265(11):1425–30.

331. Sennaroğlu L, Bajin MD. Incomplete partition type III: a rare and difficult cochlear implant surgical indication. Auris Nasus Larynx 2018;45(1):26–32.

332. Quesada JL, Cammaroto G, Bonanno L, et al. Cerebrospinal fluid leak during stapes surgery: gushing leaks and oozing leaks, two different phenomena. Ear Nose Throat J 2017;96(8):302–10.

333. Cremers CW. How to prevent a stapes gusher. Adv Otorhinolaryngol 2007;65:278–84.

334. Anniko M, Wikström SO, Wróblewski R. Microanalytic and light microscopic studies on the developing otic capsule. Acta Otolaryngol 1987;104(5–6):429–38.

335. Rask-Andersen H, Liu W, Erixon E, et al. Human cochlea: anatomical characteristics and their relevance for cochlear implantation. Anat Rec (Hoboken) 2012;295(11):1791–811.

336. Kamakura T, Nadol JB Jr. Evidence of osteoclastic activity in the human temporal bone. Audiol Neurootol 2017;22(4–5):218–25.

337. Frisch T, Bloch SL, Sørensen MS. Prevalence, size and distribution of microdamage in the human otic capsule. Acta Otolaryngol 2015;135(8):771–5.

338. Van Rompaey V, Potvin J, van den Hauwe L, et al. Third mobile window associated with suspected otosclerotic foci in two patients with an air-bone gap. J Laryngol Otol 2011;125(1):89–92.

339. Santos F, McCall AA, Chien W, et al. Otopathology in osteogenesis imperfecta. Otol Neurotol 2012; 33(9):1562–6.

340. Zatoński T, Temporale H, Krecicki T. Hearing and balance in metabolic bone diseases. Pol Merkur Lekarski 2012;32(189):198–201 [in Polish].

341. Bloch SL. On the biology of the bony otic capsule and the pathogenesis of otosclerosis. Dan Med J 2012;59(10):B4524.

342. Babcock TA, Liu XZ. Otosclerosis: from genetics to molecular biology. Otolaryngol Clin North Am 2018; 51(2):305–18.

343. Chole RA, McKenna M. Pathophysiology of otosclerosis. Otol Neurotol 2001;22(2):249–57.

344. Rudic M, Keogh I, Wagner R, et al. The pathophysiology of otosclerosis: review of current research. Hear Res 2015;330(Pt A):51–6.

345. Marshall AH, Fanning N, Symons S, et al. Cochlear implantation in cochlear otosclerosis. Laryngoscope 2005;115:1728–33.

346. Lee TC, Aviv RI, Chen JM, et al. CT grading of otosclerosis. AJNR Am J Neuroradiol 2009;30(7): 1435–9.

347. Sakai O, Curtin HD, Fujita A, et al. Otosclerosis: computed tomography and magnetic resonance findings. Am J Otolaryngol 2000;21:116–8.

348. Veillon F, Stierle JL, Dussaix J, et al. Otosclerosis imaging: matching clinical and imaging data. J Radiol 2006;87(11 Pt 2):1756–64 [in French].

349. Cureoglu S, Baylan MY, Paparella MM. Cochlear otosclerosis. Curr Opin Otolaryngol Head Neck Surg 2010;18(5):357–62.

350. Linthicum FH Jr, Filipo R, Brody S. Sensorineural hearing loss due to cochlear otospongiosis: theoretical considerations of etiology. Ann Otol Rhinol Laryngol 1975;84(4 Pt 1):544–51.

351. Quesnel AM, Moonis G, Appel J, et al. Correlation of computed tomography with histopathology in otosclerosis. Otol Neurotol 2013;34:22–8.

352. Makarem AO, Linthicum FH. Cavitating otosclerosis. Otol Neurotol 2008;29(5):730–1.

353. Makarem AO, Hoang TA, Lo WW, et al. Cavitating otosclerosis: clinical, radiologic, and histopathologic correlations. Otol Neurotol 2010;31(3): 381–4.

354. Bou-Assaly W, Mukherji S, Srinivasan A. Bilateral cavitary otosclerosis: a rare presentation of otosclerosis and cause of hearing loss. Clin Imaging 2013;37:1116–8.

355. Puac P, Rodríguez A, Lin HC, et al. Cavitary plaques in otospongiosis: CT findings and clinical implications. AJNR Am J Neuroradiol 2018;39(6): 1135–9.

356. Pippin KJ, Muelleman TJ, Hill J, et al. Prevalence of internal auditory canal diverticulum and its association with hearing loss and otosclerosis. AJNR Am J Neuroradiol 2017;38(11):2167–71.

357. Abdel-Ghany AF, Osman NM, Botros SM. Correlation between the size, CT density of otosclerotic foci, and audiological tests in cases of otosclerosis. Int Adv Otol 2014;10(2):156–61.

358. Richard C, Linthicum FH Jr. An unexpected third window in a case of advanced cavitating otosclerosis. Otol Neurotol 2012;33(6):e47–8.

359. Nemati S, Ebrahim N, Kaemnejad E, et al. Middle ear exploration results in suspected otosclerosis cases: are ossicular and footplate area anomalies rare? Iran J Otorhinolaryngol 2013;25(72):155–60.

360. Cassano P, Decandia N, Cassano M, et al. Perilymphatic gusher in stapedectomy: demonstration of a fistula of internal auditory canal. Acta Otorhinolaryngol Ital 2003;23(2):116–9.

361. Ramírez Camacho R, Arellano B, García Berrocal JR. Perilymphatic gushers: myths and reality. Acta Otorrinolaringol Esp 2000;51(3):193–8 [in Spanish].

362. Couvreur P, Baltazart B, Lacher G, et al. Perilymphatic effusion as a complication of otosclerosis. Rev Laryngol Otol Rhinol (Bord) 2003;124(1):31–7 [in French].

363. Carlson ML, Van Abel KM, Pelosi S, et al. Outcomes comparing primary pediatric stapedectomy for congenital stapes footplate fixation and juvenile otosclerosis. Otol Neurotol 2013;34(5):816–20.

364. Marini JC, Forlino A, Bächinger HP, et al. Osteogenesis imperfecta. Nat Rev Dis Primers 2017;3:17052.

365. Martin E, Shapiro JR. Osteogenesis imperfecta: epidemiology and pathophysiology. Curr Osteoporos Rep 2007;5(3):91–7.

366. Swinnen FK, Casselman JW, De Leenheer EM, et al. Temporal bone imaging in osteogenesis imperfecta patients with hearing loss. Laryngoscope 2013;123(8):1988–95.

367. Schrauwen I, Khalfallah A, Ealy M, et al. COL1A1 association and otosclerosis: a meta-analysis. Am J Med Genet A 2012;158A(5):1066–70.

368. Abidin AZ, Jameson J, Molthen R, et al. Classification of micro-CT images using 3D characterization of bone canal patterns in human osteogenesis imperfecta. Proc SPIE Int Soc Opt Eng 2017;10134 [pii:1013413].

369. Swinnen FK, De Leenheer EM, Goemaere S, et al. Association between bone mineral density and hearing loss in osteogenesis imperfecta. Laryngoscope 2012;122(2):401–8.

370. Pereira da Silva A, Feliciano T, Figueirinhas R, et al. Osteogenesis imperfecta and hearing loss–description of three case reports. Acta Otorrinolaringol Esp 2013;64(6):423–7.

371. Swinnen FK, Dhooge IJ, Coucke PJ, et al. Audiologic phenotype of osteogenesis imperfecta: use in clinical differentiation. Otol Neurotol 2012;33(2):115–22.

372. Swinnen FK, Coucke PJ, De Paepe AM, et al. Osteogenesis Imperfecta: the audiological phenotype lacks correlation with the genotype. Orphanet J Rare Dis 2011;6:88.

373. Pillion JP, Vernick D, Shapiro J. Hearing loss in osteogenesis imperfecta: characteristics and treatment considerations. Genet Res Int 2011;2011:983942.

374. Swinnen FK, De Leenheer EM, Coucke PJ, et al. Audiometric, surgical, and genetic findings in 15 ears of patients with osteogenesis imperfecta. Laryngoscope 2009;119(6):1171–9.

375. Pillion JP, Shapiro J. Audiological findings in osteogenesis imperfecta. J Am Acad Audiol 2008;19(8):595–601.

376. Mnari W, Hafsa C, Salem R, et al. Osteogenesis imperfecta and hearing loss in childhood. Arch Pediatr 2008;15(11):1663–6 [in French].

377. Ting TH, Zacharin MR. Hearing in bisphosphonate-treated children with osteogenesis imperfecta: our experience in thirty six young patients. Clin Otolaryngol 2012;37(3):229–33.

378. Swinnen FK, De Leenheer EM, Coucke PJ, et al. Stapes surgery in osteogenesis imperfecta: retrospective analysis of 34 operated ears. Audiol Neurootol 2012;17(3):198–206.

379. Vincent R, Wegner I, Stegeman I, et al. Stapedotomy in osteogenesis imperfecta: a prospective study of 32 consecutive cases. Otol Neurotol 2014;35(10):1785–9.

380. Kontorinis G, Lenarz T, Mojallal H, et al. Power stapes: an alternative method for treating hearing loss in osteogenesis imperfecta? Otol Neurotol 2011;32(4):589–95.

381. Denoyelle F, Daval M, Leboulanger N, et al. Stapedectomy in children: causes and surgical results in 35 cases. Arch Otolaryngol Head Neck Surg 2010;136(10):1005–8.

382. Rotteveel LJ, Beynon AJ, Mens LH, et al. Cochlear implantation in 3 patients with osteogenesis imperfecta: imaging, surgery and programming issues. Audiol Neurootol 2008;13(2):73–85.

383. Sasaki-Adams D, Kulkarni A, Rutka J, et al. Neurosurgical implications of osteogenesis imperfecta in children. Report of 4 cases. J Neurosurg Pediatr 2008;1(3):229–36.

384. Feller L, Wood NH, Khammissa RA, et al. The nature of fibrous dysplasia. Head Face Med 2009;5:22.

385. Lee SE, Lee EH, Park H, et al. The diagnostic utility of the GNAS mutation in patients with fibrous dysplasia: meta-analysis of 168 sporadic cases. Hum Pathol 2012;43(8):1234–42.

386. Akil O, Hall-Glenn F, Chang J, et al. Disrupted bone remodeling leads to cochlear overgrowth and hearing loss in a mouse model of fibrous dysplasia. PLoS One 2014;9(5):e94989.

387. Bousson V, Rey-Jouvin C, Laredo JD, et al. Fibrous dysplasia and McCune-Albright syndrome: imaging for positive and differential diagnoses, prognosis, and follow-up guidelines. Eur J Radiol 2014;83(10):1828–42.

388. Atalar MH, Salk I, Savas R, et al. CT and MR imaging in a large series of patients with craniofacial fibrous dysplasia. Pol J Radiol 2015;80: 232–40.

389. Fusconi M, Conte M, Pagliarella M, et al. Fibrous dysplasia of the maxilla: diagnostic reliability of the study image. Literature review. J Neurol Surg B Skull Base 2013;74(6):364–8.

390. Karino S, Yamasoba T, Kashio A, et al. Fibrous dysplasia of the temporal bone: assessment by three-dimensional helical CT imaging. Otolaryngol Head Neck Surg 2005;133(4):643.

391. Nager GT, Kennedy DW, Kopstein E. Fibrous dysplasia: a review of the disease and its manifestations in the temporal bone. Ann Otol Rhinol Laryngol Suppl 1982;92:1–52.

392. Mierzwiński J, Kosowska J, Tyra J, et al. Different clinical presentation and management of temporal bone fibrous dysplasia in children. World J Surg Oncol 2018;16(1):5.

393. Frisch CD, Carlson ML, Kahue CN, et al. Fibrous dysplasia of the temporal bone: a review of 66 cases. Laryngoscope 2015;125(6):1438–43.

394. Megerian CA, Sofferman RA, McKenna MJ, et al. Fibrous dysplasia of the temporal bone: ten new cases demonstrating the spectrum of otologic sequelae. Am J Otol 1995;16(4):408–19.

395. Lustig LR, Holliday MJ, McCarthy EF, et al. Fibrous dysplasia involving the skull base and temporal bone. Arch Otolaryngol Head Neck Surg 2001; 127(10):1239–47.

396. Boyce AM, Brewer C, DeKlotz TR, et al. Association of Hearing Loss and Otologic Outcomes With Fibrous Dysplasia. JAMA Otolaryngol Head Neck Surg 2018;144(2):102–7.

397. Fandiño M, Bhimrao SK, Saxby AJ, et al. Fibrous dysplasia of the temporal bone: systematic review of management and hearing outcomes. Otol Neurotol 2014;35(10):1698–706.

398. Moreau S, Bourdon N, Goullet de Rugy M, et al. [Temporal fibrous dysplasia with labyrinthine involvement. Apropos of a case and review of the literature]. Ann Otolaryngol Chir Cervicofac 1997; 114(4):140–3.

399. Yu Hon Wan A, Chi Fai Tong M. Fibrous dysplasia of the temporal bone presenting with facial nerve palsy and conductive hearing loss. Otol Neurotol 2008;29(7):1039–40.

400. Chinski A, Beider B, Cohen D. Fibrous dysplasia of the temporal bone. Int J Pediatr Otorhinolaryngol 1999;47(3):275–81.

401. Pouwels AB, Cremers CW. Fibrous dysplasia of the temporal bone. J Laryngol Otol 1988;102(2): 171–2.

402. Tochino R, Sunami K, Yamane H. Fibrous dysplasia of the temporal bone with cholesteatoma. Acta Otolaryngol Suppl 2004;(554):47–9.

403. Papadakis CE, Skoulakis CE, Prokopakis EP, et al. Fibrous dysplasia of the temporal bone: report of a case and a review of its characteristics. Ear Nose Throat J 2000;79(1):52–7.

404. Morrissey DD, Talbot JM, Schleuning AJ 2nd. Fibrous dysplasia of the temporal bone: reversal of sensorineural hearing loss after decompression of the internal auditory canal. Laryngoscope 1997 Oct;107(10):1336–40.

405. Djerić D, Stefanović P. Fibrous dysplasia of the temporal bone and maxillofacial region associated with cholesteatoma of the middle ear. Auris Nasus Larynx 1999;26(1):79–81.

406. Liu YH, Chang KP. Fibrous Dysplasia of the Temporal Bone with External Auditory Canal Stenosis and Secondary Cholesteatoma. J Int Adv Otol 2016; 12(1):125–8.

407. Blanchard M, Abergel A, Williams MT, et al. Aneurysmal bone cyst within fibrous dysplasia causing labyrinthine fistula. Otol Neurotol 2011; 32(2):e11.

408. Mardekian SK, Tuluc M. Malignant sarcomatous transformation of fibrous dysplasia. Head Neck Pathol 2015;9(1):100–3.

409. Lee JS, FitzGibbon EJ, Chen YR, et al. Clinical guidelines for the management of craniofacial fibrous dysplasia. Orphanet J Rare Dis 2012; 7(Suppl 1):S2.

410. Sataloff RT, Graham MD, Roberts BR. Middle ear surgery in fibrous dysplasia of the temporal bone. Am J Otol 1985;6(2):153–6.

411. Gruener G, Camacho P. Paget's disease of bone. Handb Clin Neurol 2014;119:529–40.

412. Hullar TE, Lustig LR. Paget's disease and fibrous dysplasia. Otolaryngol Clin North Am 2003;36(4): 707–32.

413. Bahmad F Jr, Merchant SN. Paget disease of the temporal bone. Otol Neurotol 2007;28(8):1157–8.

414. Nager GT. Paget's disease of the temporal bone. Ann Otol Rhinol Laryngol 1975;84(4 Pt 3 Suppl 22):1–32.

415. Van der Stappen A, Degryse H, van den Hauwe L. Paget disease of the skull and temporal bone. JBR-BTR 2005;88(3):156–7.

416. Teufert KB, Linthicum F Jr. Paget disease and sensorineural hearing loss associated with spiral ligament degeneration. Otol Neurotol 2005;26(3): 387–91 [discussion: 391].

417. Marcos Pérez SM, Montes Plaza JM, Valda Rodrigo J, et al. Paget's disease with temporal bone involvement, hypoacusis and vertigo. Apropos a case. Acta Otorrinolaringol Esp 1992; 43(4):232–4 [in Spanish].

418. Lenarz T, Hoth S, Frank K, et al. Hearing disorders in Paget's disease. Laryngol Rhinol Otol (Stuttg) 1986;65(4):213–7 [in German].

419. Meng L, Zhou HF, Wang JL. Report of a case with Paget disease with bilateral progressive hearing loss as the first symptom. Zhonghua Er Bi Yan Hou Tou Jing Wai Ke Za Zhi 2009;44(7):602–3 [in Chinese].

420. Monsell EM, Cody DD, Bone HG, et al. Hearing loss in Paget's disease of bone: the relationship between pure-tone thresholds and mineral density of the cochlear capsule. Hear Res 1995;83:114–20.

421. Nabili V, Buckner AD, Niparko JK. Radiology quiz case. Labyrinthine obliteration due to Paget disease. Arch Otolaryngol Head Neck Surg 2001; 127(9):1137–9.

422. Rüedi L. Are there cochlear shunts in Paget's and Recklinghausen's disease? Acta Otolaryngol 1968;65(1):13–24.

423. Hernández Madorrán JM, Urrutikoetxea Sarriegui A, Sanjosé Torices J, et al. Bony alterations of the otic capsule: a report case of Paget disease. An Otorrinolaringol Ibero Am 1995;22(1): 31–40 [in Spanish].

424. Lee IW, Goh EK, Kong SK, et al. A case of cochlear implantation in a patient with Paget disease. Am J Otolaryngol 2011;32(4):353–4.

425. Singer FR. Paget disease: when to treat and when not to treat. Nat Rev Rheumatol 2009;5(9): 483–9.

426. Silverman SL. Paget disease of bone: therapeutic options. J Clin Rheumatol 2008;14(5):299–305.

427. Kotowicz MA. Paget disease of bone. Diagnosis and indications for treatment. Aust Fam Physician 2004;33(3):127–31.

428. Swartz JD. The otodystrophies: diagnosis and differential diagnosis. Semin Ultrasound CT MR 2004;25(4):305–18.

429. Erkoç MF, Bulut S, İmamoğlu H, et al. CT assessment of bone remodeling in the otic capsule in chronic renal failure: association with hearing loss. AJR Am J Roentgenol 2013;200(2):396–9.

430. Brooks JK, Rivera-Ramirez LE, Errington LW, et al. Synchronous Paget disease of bone and hyperparathyroidism: report of a case with extensive craniofacial involvement. Oral Surg Oral Med Oral Pathol Oral Radiol Endod 2011;111(4): e19–24.

431. Murphey MD, Sartoris DJ, Quale JL, et al. Musculoskeletal manifestations of chronic renal insufficiency. Radiographics 1993;13(2):357–79.

432. Abid F, Lalani I, Zakaria A, et al. Cranial nerve palsies in renal osteodystrophy. Pediatr Neurol 2007;36(1):64–5.

433. Marsot-Dupuch K, Quillard J, Meyohas MC. Head and neck lesions in the immunocompromised host. Eur Radiol 2004;14(Suppl 3):E155–67.

434. Morris MS, Prasad S. Otologic disease in the acquired immunodeficiency syndrome [review]. Ear Nose Throat J 1990;69(7):451–3.

435. Darmstadt GL, Harris JP. Luetic hearing loss: clinical presentation, diagnosis, and treatment [review]. Am J Otolaryngol 1989;10(6):410–21.

436. Guttenplan M, Hendrix RA. Otosyphilis: a practical guide to diagnosis and treatment [review]. Trans Pa Acad Ophthalmol Otolaryngol 1989;41:834–8.

Arterial Anomalies of the Middle Ear
A Pictorial Review with Clinical-Embryologic and Imaging Correlation

Anne Marie Sullivan, MD[a], Hugh D. Curtin, MD[b], Gul Moonis, MD[c],*

KEYWORDS

- Persistent stapedial artery • Aberrant internal carotid artery • Embryology • CT temporal bone

KEY POINTS

- High-resolution CT of the temporal bone can accurately detect the presence of the arterial anomalies, namely the aberrant internal carotid artery (ICA) and the persistent stapedial artery (PSA).
- Although the imaging appearance of aberrant ICA is classic, there are four known types of persistent stapedial artery, each with its unique imaging findings, which have rarely been distinguished in previous clinical articles.
- Aberrant ICA and PSA can coexist, and there are cases of bilateral arterial anomalies reported in the literature.
- Review of the embryology of middle ear arterial anatomy and CT features specific to each type of variation enhances detection of these anomalies.

INTRODUCTION

Arterial anomalies of the temporal bone are rare, but critical, variations of anatomy that are important to detect on imaging studies. These anomalies are often detected incidentally, but can cause pulsatile tinnitus, conductive hearing loss, and/or vertigo, or present with a retrotympanic mass. Failure to detect these anomalies preoperatively can lead to profuse, life-threatening hemorrhage, death, or stroke during middle ear surgery. High-resolution computed tomography (CT) of the temporal bone can accurately detect the presence of the arterial anomalies, namely the aberrant internal carotid artery (ICA) and the persistent stapedial artery (PSA). Although the imaging appearance of aberrant ICA is classic, there

are four known types of PSA, each with its unique imaging findings, which have rarely been distinguished in previous clinical articles. Aberrant ICA and PSA can coexist, and there are cases of bilateral arterial anomalies reported in the literature. Review of the embryology of middle ear arterial anatomy and CT features specific to each type of variation enhance detection of these anomalies.

EMBRYOLOGY

During embryogenesis, the stapedial artery supplies most neural structures of the head and neck; however, it's role in development is completed by the 10th week of gestation as the external carotid system assumes this role.

Disclosure Statement: NA.
[a] Department of Radiology, CRA Medical Imaging, 5008 Brittonfield Parkway Suite 100, East Syracuse, NY 13057, USA; [b] Department of Radiology, Massachusetts Eye and Ear Infirmary, 243 Charles Street, Boston, MA 02114, USA; [c] Department of Radiology, Columbia University Medical Center, 622 West 168th Street, PB-1-301, New York, NY 10032, USA
* Corresponding author.
E-mail address: Gm2640@cumc.columbia.edu

Neuroimag Clin N Am 29 (2019) 93–102
https://doi.org/10.1016/j.nic.2018.09.010
1052-5149/19/© 2018 Elsevier Inc. All rights reserved.

In the human embryo, there are six aortic arches that develop in a cranial to caudal sequence arising from the truncus arteriosus.[1] The first and second arches join the external carotid artery (ECA) and ICA. The ventral aspect of the first arch becomes the pharyngeal artery (external carotid system) and combines with the dorsal part of the second arch that has been replaced by the hyoid artery (internal carotid system), which has an anastomosis with the inferior tympanic artery, a branch of the external carotid system. The stapedial artery then arises from the hyoid artery (thus, the stapedial artery and its branches initially originate from the internal carotid system) and courses through the stapes crura shaping the stapes primordium and coursing alongside the facial nerve. The stapedial artery then ends in three branches accompanying the branches of the trigeminal nerve.[1] The supraorbital branch (dorsal division) extends into the orbit and remains as the lacrimal artery and forms portions of the middle meningeal artery.[1,2] The infraorbital and the mandibular branches stem from a common trunk (ventral division)[1] and form the infraorbital and the inferior alveolar arteries. Before the separation of the ventral division into the infraorbital and mandibular branches, an anastomoses develops between the stapedial artery and the ECA via the pharyngeal artery.[1] The foramen spinosum forms at the anastomotic site. After the stapedial artery degenerates at the 10th week of gestation,[3] this anastomosis becomes the internal maxillary artery and the middle meningeal artery, a branch of the internal maxillary artery, now arises from the external carotid system rather than the internal carotid system as do all the aforementioned branches of the former stapedial artery. The remnant of the hyoid artery becomes the caroticotympanic artery. The inferior tympanic artery becomes a branch of the ascending pharyngeal artery.

Therefore, the stapedial artery is a normally a transient artery that acts as a collateral vessel between the internal and external carotid system and then regresses (Fig. 1).

ABERRANT INTERNAL CAROTID ARTERY

The first case of aberrant ICA was reported by Max[4] in 1899. Since then, numerous cases have been reported but the true incidence of aberrant ICA is not known.[5]

The normal ICA arises from the common carotid artery in the mid-neck and courses superiorly, entering the skull through the vertical carotid canal and then taking an anteromedial bend to extend through the horizontal carotid canal. The ICA then ascends superior to the foramen lacerum and extends into the carotid sinus and terminating superior and lateral to the anterior clinoid process. The normal ICA courses inferior to the cochlear promontory and is separated from the middle ear by the carotid plate, a thin bony covering. A normally tiny branch of the ICA, the caroticotympanic artery, enters the middle ear through the carotid plate. This artery anastomoses with the normally tiny inferior tympanic artery, a branch of the ascending pharyngeal artery, which normally arises from the ECA. The ordinarily tiny arteries join over the cochlear promontory, and this union is not normally visible by high-resolution CT (Fig. 2).

The aberrant ICA occurs when the cervical portion of the internal carotid is absent, which results in formation of a collateral pathway. In this case, the normally diminutive inferior tympanic and caroticotympanic (called the hyoid artery when enlarged) arteries enlarge, still joining over the cochlear promontory, but now easily visible by high-resolution CT. The inferior tympanic artery essentially "replaces" the normal ICA, entering the cranial vault via an enlarged tympanic canaliculus, coursing through the hypotympanum, uniting with the hyoid artery, and then entering the horizontal carotid canal. The normal vertical carotid canal is absent, and there is no carotid plate separating the artery from the middle ear cavity (Fig. 3).

PERSISTENT STAPEDIAL ARTERY

The first case of PSA was described by Hrytl in 1836.[6] The histopathologic incidence is reported as 0.48%,[7] and the incidence at stapes surgery has been found to be 0.01% to 0.02%.[8] The stapedial artery can persist as four distinct types,[3] and these reported incidences include all variations of PSA. The incidence of each type has not been reported to our knowledge, although it is believed that the PSA arising from the inferior tympanic artery with an aberrant ICA (aberrant carotid-stapedial artery) is the most common type. The PSA is unilateral or bilateral and can occur with or without an aberrant ICA.

There are certain imaging features that each type of PSA has in common. In all types of PSA, the foramen spinosum, which normally contains the middle meningeal artery, is absent. Three percent of the population has a congenitally absent foramen spinosum[9] because of aberrant origin of the middle meningeal artery from either the ophthalmic artery[10] or the PSA, so additional findings confirming PSA must be sought. The PSA is seen as a soft tissue density passing through the stapes crura regardless of the PSA

A

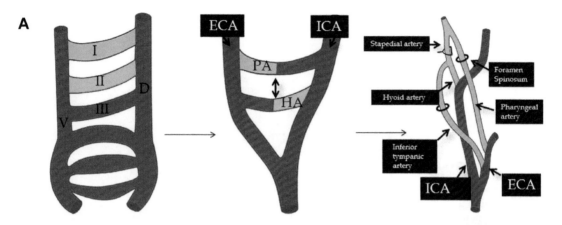

The six aortic arches form in a cranio-caudal sequence between the ventral (V) and dorsal (D) aorta. The first three (I, II, III) arches are the basis for the carotid system.	The first and second arches join the external (ECA) and internal (ICA) carotid arteries. The ventral aspect of the 1st arch (pharyngeal artery, PA) combines with the dorsal part of the 2nd arch (hyoid artery, HA)	The stapedial artery (SA) arises from the HA and extends through the stapes, and joins the PA. The foramen spinosum forms at the anastomosis between the SA and PA. Distally the SA becomes the middle meningeal artery. The inferior tympanic artery has an anastomosis with the HA.

B

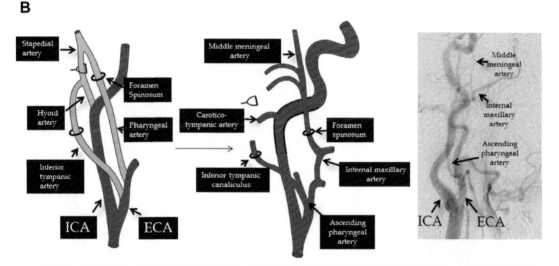

The stapedial artery normally disappears by the 10th week in utero after transferring the middle meningeal artery from the internal carotid to the external carotid system as a branch of the internal maxillary artery. The remnant of the hyoid artery becomes the carotico-tympanic artery. The inferior tympanic artery becomes a branch of the ascending pharyngeal artery.

Fig. 1. (A, B) Embryology and normal anatomy of the arterial system of the middle ear.

variant that is present. When any type PSA is present, the artery either enters the tympanic segment of the facial canal, widening the canal, or travels just lateral to the tympanic segment of the facial nerve. The PSA enters the middle cranial fossa via an opening lateral and posterior to the genu of the facial nerve. In addition to these shared features, each type of PSA has its own unique CT

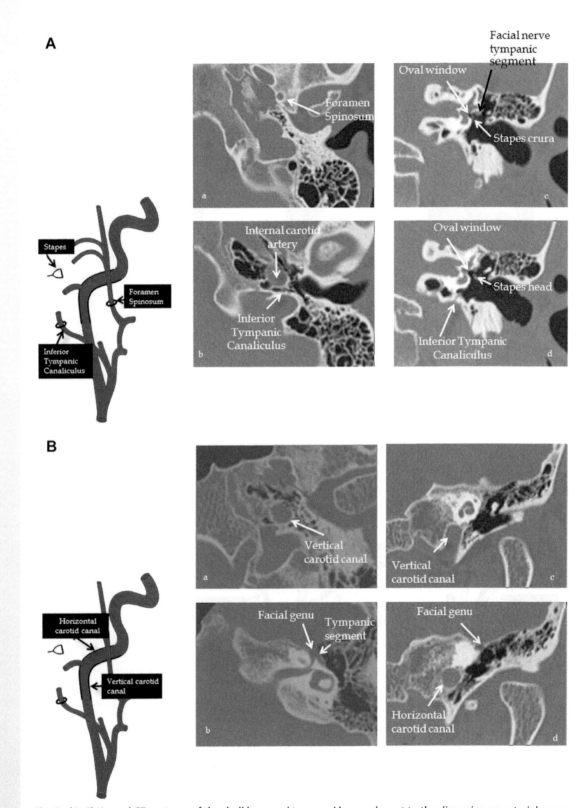

Fig. 2. (*A*, *B*) Normal CT anatomy of the skull base and temporal bone relevant to the discussion on arterial anomalies of the middle ear. The inferior tympanic canaliculus is normally a thin channel as noted in (*A*). Also note the normal foramen spinosum, the normal carotid canal and the normal tympanic segment of the facial N on both coronal and axial images.

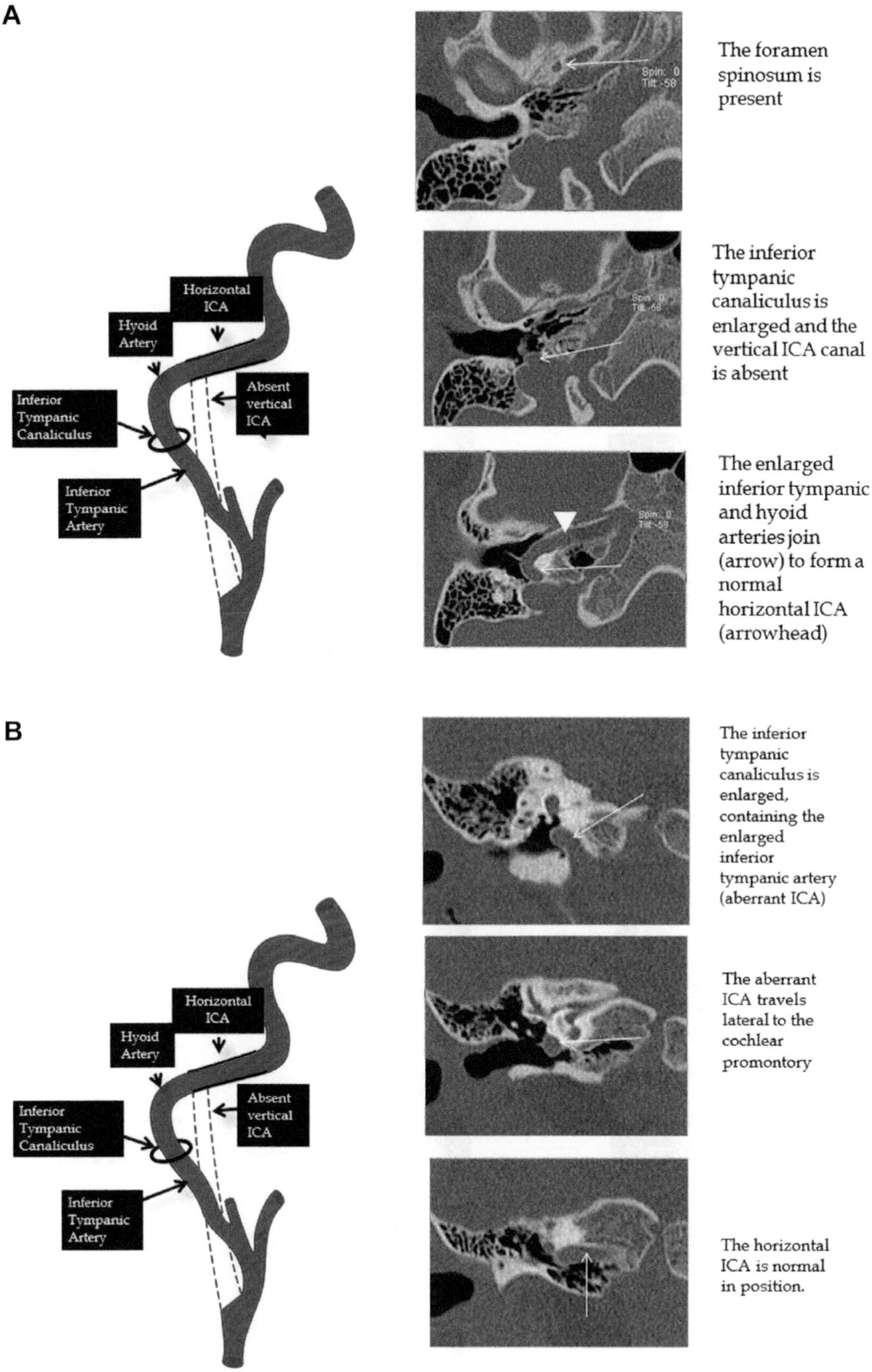

A

- The foramen spinosum is present
- The inferior tympanic canaliculus is enlarged and the vertical ICA canal is absent
- The enlarged inferior tympanic and hyoid arteries join (arrow) to form a normal horizontal ICA (arrowhead)

B

- The inferior tympanic canaliculus is enlarged, containing the enlarged inferior tympanic artery (aberrant ICA)
- The aberrant ICA travels lateral to the cochlear promontory
- The horizontal ICA is normal in position.

Fig. 3. (A) Aberrant ICA. Axial CT images through the temporal bone. When an aberrant ICA is present, the normal cervical ICA is absent and the inferior tympanic and the caroticotympanic (known as hyoid artery when enlarged) arteries are enlarged and then rejoin to form the horizontal ICA. (B) Aberrant ICA. Coronal CT images through the temporal bone. The aberrant ICA courses through the middle ear along the cochlear promontory and appears as a retrotympanic red mass. The clinical differential is paraganglioma (glomus tympanicum) and imaging is crucial to distinguish these entities before intervention.

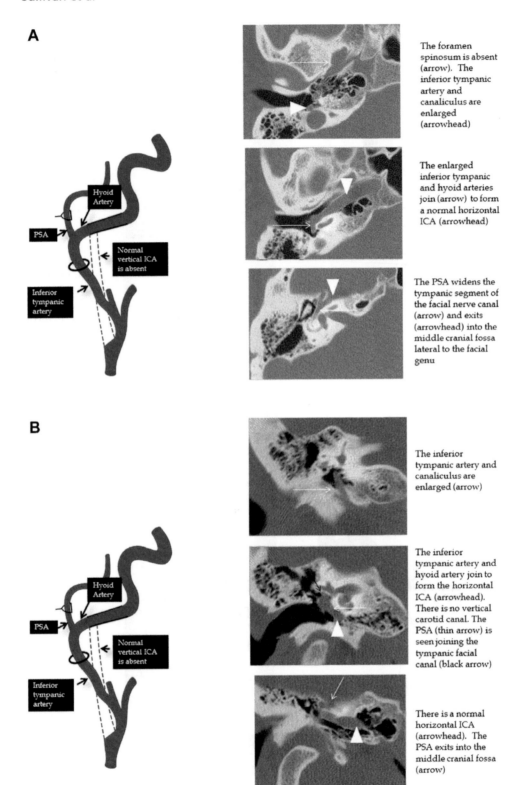

Fig. 4. (*A*) PSA arising from inferior tympanic artery with an aberrant ICA. Axial CT images demonstrate the PSA arising from the aberrant ICA (enlarged inferior tympanic and hyoid arteries). This variant is also known as an aberrant carotid-stapedial artery. (*B*) Coronal CT images from the same patient. In this variant, there is agenesis of the cervical portion of the ICA. In contradistinction, a small-caliber vertical ICA is present when the PSA arises from a "fenestrated" ICA. ([A] *Courtesy of* Dr Christine Glastonbury, San Francisco, CA.)

findings that render distinction of the specific PSA variant possible.

Persistent Stapedial Artery Arising from Inferior Tympanic Artery with an Aberrant Internal Carotid Artery

This type of PSA is also known as an aberrant carotid-stapedial artery. The distinguishing feature of this PSA variant is that the PSA arises directly from an aberrant ICA, which has a course identical to an isolated aberrant ICA as described previously. In this case, the vertical carotid canal and foramen spinosum are absent, enlarged hyoid and inferior tympanic arteries form the aberrant ICA, and the PSA arises from the enlarged inferior tympanic artery just proximal to where this artery joins the hyoid artery. The inferior tympanic canaliculus is enlarged. The PSA passes through the stapes crura and either enters the tympanic facial

canal or travels just lateral to the canal. The horizontal carotid is normal (**Fig. 4**).

Persistent Stapedial Artery Arising from Inferior Tympanic Artery Without an Aberrant Internal Carotid Artery

This type of PSA is also known as the pharyngostapedial artery. In this case, the ICA has a normal course, and the PSA arises from an inferior tympanic artery with a normal caliber. The hyoid artery has regressed, but the stapedial artery persists as a branch of the inferior tympanic artery, which arises from the pharyngeal artery, a branch of the ECA. The foramen spinosum is absent. The inferior tympanic artery is followed through the inferior tympanic canaliculus, located just anterior to the jugular foramen. The PSA arises from the inferior tympanic artery and is seen along the cochlear promontory and passing through the stapes crura.

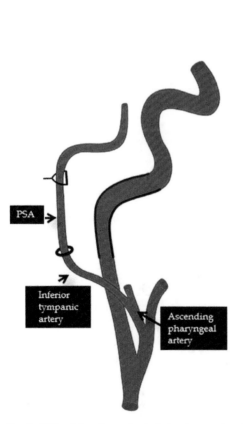

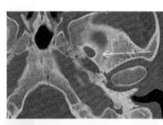
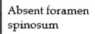
Absent foramen spinosum

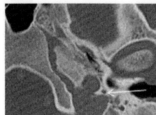
The inferior tympanic artery passes through the inferior tympanic canaliculus

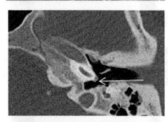
The PSA courses through the middle ear along cochlear promontory

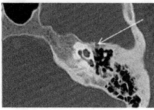
The PSA exits into the middle cranial fossa posterior and lateral to the facial genu.

Fig. 5. PSA arising from the inferior tympanic artery without an aberrant ICA. Axial CT images. The PSA arises from a normal size inferior tympanic artery, a branch of the ascending pharyngeal artery originating from the ECA. The internal carotid artery has a normal course. This variation is also known as a pharyngostapedial artery.

As in all PSA variants, the PSA either enters the tympanic facial canal or travels just lateral to the canal (Fig. 5).

Persistent Stapedial Artery Arising from the Caroticotympanic Artery

This variant is also known as the hyoid-stapedial artery. The ventral division of the stapedial artery does not anastomose with the external carotid system as it normally should. Therefore, the hyoid artery persists and rather than the hyoid remnant becoming the normal caroticotympanic artery, the PSA arises directly from the caroticotympanic artery, called the hyoid artery in this case. On CT, the caroticotympanic artery is seen arising from the ICA just proximal to the junction of the vertical and horizontal portions of the ICA and continues through the middle ear through the stapes crura

as the PSA. Again, the foramen spinosum is absent and the PSA travels either within or just lateral to the facial nerve canal (Fig. 6).

Persistent Stapedial Artery Arising from a "Fenestrated" or "Duplicated" Internal Carotid Artery

This variant is also known as the pharyngohyostapedial artery. The vertical ICA is present, but small in caliber, and the PSA arises from enlarged hyoid and inferior tympanic arteries, which join as seen with an aberrant ICA. In this case, the ascending pharyngeal artery arises from the ICA rather than the ECA, ascends toward the skull base as an enlarged inferior tympanic artery, and joins the hyoid artery over the cochlear promontory. Although this appearance has previously been described as ICA "fenestration" or

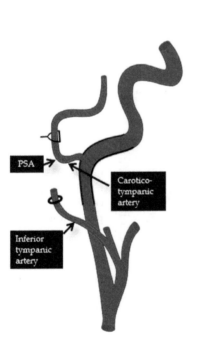

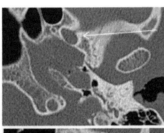

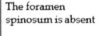
The foramen spinosum is absent

The carotico-tympanic artery arises from the ICA and courses toward the middle ear

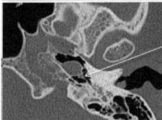
The PSA is seen at the oval window within the stapes crura

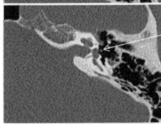
The PSA enters and widens the facial canal, exiting into the middle cranial fossa posterior to the facial genu

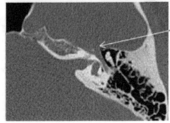

Fig. 6. PSA arising from the caroticotympanic artery. Axial CT images. The internal carotid artery has a normal course, and the PSA arises from the caroticotympanic artery near the junction of the vertical and horizontal portions of the ICA. This variation is also known as the hyoid-stapedial artery.

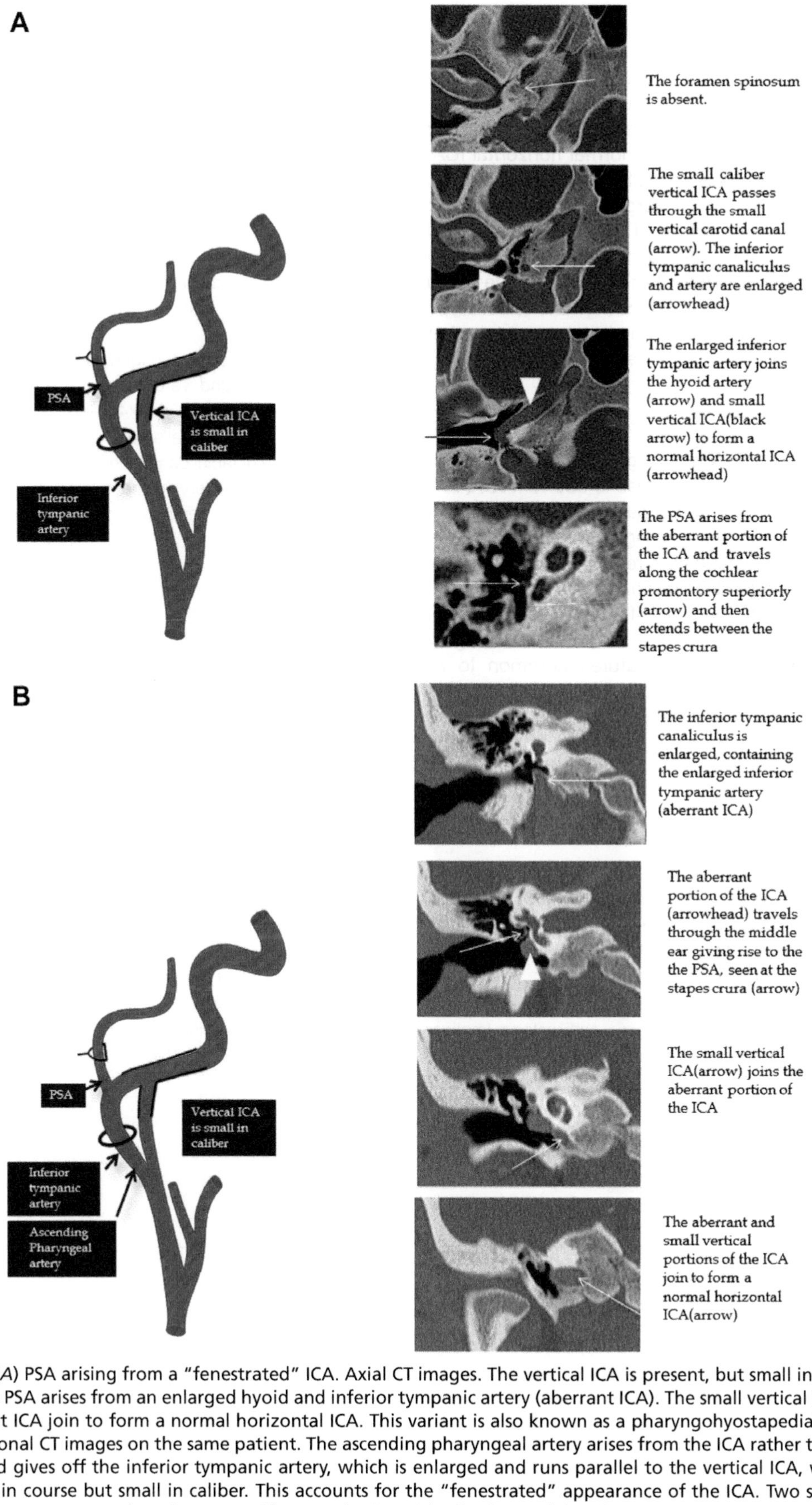

A

The foramen spinosum is absent.

The small caliber vertical ICA passes through the small vertical carotid canal (arrow). The inferior tympanic canaliculus and artery are enlarged (arrowhead)

The enlarged inferior tympanic artery joins the hyoid artery (arrow) and small vertical ICA(black arrow) to form a normal horizontal ICA (arrowhead)

The PSA arises from the aberrant portion of the ICA and travels along the cochlear promontory superiorly (arrow) and then extends between the stapes crura

B

The inferior tympanic canaliculus is enlarged, containing the enlarged inferior tympanic artery (aberrant ICA)

The aberrant portion of the ICA (arrowhead) travels through the middle ear giving rise to the the PSA, seen at the stapes crura (arrow)

The small vertical ICA(arrow) joins the aberrant portion of the ICA

The aberrant and small vertical portions of the ICA join to form a normal horizontal ICA(arrow)

Labels in diagram A: PSA; Vertical ICA is small in caliber; Inferior tympanic artery

Labels in diagram B: PSA; Vertical ICA is small in caliber; Inferior tympanic artery; Ascending Pharyngeal artery

Fig. 7. (*A*) PSA arising from a "fenestrated" ICA. Axial CT images. The vertical ICA is present, but small in caliber, and the PSA arises from an enlarged hyoid and inferior tympanic artery (aberrant ICA). The small vertical ICA and aberrant ICA join to form a normal horizontal ICA. This variant is also known as a pharyngohyostapedial artery. (*B*). Coronal CT images on the same patient. The ascending pharyngeal artery arises from the ICA rather than the ECA and gives off the inferior tympanic artery, which is enlarged and runs parallel to the vertical ICA, which is normal in course but small in caliber. This accounts for the "fenestrated" appearance of the ICA. Two separate vessels are present so there is no true "fenestration" or "duplication" of the ICA.

"duplication,"[11–13] two separate vessels are present[2] so there is no true "fenestration" or "duplication" of the ICA. The small vertical ICA and the hyoid artery join to form a normal horizontal ICA. CT findings include a small vertical carotid canal and artery and an enlarged inferior tympanic canaliculus and artery. The PSA is identified arising from the enlarged inferior tympanic artery just proximal to where this artery joins the hyoid artery, and, as in all types of PSA, is followed through the middle ear and stapes crura to either join or run parallel to the facial canal (**Fig. 7**).

SUMMARY

The clinical differential diagnosis of a red and/or pulsatile retrotympanic mass is aberrant ICA, any type of PSA, glomus tympanicum, and dehiscent jugular bulb. By recognizing the features of aberrant ICA and PSA on high-resolution CT, these entities are easily distinguished by the radiologist. The PSA is further classified by type because each type demonstrates a unique set of imaging features in addition to features common to all types. Although rarely encountered, it is important to reliably and consistently detect these anomalies because failure to do so can lead to disastrous surgical outcomes.

REFERENCES

1. Altmann F. Anomalies of the internal carotid artery and its branches, their embryological and comparative anatomical significance: a report of a new case of persistent stapedial artery in man. Laryngoscope 1947;57:313–39.
2. Lefrournier V, Vasdev A, Bessou P, et al. A persistent pharyngohyostapedial artery: embryologic implications. AJNR Am J Neuroradiol 1999;20:271–4.
3. Hitier M, Zhang M, Labrousse M, et al. Persistent stapedial arteries in human: from phylogeny to surgical consequences. Surg Radiol Anat 2013;35:883–91.
4. Max E. Die bedeutung arteria carotitis interna in der hals nasan ohrenheilkinde. Msch Ohrenheilk 1899; 33:251.
5. Rolla JD, Urbanb MA, Theodore C, et al. Bilateral aberrant internal carotid arteries with bilateral persistent stapedial arteries and bilateral duplicated internal carotid arteries. AJNR Am J Neuroradiol 2003;24:762–5.
6. Hyrtl J. Neve Beobachtongen aus dem Gebiete der Menschlichen und Vergleichenden Anatomie. Med Jahrb Oesterreich 1836;10:457–66.
7. Moreano EH, Puparella MM, Zelterman D, et al. Prevalence of facial canal dehiscence and of persistent stapedial artery in the human middle ear: a report of 1000 temporal bones. Laryngoscope 1994;104:309–20.
8. Govaerts PJ, Marquet TF, Cremers CWRJ, et al. Persistent stapedial artery: does it prevent successful surgery? Ann Otol Rhinol Laryngol 1993;102: 724–8.
9. Ginsberg LE, Pruett SW, Chen MY, et al. Skull-base foramina of the middle cranial fossa: reassessment of normal variation with high-resolution CT. AJNR Am J Neuroradiol 1994;15(2):283–91.
10. Greig DM. Congenital anomalies of the foramen spinosum. Edinb Med J 1929;36:363–71.
11. Killien FC, Wyler AR, Cromwell LD. Duplication of the internal carotid artery. Neuroradiology 1980;19: 101–2.
12. Koenigsberg RA, Zito JL, Patel M, et al. Fenestration of the internal carotid artery: a rare mass of the hypotympanum associated with persistence of the stapedial artery. AJNR Am J Neuroradiol 1995;16:908–10.
13. Chess MA, Barsotti JB, Chang JK, et al. Duplication of the extracranial internal carotid artery. AJNR Am J Neuroradiol 1995;16:1545–7.

Imaging of Pediatric Hearing Loss

Karuna V. Shekdar, MD*, Larissa T. Bilaniuk, MD

KEYWORDS

- Pediatric hearing loss • CT temporal bone • MR imaging temporal bone • Cholesteatoma
- External auditory canal atresia • Enlarged vestibular aqueduct • Cochlear malformation

KEY POINTS

- Computed tomography is the imaging modality of choice in pediatric patients with conductive hearing loss, temporal bone trauma, or suspected third window disorder.
- Magnetic resonance (MR) imaging with high-resolution heavily T2-weighted sequences provides excellent detail and superior delineation of inner ear structures, especially the cochlear nerve, cochlea, vestibule, and semicircular canals. MR imaging also helps in identification of intracranial findings, particularly following meningitis and in various syndromes with intracranial manifestations and brainstem disorders that may result in hearing loss.
- Enlarged vestibular aqueduct is the most common imaging finding in sensorineural hearing loss (SNHL) in children, which is usually bilateral and commonly associated with cochlear malformations, especially type II incomplete partition in up to 85% of cases.
- Cochlear nerve hypoplasia or absence is diagnosed in up to 18% of patients with SNHL, and MR imaging is the modality of choice for detection of cranial nerve hypoplasia or aplasia.
- CHARGE syndrome, Pendred syndrome, Waardenburg syndrome, and branchio-oto-renal syndrome are some common syndromes associated with congenital SNHL.

INTRODUCTION

Hearing loss is one of the most common congenital sensory impairments, with 6 in 1000 children being diagnosed with hearing loss by the age of 18 years.[1] With the implementation of universal screening of newborn infants for hearing loss, it is now possible to diagnose hearing loss as early as at age 2 to 3 months.[2] In addition to a complete physical examination, the diagnostic work-up of hearing loss in children includes imaging studies, laboratory testing, and genetic testing.[3] This article discusses the role of imaging in the evaluation of pediatric patients with conductive, sensorineural, and mixed hearing loss, and describes the pertinent imaging findings in some of the common causes of pediatric hearing loss.

IMAGING MODALITIES

Historically, radiographs were used to identify temporal bone anomalies. With advances in imaging technology, the utility of radiographs is limited. Computed tomography (CT) of the temporal bones is the imaging modality of choice in patients with conductive hearing loss because it can evaluate the external auditory canal, tympanic membrane, osseous structures including the ossicles, the air-filled middle ear cavity, and the bony margins of the inner ear structures including the cochlea, vestibule, and semicircular canals, internal acoustic

Conflict of Interest/Author Disclaimer: None.

Department of Radiology, Perelman School of Medicine at University of Pennsylvania, The Children's Hospital of Philadelphia, 34 Civic Center Boulevard, Philadelphia, PA 19104, USA
* Corresponding author. The Children's Hospital of Philadelphia, 2121- Neuroradiology Office Suites, #2115 Wood Building, 34 Civic Center Boulevard, Philadelphia, PA 19104.
E-mail address: shekdar@email.chop.edu

canal, and the vestibular aqueduct.[4] CT of the temporal bones has the advantage of short acquisition times and excellent visualization of bony anatomy, with the penalty of a small doses of ionizing radiation.[5] CT is the imaging modality of choice in pediatric patients with conductive hearing loss, suspected superior semicircular canal dehiscence, or temporal bone trauma. Subcentimeter slice thickness, noncontrast, axial CT acquisition with a high-resolution bone algorithm through the temporal bones with coronal reformations is the recommended protocol for hearing loss. Additional reformats in other planes (eg, Stenvers and Pöschl) can be produced to facilitate visualization of structures such as the semicircular canals and vestibular aqueduct.

Magnetic resonance (MR) imaging offers benefits (compared with CT) in delineating inner ear structures, including the entire course of the cochlear nerve, the cochlea, vestibule, and semicircular canals, and the endolymphatic sac and duct.[6] In patients with sensorineural hearing loss (SNHL), therefore, MR imaging should be strongly considered, although in some cases both MR imaging and CT of the temporal bones may need to be performed and the information obtained from MR imaging and CT is complementary.[7]

MR imaging of the temporal bone and internal auditory canal (IAC) offers excellent soft tissue detail with multiplanar imaging capability. Noncontrast heavily T2-weighted MR imaging has been shown to be highly sensitive and specific for detection of structural abnormalities related to sensorineural hearing loss.[8,9] In the absence of suspicion for neoplastic, infectious, or inflammatory processes, intravenous contrast is not necessary. In a newborn or young infant, an adequate MR imaging study can often be obtained without sedation, using the feed-and-wrap technique. Otherwise, in toddlers and young children, sedation is usually required.

The goals of imaging for pediatric hearing loss are:

- Identify structural causes of hearing loss
- Search for additional abnormalities that may help reveal an underlying syndrome
- Assess whether the patient is a surgical candidate
- Help determine cochlear implantation feasibility and laterality
- Report anatomic risk factors in the context of surgical planning

Hearing loss may be classified as follows:

- Conductive, caused by limitation of sound wave transmission from the external environment to the inner ear. The pathophysiology is thus usually mechanical, related to structures from the pinna, tympanic membrane, middle ear, through the ossicles.
- Sensorineural, caused by limitation in transmission of neural impulses from the inner ear to the brain. The pathophysiology lies in the inner ear structures (cochlea, vestibule, semicircular canals), through the cochlear nerve, to the brainstem nucleus.
- Mixed, a combination of conductive and sensorineural hearing loss.

CONDUCTIVE HEARING LOSS
Acute Otitis Media, Chronic Otitis Media, and Cholesteatoma

The most common cause of intermittent, mild to moderate acquired hearing loss in infants and young children is conductive hearing loss (CHL) associated with otitis media (OM) and middle ear effusions.[10] Almost 75% of the affected children experience at least 1 episode of OM by age 6 years. Other acquired causes of CHL include acquired cholesteatoma and trauma. Congenital CHL can result from external auditory canal atresia, congenital cholesteatoma, and ossicular malformations. High-resolution CT of the temporal bone plays an important role in identifying structural abnormalities in CHL.

Acute OM causes CHL by limiting mobility of the tympanic membrane and ossicles, which results in decreased sound transmission through the middle ear.[10] Most patients with CHL caused by OM do not require imaging work-up, because there is resolution of transient CHL as a middle ear effusion resolves.[11] In patients with acute OM that does not respond to medical treatment, a myringotomy tube insertion may be needed.[11]

Chronic OM (COM) is characterized by persistent OM with tympanic membrane perforation, with or without formation of cholesteatoma. Cholesteatoma is a focus of keratin surrounded by stratified squamous epithelium and is often referred to as skin in the wrong place. It often occurs in the middle ear and can be congenital or acquired.[12] Cholesteatomas cause CHL either because of mass effect on the ossicular chain or by erosion of the ossicles.[13]

Congenital cholesteatomas develop from embryonic epithelial rests, which can be located anywhere in the temporal bone; for example, the middle ear, petrous apex, mastoid, tympanic membrane, or external auditory canal. Middle ear congenital cholesteatomas represent approximately 2% of all middle ear cholesteatomas.[14] Congenital cholesteatomas can be associated

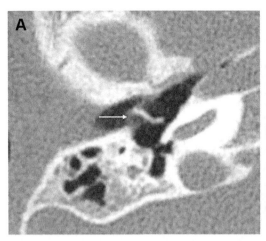
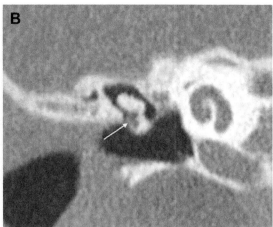

Fig. 1. Retraction pocket. Axial (*A*) and coronal (*B*) CT images of the temporal bone reveal a small nodular soft tissue focus (*arrows*) within Prussak space (the inferior portion of the lateral epitympanic recess), likely to represent a retraction pocket.

with external auditory canal atresia and sometimes with first branchial remnants.

Acquired cholesteatomas can be subdivided into primary and secondary acquired cholesteatomas. A primary acquired cholesteatoma develops behind an apparently intact tympanic membrane typically in the region of pars flaccida; it is therefore also referred to as attic cholesteatoma and accounts for 80% of all middle ear cholesteatomas. Keratin accumulates in a pouch formed from an abnormal folding of the tympanic membrane, termed a retraction pocket, which extends medially into the middle ear space[13] (**Fig. 1**). A secondary acquired cholesteatoma grows into the middle ear cavity through a perforated tympanic membrane, typically through the pars tensa and rarely through the pars flaccida, and may cause ossicular erosion (**Fig. 2**). A large cholesteatoma can extend into the mastoid air cells (**Fig. 3**). Cholesteatomas

associated with COM are secondary acquired cholesteatomas.[13] Acquired cholesteatomas often present with otorrhea and chronic ear infection.

High-resolution CT is the modality of choice in imaging acquired and congenital cholesteatomas. Typical HRCT findings of a cholesteatoma include a soft tissue lesion associated with bone erosion.[13] The bone erosions typically involve the middle ear ossicles, and sometimes the scutum and the tympanic tegmen. However, erosions may be absent when the cholesteatoma is small; hence, the absence of bony erosion does not exclude cholesteatoma. CT offers detailed assessment of the middle ear cavity, ossicles, and mastoid structures because of its high spatial resolution and excellent delineation of bone and air. Presence of labyrinthine fistula or tegmental defects can be assessed with high-resolution CT. Some limitations of CT imaging in cholesteatomas are the low specificity and

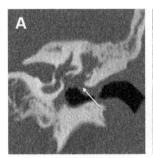
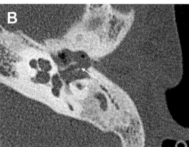
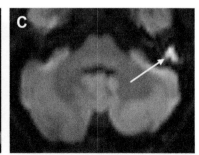

Fig. 2. Left middle ear cholesteatoma. Coronal (*A*) and axial (*B*) CT images of the temporal bone in a patient with a history of recurrent otitis media. There is abnormal soft tissue filling the entire middle ear cavity eroding the scutum (*arrow* in *A*), encasing the ossicles (*arrow* in *B*), with demineralization/early erosions and nonvisualization of the stapes. Axial diffusion-weighted MR image (*C*) shows restricted diffusion (*arrow*) within the area of soft tissue, consistent with a cholesteatoma.

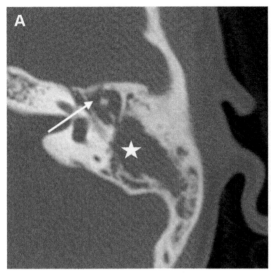
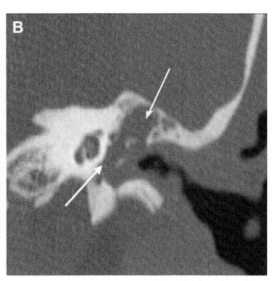

Fig. 3. Large cholesteatoma with extension into the mastoid. Axial (*A*) and coronal (*B*) CT images of the temporal bone reveal a large opacity (*arrows*) representing cholesteatoma extending into the mastoid (*asterisk*).

difficulty differentiating cholesteatoma from granulation tissue, fluid/effusion, or other soft tissue lesions in the chronically inflamed middle ear and mastoid.[13] Preoperative CT has been shown to be useful in detection of tegmen erosion, semicircular canal erosion, and facial canal dehiscence, which are findings that affect surgical planning.

There is a high rate of residual as well as recurrent cholesteatomas in patients undergoing primary cholesteatoma surgery. Historically, a second-look surgery is performed in these cases. However, with the increased diagnostic capability of high-resolution CT, temporal bone imaging can be used in place of this second-stage surgery. **Fig. 4** shows CT findings in a case of recurrent cholesteatoma following canal wall up tympanomastoidectomy.

Diffusion-weighted (DW) MR imaging has yielded very good results in differentiating

cholesteatomas from noncholesteatomatous soft tissues.[15] **Fig. 5** shows diffusion restriction in the soft tissue of the middle ear cavity making it consistent with a recurrent cholesteatoma. Non–echo-planar DW MR imaging to detect cholesteatomas has shown sensitivity of 77% to 100% and specificity of 100%, with positive predictive value 100% and negative predictive value of 75% to 100%.[15] The use of DW MR imaging to identify cholesteatomas is limited to cholesteatomas that are greater than 5 mm in size, and it should be recognized that the anatomic localization of the DW MR images is limited.[13,15]

External Auditory Canal Atresia

External auditory canal (EAC) atresia or congenital aural atresia is characterized by complete or incomplete atresia of the external auditory canal,

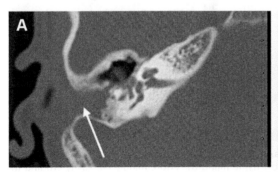
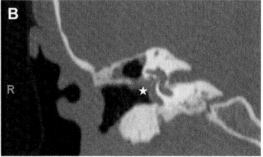

Fig. 4. Recurrent cholesteatoma. Axial (*A*) and coronal (*B*) CT images through the temporal bone show soft tissue in the mesotympanum and hypotympanum (*asterisk* in *B*). The patient has had canal wall up tympanomastoidectomy (*arrow* in *A*).

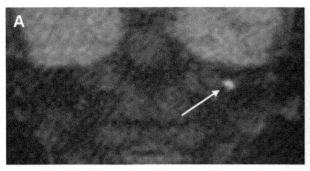

Fig. 5. Cholesteatoma on DW MR imaging. Coronal (*A*) and axial (*B*) non–echo-planar DW MR images. There is restricted diffusion (*white arrows*) in the middle ear consistent with a cholesteatoma.

which may be bony or membranous. It may be isolated or occur in the setting of an associated syndrome. The incidence of EAC atresia is approximately 1 in 10,000 to 20,000 live births.[16] Bilateral involvement is seen in approximately one-third of patients.[16]

A spectrum of findings is noted in EAC atresia.[17] Findings in the middle ear cavity and ossicles are variable. The IAC and inner ear structures are typically normal because they develop earlier in gestation from a different neurologic source and process. Congenital cholesteatoma formation may occur behind the atresia plate in the middle ear in patients with EAC atresia.[17,18]

High-resolution CT is the modality of choice for assessing EAC atresia. A specific checklist (Jahrsdoerfer grading scale) should be looked at and specifically mentioned in reports because this affects surgical reconstruction in EAC atresia.[17–19] The middle ear cavity space typically should be greater than 3 mm for successful surgery. A spectrum of ossicular abnormalities is noted with EAC atresia. The malleus may have a rudimentary handle caused by absence of the normal tympanic membranes. The malleus and incus may be fused together in a boomerang shape. Stapes may be normal/dysmorphic or absent. The presence of a normal stapes is given the highest score in preoperative imaging, which determines surgical outcome. It is important to visualize the oval and round windows that need to be present for successful surgery. The course of the internal carotid artery and the jugular bulb needs to be noted because an anomalous course can be hazardous for surgery. The course of the facial nerve is typically abnormally anterior; this should be noted to avoid damage during the reconstruction procedure.[17,18,20]

Ossicular Malformations

Malformations of the ossicular chain are rare causes of CHL in the pediatric population. Among all the ossicular malformations, malleus fixation, stapes fixation, and incudostapedial discontinuity are the most common anomalies[16] (**Figs. 6** and **7**).

A rare cause of CHL is a high-riding jugular bulb, in which case the hearing loss may be attributable to the jugular bulb contacting the tympanic membrane and obstructing the round window. These patients with jugular bulb anomalies may present with symptoms such as tinnitus or CHL.[21]

Otosclerosis is rare in the pediatric population. Lucent foci near the fissula ante fenestram has been described in a small study in children.[22]

SENSORINEURAL HEARING LOSS

The incidence of sensorineural hearing loss (SNHL) is 1 to 2 newborns per 1000 births in the United States each year.[1,2] The SNHL in children can range from profound congenital bilateral deafness to mild unilateral hearing loss. Several significant factors, such as age of onset, laterality (unilateral or bilateral), severity, and associated genetic or syndromic factors affect the imaging work-up.

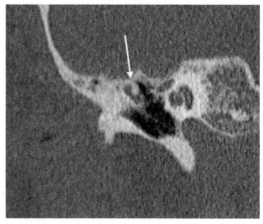

Fig. 6. Malleus fixation. Coronal CT image in a 4-year-old boy shows fixation of the malleus to the tegmen tympani (*white arrow*).

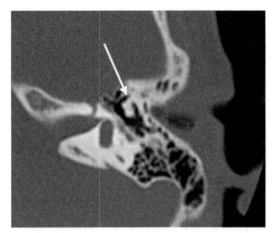

Fig. 7. Malleus fixation. Axial CT image reveals close approximation of the head of the malleus to the lateral wall of the mesotympanum, suggesting fixation (*white arrow*).

There has been significant improvement in the understanding of molecular genetics and genetic testing in the past 2 decades.[23] Mutations of the gap junction beta 2 (GJB2) gene results in abnormalities of the connexin 26 protein.[24,25] The *GJB2* gene mutation related form of hearing loss has been implicated as the cause of hearing loss in up to 40% of SNHL.[24] Those patients with bilateral SNHL who screen negative for deafness-causing mutations should get imaging because the diagnostic yield of imaging studies in this set of patients is significantly high, especially if there is severe to profound congenital SNHL.

A broad spectrum of imaging findings can be seen with SNHL in children. This article describes some of the most common findings in pediatric SNHL.

Large Vestibular Aqueduct

Large vestibular aqueduct (LVA) represents one of the most common abnormalities detected on CT or MR imaging in patients with SNHL. An enlarged vestibular aqueduct can be isolated, but almost 75% of patients have associated cochlear or vestibular anomalies.[26] Associated cochlear anomalies can range from mild asymmetry of the modiolus to gross dysplasia (**Figs. 8–10**).

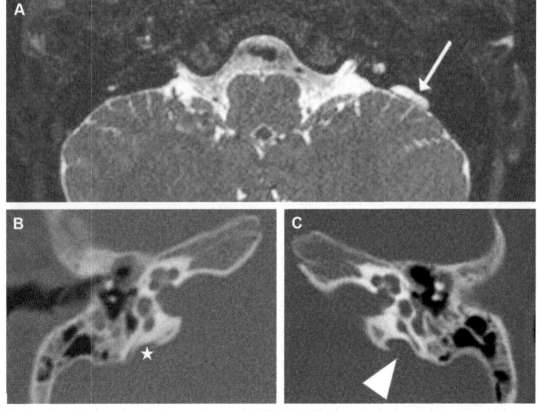

Fig. 8. Unilateral enlarged vestibular aqueduct on the left. (*A*) Axial high-resolution heavily T2-weighted MR image shows enlargement of the left endolymphatic sac (*white arrow*). (*B, C*) Axial CT images of same patient show enlarged left vestibular aqueduct (*arrowhead* in *C*) compared with the normal right vestibular aqueduct (*asterisk* in *B*).

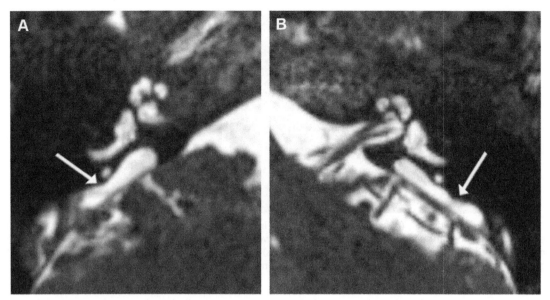

Fig. 9. Bilateral enlarged vestibular aqueduct. Axial heavily T2-weighted MR images show markedly enlarged right (A) and left (B) endolymphatic sacs and ducts (arrows). The cochleae appear normal.

On HRCT the vestibular aqueduct is considered enlarged when the diameter midway between the common crus and the external aperture is greater than 1 mm or if the diameter at the aperture is greater than 2 mm.[27] More recently, it has been shown that measurement of the vestibular aqueduct is more accurately performed in the Pöschl plane than in the axial plane, likely providing a better estimate of whether there is true LVA.[28]

High-resolution CT of the temporal bones can assess the bony enlargement of the vestibular aqueduct; however, the associated cochlear and vestibular abnormalities are better assessed on axial thin-section high-resolution T2-weighted MR images.[26,29] Genetic testing for SLC26A4 mutation is recommended.[30] The vestibule and the semicircular canals may be normal to mildly enlarged or rarely dysplastic.[26] A massively enlarged vestibular aqueduct is a frequently seen

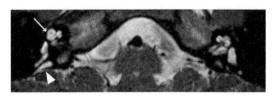

Fig. 10. Right enlarged vestibular aqueduct and incomplete partition type II (IP-II) anomaly. Axial heavily T2-weighted MR image shows a markedly enlarged right endolymphatic duct (arrowhead), and associated IP-II anomaly on the ipsilateral right side (arrow).

finding in Pendred syndrome, which is characterized by congenital SNHL and goiter[31] (Fig. 11).

Patients with enlarged vestibular aqueducts and SNHL typically experience sudden onset of hearing loss, which fluctuates in severity. The SNHL in these patients can be aggravated by minor head injury, biometric pressure changes, or activity that may cause increased intracranial pressure. Hence, children with LVA are cautioned to avoid situations in which head trauma is a significant possibility, such as contact sports.

Inner Ear Anomalies

Cochlear anomalies have been detected in 4% of patients with SNHL. The spectrum of cochlear deformities is linked to the gestational age at which the development was interrupted or an insult occurred. Many syndromes with associated inner ear malformations have been described elsewhere in articles about syndromes with hearing loss. This article discusses some of the common malformations, which have been exquisitely described by the classification system developed by Sennaroglu and Saatci.[32]

Cochlear aplasia or complete absence of the cochlea is likely caused by arrest in development as early as third to fifth week of gestation.[33] The vestibule and semicircular canals are often malformed but may be normal (Fig. 12). Dense bone is present at the expected site of cochlea on CT and may mimic labyrinthitis ossificans.[34]

Common cavity malformation or incomplete partition of the cochlea type I is a common cavity

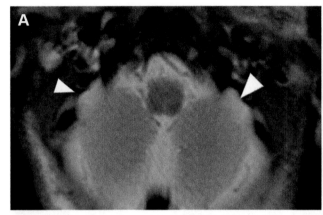
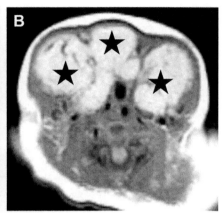

Fig. 11. Pendred syndrome. (*A*) Axial T2-weighted MR image through the temporal bones shows bilateral enlarged endolymphatic sacs (*arrowheads*). (*B*) Axial T1-weighted MR image through the lower neck shows a multilobulated T1-hyperintense soft tissue mass (*asterisks*) encasing the trachea, inseparable from the thyroid gland, in keeping with goiter. These findings are consistent with Pendred syndrome.

malformation defined by the absence of the normal differentiation between the cochlea and vestibule (see **Fig. 12**). This condition usually results from an insult in the fourth week of gestation and accounts for about 25% of all cochlear malformations.[32,33] The semicircular canals also are frequently malformed but are sometimes normal (**Fig. 13**).

Type II incomplete partition (Mondini deformity) is the most common type of cochlear malformation, accounting for greater than 50% of cochlear anomalies.[32] The cochlea consists of 1.5 turns and the interscalar septum and osseous spiral lamina are absent. The basal turn of the cochlea appears normal but the middle and apical turns coalesce to form a bulbous apex (see **Fig. 10**).[29] The modiolus is present only at the level of the basal turn. Type II incomplete partition is commonly associated with LVA.[26]

Vestibular malformations are commonly encountered along with malformations of the semicircular canals and cochlea. The most

common vestibular abnormality is dilatation of the vestibule with partial or complete assimilation of the semicircular canals into the vestibule (**Fig. 14**). Dysplasia of the semicircular canals is more common than aplasia. Absence of all the semicircular canals commonly occurs in patients with CHARGE (coloboma, heart abnormalities, choanal atresia, retardation of growth, genital and ear anomalies) syndrome.[35](**Fig. 15**). Isolated aplasia of the posterior semicircular canal has

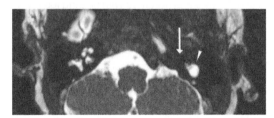

Fig. 12. Cochlear aplasia. Axial heavily T2-weighted MR image in a patient with profound left unilateral sensorineural hearing loss. There is left cochlear aplasia (*arrow*), with dysplastic bulbous vestibule and semicircular canals (*arrowhead*). The left cochlear nerve is absent (not shown).

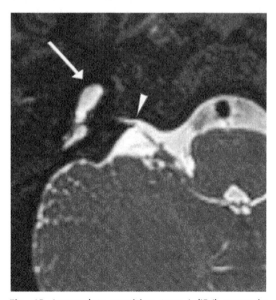

Fig. 13. Incomplete partition type I (IP-I) anomaly. Axial heavily T2-weighted MR image through the right temporal bone shows a dysplastic amorphous cystic cochlea compatible with IP-I anomaly (*arrow*), also referred to as common cavity malformation, with a small right IAC (*arrowhead*).

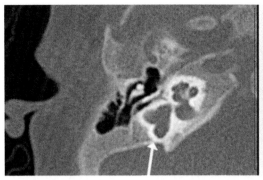
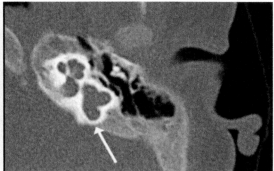

Fig. 14. Enlarged dysplastic vestibules and semicircular canals. Axial CT images show enlarged dysplastic vestibules and semicircular canals bilaterally (*arrows*).

been described in patients with Waardenburg syndrome and Alagille syndrome.[33,36]

Cochlea Vestibular Nerve Deficiency

Cochlear nerve deficiency (CND) is defined as either an absent or hypoplastic cochlear nerve (**Fig. 16**). CND is diagnosed in 12% to 18% of patients with SNHL.[33,37] In patients with CND, the IAC may also be hypoplastic (see **Fig. 13**). CND may be unilateral or bilateral. CND may be isolated or may be associated with other inner ear abnormalities. MR imaging is the modality that allows

visualization of the cochlear nerve as well as the associated inner ear malformations.

Infection and Hearing Loss

Hearing loss following meningitis is the most common cause of acquired bilateral SNHL in the pediatric population.[38] This condition is usually a result of postmeningitis scarring and labyrinthine ossification. During the acute stage, imaging may be normal on CT, whereas MR imaging reveals intense enhancement of the cochlea; in later stages, fibrosis is shown by loss of fluid signal in

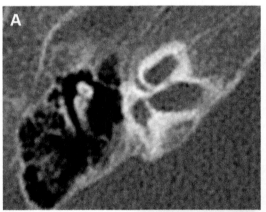
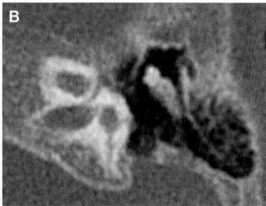
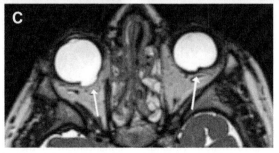

Fig. 15. CHARGE syndrome. (*A*, *B*) Axial CT images through the right and left temporal bones show absent semicircular canals. (*C*) Axial T2-weighted MR image through the orbits shows bilateral colobomas (*arrows*).

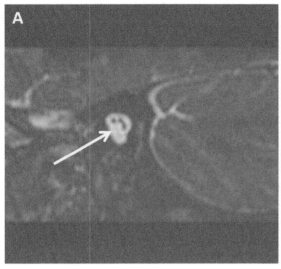

Fig. 16. Cochlear nerve hypoplasia. (*A, B*) Sagittal oblique reformats from a heavily T2-weighted MR sequence through the right (*A*) and left (*B*) IACs. There is a markedly hypoplastic right cochlear nerve (*arrow* in *A*). The left cochlear nerve is normal (*arrowhead* in *B*).

the cochlea[38] (**Fig. 17**). The ossifying stage can be seen on both CT and MR. The ideal time for cochlear implantation is before fibrosis or scarring.

Prenatal infectious causes such as TORCH (toxoplasmosis, other [syphilis, varicella-zoster, parvovirus B_{19}], rubella, cytomegalovirus, and herpes) infections account for about 3% of patients with bilateral SNHL. Intracranial findings of cytomegalovirus are more classic than the presence of inner ear structural abnormalities. Intracranial abnormalities include calcifications, ventriculomegaly, white matter abnormalities, migrational abnormalities, and in some cases extensive areas of insult and parenchymal destruction.

Mass Lesions and Hearing Loss

Vestibular schwannomas are more common in the adult population. Bilateral vestibular schwannomas of neurofibromatosis[2] (NF2) can sometimes present only with SNHL in children (**Fig. 18**).

MIXED HEARING LOSS
Syndromic Causes

The possibility of syndromic mixed hearing loss, such as X-linked stapes gusher syndrome, should

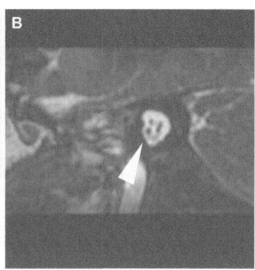

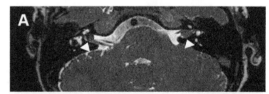

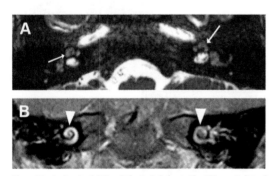

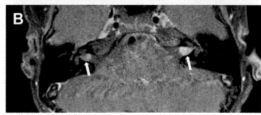

Fig. 17. Labyrinthitis. (*A*) Axial heavily T2-weighted MR image shows loss of normal fluid signal in bilateral cochleae (*arrows*). (*B*) Coronal contrast-enhanced T1-weighted MR image shows enhancement in bilateral cochleae (*arrowheads*). Findings are compatible with labyrinthitis, a sequela of the patient's meningitis.

Fig. 18. Bilateral vestibular schwannomas in NF2. (*A*) Axial heavily T2-weighted MR image shows lobulated masses in the IACs bilaterally (*arrowheads*). (*B*) Axial contrast-enhanced T1-weighted MR image shows enhancement of these masses (*arrows*), compatible with bilateral vestibular schwannomas in the setting of NF2.

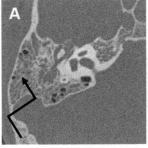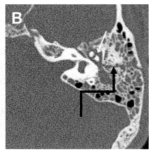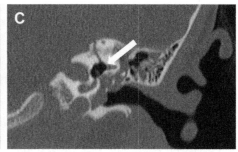

Fig. 19. Temporal bone fractures. (A, B) Axial CT images through the temporal bones show bilateral longitudinal fractures (black arrows), with abnormal widening of the left incudomalleal joint (white arrow in B). (C) Coronal CT image in a different patient, showing a fracture traversing the otic capsule, and air in the vestibule (arrow).

be considered in patients presenting with mixed hearing loss. This syndrome is rare but represents about 50% of all cases of X-linked hearing loss.[39] Family history is negative in about one-third of patients. This syndrome should be considered in all male patients with congenital mixed hearing loss. HRCT reveals hypoplasia of the cochlea, corkscrew appearance of the cochlea, absence of bony modiolus, enlarged IACs, and abnormal labyrinthine facial nerve canal courses.[40] It is important to identify this condition before operative intervention to avoid possible significant complications such as perilymph or cerebrospinal fluid fistula.

Trauma

Temporal bone fractures can be classified as a longitudinal or transverse, with longitudinal fractures being more common, accounting for almost 90% of fractures.[41] If there is disruption of the ossicular chain, this may result in sudden CHL. However, if there is violation of the otic capsule with pneumolabyrinth, there may be associated SNHL (Fig. 19).

SUMMARY

High-resolution temporal bone CT and MR imaging are valuable tools in the evaluation of pediatric hearing loss. CT plays an important role in the evaluation of pediatric patients with CHL and is the imaging modality of choice for evaluation of osseous abnormalities, including the middle ear ossicular chain, EAC, posttraumatic sequelae, and inner ear dysplasia. MR imaging is the imaging of choice for evaluation of sensorineural hearing loss. MR imaging is superior to CT in the evaluation of the membranous labyrinth, including the internal structure and contour of the cochlea, vestibule, semicircular canals, endolymphatic duct and sac, the IAC, the cochlear nerve, the brainstem, and other intracranial abnormalities associated with hearing loss. CT

and MR imaging provide complementary information and are often used in conjunction in the preoperative evaluation of pediatric candidates for cochlear implantation. Imaging plays a vital role in the diagnosis and management of pediatric hearing loss.

REFERENCES

1. Harrison M, Roush J, Wallace J. Trends in age of identification and intervention in infants with hearing loss. Ear Hear 2003;24(1):89–95.
2. Russ SA, Hanna D, DesGeorges J, et al. Improving follow-up to newborn hearing screening: a learning-collaborative experience. Pediatrics 2010;126(Suppl 1):S59–69.
3. American Academy of Pediatrics, Joint Committee on Infant Hearing. Year 2007 position statement: principles and guidelines for early hearing detection and intervention programs. Pediatrics 2007;120: 898–921.
4. DeMarcantonio M, Choo DI. Radiographic evaluation of children with hearing loss. Otolaryngol Clin North Am 2015;48(6):913–32.
5. Pearce MS, Salotti JA, Little MP, et al. Radiation exposure from CT scans in childhood and subsequent risk of leukaemia and brain tumours: a retrospective cohort study. Lancet 2012;380(9840): 499–505.
6. Prosser JD, Cohen AP, Greinwald JH. Diagnostic evaluation of children with sensorineural hearing loss. Otolaryngol Clin North Am 2015;48(6): 975–82.
7. Licameli G, Kenna MA. Is computed tomography (CT) or magnetic resonance imaging (MRI) more useful in the evaluation of pediatric sensorineural hearing loss? Laryngoscope 2010;120(12): 2358–9.
8. Huang BY, Zdanski C, Castillo M. Pediatric sensorineural hearing loss, part 2: syndromic and acquired causes. AJNR Am J Neuroradiol 2012;33(3): 399–406.

9. Huang BY, Zdanski C, Castillo M. Pediatric sensori-neural hearing loss, part 1: practical aspects for neuroradiologists. AJNR Am J Neuroradiol 2012; 33(2):211–7.

10. Roizen NJ. Etiology of hearing loss in children. Nongenetic causes. Pediatr Clin North Am 1999; 46(1):49–64, x.

11. Lieberthal AS, Carroll AE, Chonmaitree T, et al. The diagnosis and management of acute otitis media. Pediatrics 2013;131(3):e964–99.

12. Leighton SE, Robson AK, Anslow P, et al. The role of CT imaging in the management of chronic suppura-tive otitis media. Clin Otolaryngol Allied Sci 1993; 18(1):23–9.

13. Barath K, Huber AM, Stampfli P, et al. Neuroradi-ology of cholesteatomas. AJNR Am J Neuroradiol 2011;32(2):221–9.

14. Zhang X, Yuan H, Shen W, et al. Congenital choles-teatoma of middle ear: 20 patients' clinical symp-toms and imaging features. Lin Chung Er Bi Yan Hou Tou Jing Wai Ke Za Zhi 2014;28(16):1225–8 [in Chinese].

15. Migirov L, Tal S, Eyal A, et al. MRI, not CT, to rule out recurrent cholesteatoma and avoid unnecessary second-look mastoidectomy. Isr Med Assoc J 2009;11(3):144–6.

16. Kosling S, Omenzetter M, Bartel-Friedrich S. Congenital malformations of the external and middle ear. Eur J Radiol 2009;69(2):269–79.

17. Gassner EM, Mallouhi A, Jaschke WR. Preoperative evaluation of external auditory canal atresia on high-resolution CT. AJR Am J Roentgenol 2004;182(5): 1305–12.

18. Swartz JD, Faerber EN. Congenital malformations of the external and middle ear: high-resolution CT find-ings of surgical import. AJR Am J Roentgenol 1985; 144(3):501–6.

19. Shonka DC Jr, Livingston WJ III, Kesser BW. The Jahrsdoerfer grading scale in surgery to repair congenital aural atresia. Arch Otolaryngol Head Neck Surg 2008;134(8):873–7.

20. Yu Z, Han D, Gong S, et al. Facial nerve course in congenital aural atresia–identified by preoperative CT scanning and surgical findings. Acta Otolaryngol 2008;128(12):1375–80.

21. Koo YH, Lee JY, Lee JD, et al. Dehiscent high-riding jugular bulb presenting as conductive hearing loss: a case report. Medicine (Baltimore) 2018;97(26): e11067.

22. Salomone R, Riskalla PE, Vicente Ade O, et al. Pedi-atric otosclerosis: case report and literature review. Braz J Otorhinolaryngol 2008;74(2):303–6.

23. Lalwani AK, Castelein CM. Cracking the auditory ge-netic code: nonsyndromic hereditary hearing impair-ment. Am J Otol 1999;20(1):115–32.

24. Kelsell DP, Dunlop J, Stevens HP, et al. Con-nexin 26 mutations in hereditary non-syndromic

sensorineural deafness. Nature 1997;387(6628): 80–3.

25. Griffith AJ, Wangemann P. Hearing loss associated with enlargement of the vestibular aqueduct: mechanistic insights from clinical phenotypes, ge-notypes, and mouse models. Hear Res 2011; 281(1–2):11–7.

26. Davidson HC, Harnsberger HR, Lemmerling MM, et al. MR evaluation of vestibulocochlear anomalies associated with large endolymphatic duct and sac. AJNR Am J Neuroradiol 1999;20(8):1435–41.

27. Vijayasekaran S, Halsted MJ, Boston M, et al. When is the vestibular aqueduct enlarged? A statistical analysis of the normative distribution of vestibular aqueduct size. AJNR Am J Neuroradiol 2007;28(6): 1133–8.

28. Juliano AF, Ting EY, Mingkwansook V, et al. Vestib-ular aqueduct measurements in the 45° oblique (Pöschl) plane. AJNR Am J Neuroradiol 2016; 37(7):1331–7.

29. Reinshagen KL, Curtin HD, Quesnel AM, et al. Mea-surement for detection of incomplete partition type II anomalies on MR imaging. AJNR Am J Neuroradiol 2017;38(10):2003–7.

30. Fitoz S, Sennaroglu L, Incesulu A, et al. SLC26A4 mutations are associated with a specific inner ear malformation. Int J Pediatr Otorhinolaryngol 2007; 71(3):479–86.

31. Phelps PD, Coffey RA, Trembath RC, et al. Radiolog-ical malformations of the ear in Pendred syndrome. Clin Radiol 1998;53(4):268–73.

32. Sennaroglu L, Saatci I. A new classification for coch-leovestibular malformations. Laryngoscope 2002; 112(12):2230–41.

33. Joshi VM, Navlekar SK, Kishore GR, et al. CT and MR imaging of the inner ear and brain in children with congenital sensorineural hearing loss. Radio-graphics 2012;32(3):683–98.

34. Yiin RS, Tang PH, Tan TY. Review of congenital inner ear abnormalities on CT temporal bone. Br J Radiol 2011;84(1005):859–63.

35. Morimoto AK, Wiggins RH 3rd, Hudgins PA, et al. Absent semicircular canals in CHARGE syndrome: radiologic spectrum of findings. AJNR Am J Neuro-radiol 2006;27(8):1663–71.

36. Madden C, Halsted MJ, Hopkin RJ, et al. Temporal bone abnormalities associated with hearing loss in Waardenburg syndrome. Laryngoscope 2003; 113(11):2035–41.

37. Chiang MJ, Wu CM. Cochlear nerve aplasia and hy-poplasia: diagnosis with three-dimensional mag-netic resonance imaging. Cochlear Implants Int 2004;5(Suppl 1):153–5.

38. Beijen J, Casselman J, Joosten F, et al. Magnetic resonance imaging in patients with meningitis induced hearing loss. Eur Arch Otorhinolaryngol 2009;266(8):1229–36.

39. Phelps PD, Reardon W, Pembrey M, et al. X-linked deafness, stapes gushers and a distinctive defect of the inner ear. Neuroradiology 1991; 33(4):326–30.

40. Talbot JM, Wilson DF. Computed tomographic diagnosis of X-linked congenital mixed deafness, fixation of the stapedial footplate, and perilymphatic gusher. Am J Otol 1994;15(2):177–82.

41. Dunklebarger J, Branstetter B, Lincoln A, et al. Pediatric temporal bone fractures: current trends and comparison of classification schemes. Laryngoscope 2014;124(3):781–4.

Imaging Findings in Syndromes with Temporal Bone Abnormalities

Daniel Thomas Ginat, MD, MS

KEYWORDS

• Syndrome • Temporal bone • Anomalies • Imaging

KEY POINTS

- Temporal bone imaging is often an integral part of treatment planning in patients with congenital syndromes and hearing loss.
- Although the phenotypic expression can vary from individual to individual, many syndromes have a predictable constellation of temporal bone anomalies.
- External auditory canal atresia is a hallmark of syndromes related to first and second branchial arch malformations; however, inner ear anomalies are also routinely encountered on imaging.
- Otomastoiditis tends to occur in a variety of congenital syndromes characterized by residual mesenchymal elements in the temporal bone.

INTRODUCTION

There are numerous congenital syndromes that can affect the ear and temporal bone. Many of these syndromes feature overlapping patterns of temporal bone anomalies due to similar embryologic disruptions, but may otherwise be distinguished by the presence of abnormalities in other parts of the body and specific genetic mutations. Although the diagnosis is often made clinically, imaging is useful for defining the extent of temporal bone anomalies in patients with hearing loss, which in turn can affect management. The goal of this article is to review the temporal bone imaging findings of selected congenital syndromes in the context of the underlying pathogenesis via a systematic approach.

DISCUSSION
Treacher Collins Syndrome

Treacher Collins syndrome, or mandibulofacial dysostosis, is an autosomal dominant disorder caused by TCOF1, POLR1C, or POLR1D gene mutations.[1–3] The products of these genes are involved in ribosome synthesis in the neural crest cells that form the first 2 branchial arches.[1] The phenotype of Treacher Collins syndrome is variable; however characteristic features include downward-slanting palpebral fissures, mandibular hypoplasia, external auditory canal and middle ear deformities, cleft palate, and choanal atresia. Between 30% and 50% of affected individuals have severe bilateral conductive hearing loss due to external auditory canal stenosis or atresia.[4,5] The degree of associated middle ear and mastoid cavities hypoplasia and ossicular chain anomalies tend to be severe (**Fig. 1**); consequently, most Treacher Collins patients are poor candidates for atresia surgery.[4,5] In addition, some patients may exhibit lateral semicircular canal-vestibular dysplasia, in which the bone island measures less than 3 mm in diameter, whereas the cochlea and the superior and posterior semicircular canals tend to be normal (**Fig. 2**).[4]

Disclosures: None.
Department of Radiology, University of Chicago, Pritzker School of Medicine, 5841 South Maryland Avenue, Chicago, IL 60637, USA
E-mail address: dtg1@uchicago.edu

Neuroimag Clin N Am 29 (2019) 117–128
https://doi.org/10.1016/j.nic.2018.08.004
1052-5149/19/© 2018 Elsevier Inc. All rights reserved.

neuroimaging.theclinics.com

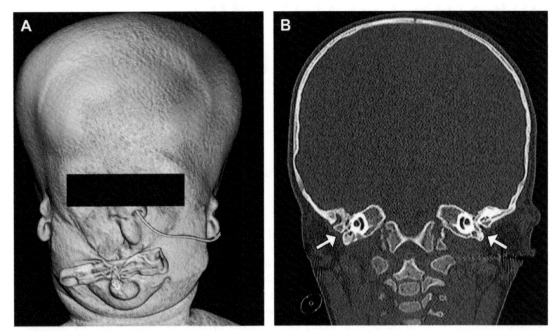

Fig. 1. Treacher Collins syndrome. Three-dimensional (3D) reconstruction (A) and coronal (B) computed tomography (CT) images demonstrate bilateral microtia and severe external auditory canal atresia (arrows in B).

Oculo-Auriculo-Vertebral Dysplasia Spectrum

Oculo-auriculo-vertebral dysplasia spectrum comprises hemifacial microsomia and Goldenhar syndrome, which represent different severities of malformations involving the development of the first and second branchial arches and beyond.

The severity of the condition can be graded based on the OMENS system, which comprises orbital asymmetry, mandibular hypoplasia, ear deformity, nerve dysfunction, and soft-tissue deficiency.[6] In particular, findings associated with oculo-auriculo-vertebral spectrum may include a variety of ear and temporal bone anomalies; ocular

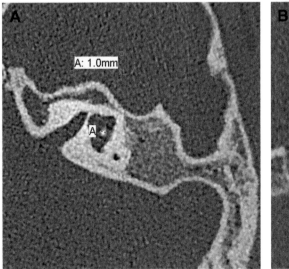
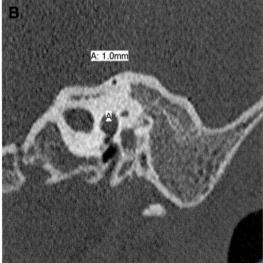

Fig. 2. Treacher Collins syndrome. Axial (A) and coronal (B) CT images shows left lateral semicircular canal-vestibular dysplasia with a small bone island (calipers). There is also absent mastoid pneumatization and a markedly hypoplastic middle ear cavity.

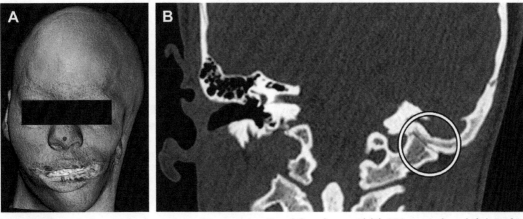

Fig. 3. Oculo-auriculo-vertebral spectrum. 3D reconstruction (*A*) and coronal (*B*) CT images show left hemifacial macrosomia with severe left microtia, external auditory canal atresia, and a hypoplastic middle ear cavity (*circle*).

epibulbar dermoids; underdevelopment of the craniofacial structures; vertebral abnormalities, including segmentation anomalies and scoliosis; and even brain malformations, such as tegmental cap anomaly and ventriculomegaly.[7] Microtia with external auditory canal atresia are the main ear and temporal bone malformations encountered in oculo-auriculo-vertebral dysplasia spectrum and can be bilateral in up to 50% of cases (Fig. 3).[7,8] However, many other ear and temporal bone anomalies can be identified on imaging (Box 1), in which inner ear abnormalities are present in one-third of patients. Although these may not be of clinical significance, some defects of the inner ear can be severe and require elaborate hearing loss therapy (Fig. 4).[9]

Klippel-Feil Syndrome

Klippel-Feil syndrome is genetically heterogeneous and is defined as a short neck with limited range of motion and low posterior hairline secondary to abnormal cervical segmentation.[10,11] Furthermore, deafness is a common feature of Klippel-Feil syndrome and may be sensorineural, conductive, or mixed. Associated findings may include microtia, external ear canal stenosis, chronic ear inflammation, anomalies of the tympanic cavity and ossicles, inner ear dysplasias, deformed internal auditory canal, and enlarged vestibular aqueduct (Fig. 5).[11] Klippel-Feil syndrome can actually be a component of other disorders, such as oculo-auriculo-vertebral dysplasia spectrum and Wildervanck syndrome.

Branchio-Oto-Renal Syndrome

Branchio-oto-renal syndrome is a rare autosomal dominant phenotype caused by mutations in the EYA1 or SIX1 genes.[12] The condition is characterized by the presence of branchial cysts or fistulae; sensorineural, conductive, or mixed hearing loss; and renal anomalies.[12] Temporal bone imaging findings may include a hypoplastic apical turn of the cochlea, aberrant facial nerve with a medially deviated tympanic segment, a funnel-shaped internal auditory canal, a patulous Eustachian tube, a small middle ear cavity, ossicular chain malformations, a dilation of the endolymphatic sac and duct, and hypoplasia of the semicircular canals (Fig. 6).[13–15]

Box 1
Variety of ear and temporal bone anomalies in oculo-auriculo-vertebral dysplasia spectrum

Enlarged eustachian tube lumen

Preauricular appendages and fistulas

Microtia or anotia

Stenosis or atresia of the external auditory canal

Underdeveloped middle ear cavity and mastoid

Dysmorphic or absent ossicles

Stenosis of the oval and round windows

Distorted and hypoplastic cochlea

Absence of the cochlear aqueduct

Underdeveloped vestibular system and absence of the semicircular canals

Anomalous endolymphatic duct

Enlargement of the vestibular aqueduct

Absent or aberrant facial nerve canal

Short and wide, narrowed, or duplicated internal auditory canal

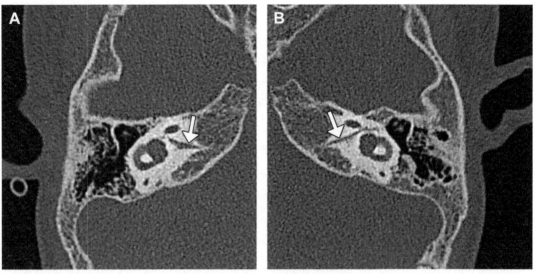

Fig. 4. Oculo-auriculo-vertebral spectrum. Axial CT images (*A*, *B*) show very narrow internal auditory canals bilaterally (*arrows*). In addition, the vestibules and lateral semicircular canals are mildly dysplastic.

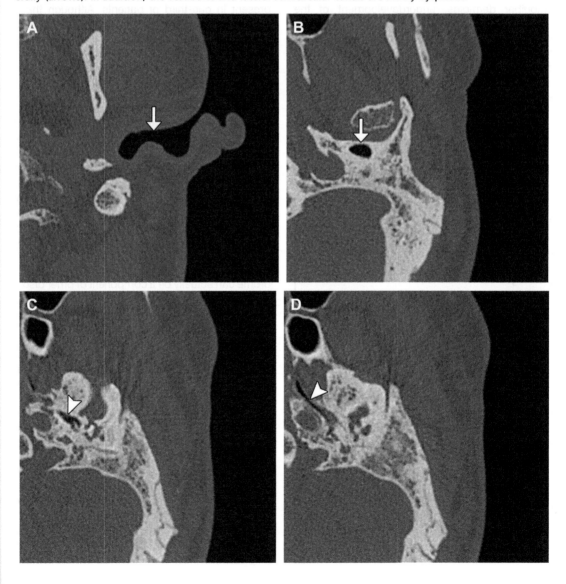

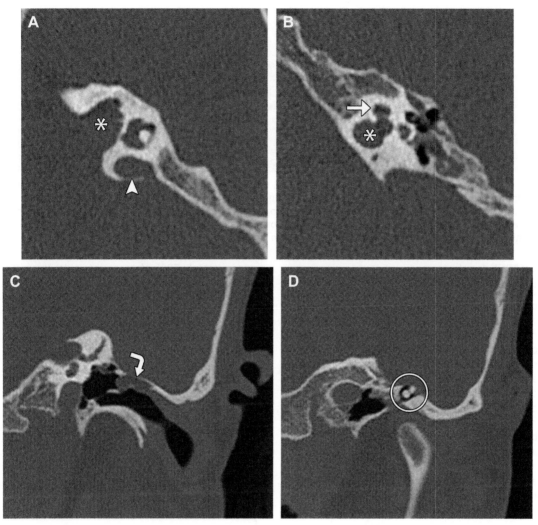

Fig. 6. Branchio-oto-renal syndrome. Axial (*A, B*) and coronal (*C, D*) CT images of the temporal bones show a short and wide left internal auditory canal (*asterisks in A and B*), an enlarged left vestibular aqueduct (*arrowhead in A*), a hypoplastic cochlea (*arrow in B*), dysmorphic lateral semicircular canal (*A*), a malformed external auditory canal with a partly duplicated segment (*curved arrow in C*), and dysmorphic right incudomalleal ossicular complex (*encircled in D*).

Pierre Robin Sequence

The Pierre Robin sequence encompasses multiple syndromes related to the abnormal development of the first and second branchial arches with the classic triad of micrognathia, cleft palate, and glossoptosis.[16] Indeed, more than 40 syndromes associated with Pierre Robin sequence have been described, the most common of which are Stickler syndrome and chromosome 22q11.2 deletion syndrome. Overall, hearing loss in Pierre Robin sequence has an incidence of more than 80% and is usually conductive and bilateral; and often associated with varying degrees of microtia, external auditory canal stenosis, and middle ear and ossicular anomalies, including the stapes.[17,18] The presence of a cleft and high arched palate confers an increased incidence of otomastoiditis, which can contribute to conductive hearing loss.[17,18] Ultimately, there can be a wide variety of anomalies in Pierre Robin sequence throughout the temporal bone that should be sought on temporal bone imaging, as exemplified in **Fig. 7** and listed in **Box 2**.[17,18]

Fig. 5. Klippel-Feil syndrome. Axial CT images (*A–D*) show the left external auditory canal (*arrows in A and B*) communicates directly with the Eustachian tube (*arrowheads in C and D*), virtually bypassing an atretic middle ear cavity with dysmorphic ossicles.

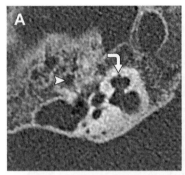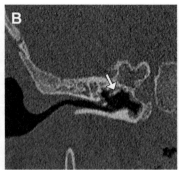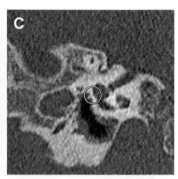

Fig. 7. Pierre Robin sequence. Axial (*A*) and coronal (*B, C*) CT images show a narrow external auditory canal (*B*); an anomalous facial nerve canal (*arrowhead in A*); an anomalous stapes (*arrow in B*) that is ankylosed to the wall of the middle ear; oval window atresia (*encircled in C*); opacification of the middle ear and mastoid (*A*), which are underdeveloped; dysplastic semicircular canals (*A*); a short and wide internal auditory canal (*A*); and a hypoplastic cochlea with absence of the modiolus (*curved arrow in A*).

CHARGE Syndrome

CHARGE syndrome is an autosomal dominant condition caused by a mutation in the CHD7 gene, which plays a role in the formation of migratory neural crest cells.[19] The syndrome is characterized by coloboma, heart defects, choanal atresia, mental retardation, genitourinary malformations, and ear anomalies, although the phenotypic expression can be quite variable.[19] Patients with CHARGE syndrome may have conductive and/or sensorineural hearing loss and a wide spectrum of temporal bone anomalies that can be encountered on imaging (**Box 3**), although the computed tomography (CT) findings do not necessarily correlate with audiogram results.[20] Some of the most common temporal bone anomalies in CHARGE syndrome include abnormalities of the semicircular canal in

approximately 70% of cases, ossicular anomalies in up to 80% of cases, and facial nerve anomalies in up to 70% of cases (**Fig. 8**). Of note, stenosis of the cochlear nerve aperture can be observed on CT in patients with CHARGE syndrome, which suggests cochlear nerve deficiency and warrants further investigation via MR imaging (**Fig. 9**). Absence of the cochlear nerve would be a contraindication to cochlear implantation.[21]

Pendred Syndrome

Pendred syndrome is an autosomal recessive disorder caused by mutations in the SLC26A4/PDS gene that encodes the anion exchanger pendrin, which is involved in the maintenance

---

Box 2
Temporal bone anomalies related to Pierre Robin sequence

Middle ear and mastoid air cell opacification, under-pneumatization, and erosions

Residual Reichert cartilage that forms a mass at the tympanic end of the fissula ante fenestram

Anomalous and ankylosed ossicles

Anomalous facial nerve with oblique course through the tympanic and mastoid segment

Oval window atresia

Enlarged lateral semicircular canal

Small, incomplete, or absent posterior semicircular canal

Hypoplastic cochlea with a deficient modiolus

Abnormal configuration of internal auditory canal

Box 3
Temporal bone anomalies related to CHARGE syndrome

Small middle ear cavities

Dysplastic and/or ankylosed ossicles

Posteriorly displaced labyrinthine segment and first genu of facial nerve

Oval and round windows stenosis or atresia

Semicircular canal absence, dysplasia, or hypoplasia, particularly the lateral and posterior

Vestibular hypoplasia or dysplasia

Cochlear dysplasia with enlarged basal turns and hypoplastic or incompletely partitioned apical turns

Cochlear nerve aperture stenosis

Cochlear nerve deficiency

Petrosquamous emissary sinus

Jugular bulb diverticulum

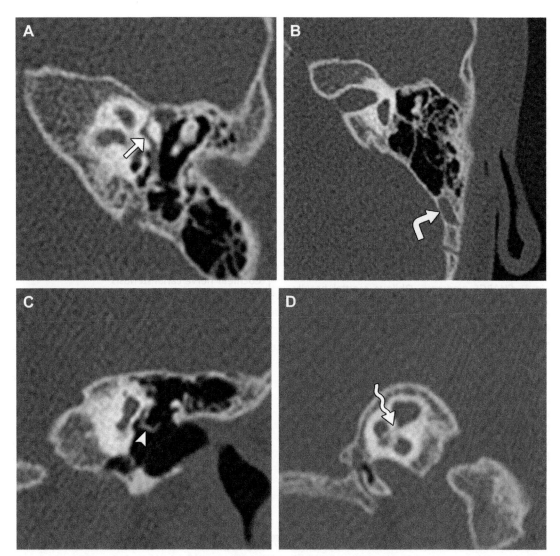

Fig. 8. CHARGE syndrome. Axial (*A, B*), coronal (*C*), and oblique sagittal (*D*) CT images show an aberrant facial nerve canal (*arrow in A*); an anomalous emissary vein (*curved arrow in B*); malformed ossicles, including fixation of a monopod stapes (*arrowhead in C*) to a dehiscence tympanic facial nerve; a dysmorphic vestibule with absence of the lateral and posterior semicircular canals; and a dysplastic cochlea with deficient distal turns, a wide basal turn, and cochlear aperture stenosis (*squiggly arrow in D*).

of the endocochlear electrical potential.[22,23] The condition is characterized by the combination of bilateral sensorineural hearing loss and goiter due to abnormal organification of iodide with or without hypothyroidism.[22,23] The hearing loss of Pendred syndrome is associated with inner ear malformations, particularly enlarged vestibular aqueducts bilaterally.[23,24] This can be accompanied by deficiency of the interscalar septum in the distal turns of the cochlea, which is an incomplete partition type 2 anomaly (**Fig. 10**).[24]

Down Syndrome

Down syndrome, or trisomy 21, is the most common chromosomal abnormality in children and is often associated with otolaryngologic issues, including chronic otitis media, sensorineural hearing loss, airway obstruction, sleep apnea, and chronic rhinosinusitis.[25] There are many potential temporal bone findings associated with Down syndrome that can be depicted on imaging (**Box 4**).[26–28] Middle and external ear abnormalities are especially prevalent, mainly consisting of

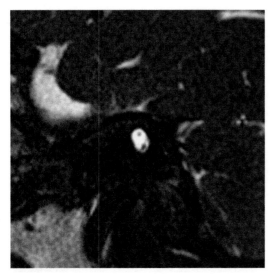

Fig. 9. CHARGE syndrome. Oblique sagittal heavily T2-weighted MR image through the internal auditory canal shows absence of the cochlear nerve. Only the facial nerve and the vestibular nerve complex are visible in cross-section.

middle ear and mastoid opacification and hypopneumatization (Fig. 11).[28] Inner ear anomalies are also rather common in patients with Down syndrome. In particular, lateral semicircular canal-vestibular dysplasia is typical (Fig. 12).[26,28] Furthermore, internal auditory canal stenosis is most strongly correlated with sensorineural hearing loss among the various temporal bone anomalies in Down syndrome due to cochlear nerve deficiency, which can be evaluated via high-resolution MR imaging.[29] If present, this finding can be a contraindication for cochlear implantation.

Trisomy 18

Trisomy 18, or Edward syndrome, is the second most common aneuploidy after trisomy 21 and is characterized by multisystem anomalies, including the craniofacial structures, the musculoskeletal system, the cardiovascular system,

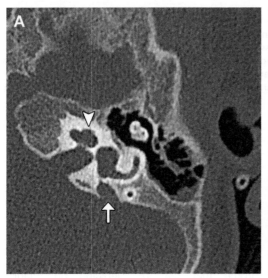
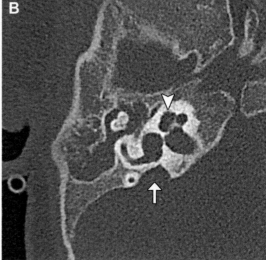

Fig. 10. Pendred syndrome. Axial CT images of the temporal bones (*A, B*) show marked dilatation of bilateral vestibular aqueducts (*arrows*) and deficiency of the cochlear turns (*arrowheads*). There is also extensive right tympanomastoid opacification.

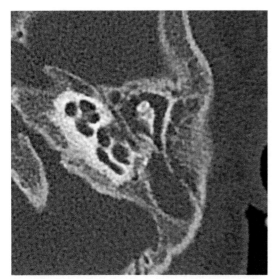

Fig. 11. Down syndrome. Axial CT image shows diffuse left otomastoid opacification and mastoid hypopneumatization.

abdominal organs, and the nervous system.[30] Less than 10% of patients with trisomy survive beyond the first year of life[30]; consequently, there is a paucity of literature regarding temporal bone imaging findings. Nevertheless, among the limited cases described, there can be multiple temporal bone anomalies, many of which are reminiscent of those typically derived from the first and second branchial arches (Box 5).[31,32] Of note, the labyrinthine structures can be affected in a peculiar manner, such as effacement of the superior semicircular canal (Fig. 13).

Box 5
Temporal bone anomalies related to Trisomy 18

External auditory canal stenosis or atresia

Aberrant tensor tympani muscle

Malformed stapes, malleus, and incus continuous with a persistent Meckel cartilage

Aberrant facial nerve with an obtuse angulation at the first genu and malpositioned geniculate ganglion

Shortened cochlea

Vestibular anomalies, such as bony and membranous blockage of the superior semicircular canal

Turner Syndrome

Turner syndrome is caused by partial or complete absence of one of the X chromosomes and is characterized by gonadal dysgenesis; short stature; coarctation of the aorta; and multiple head and neck abnormalities, such as chronic or recurrent otitis media, sensorineural and/or conductive hearing loss, dysmorphic palate, pinna deformity, pterygium colli, low posterior hairline, low-set ears, and micrognathia.[33–35] Other than tympanomastoid opacification, temporal bone imaging may reveal cochlear malformations, which can resemble incomplete partition type 2 (Fig. 14).[36]

Neurofibromatosis Type 2

Neurofibromatosis type 2 is caused by a mutation on the NF2 gene on chromosome 22, which encodes Merlin, a tumor suppressor protein.[37] The syndrome is characterized by the presence of

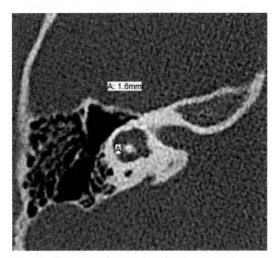

Fig. 12. Down syndrome. Axial CT image shows a small right lateral semicircular canal bone island.

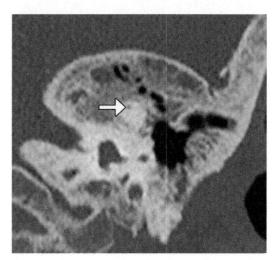

Fig. 13. Trisomy 18. Coronal CT image show ossification of the superior semicircular canal (arrow) and a generally abnormal appearance of the bone.

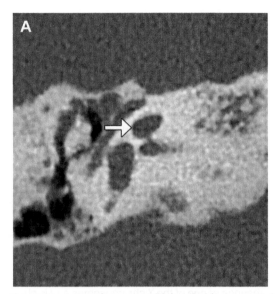
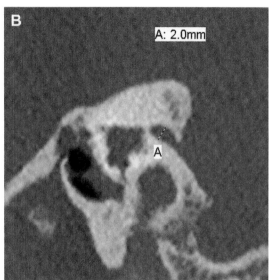

Fig. 14. Turner syndrome. Axial (*A*) and oblique sagittal (*B*) CT images show a malformed cochlea with deficiency of the modiolus and turns (*arrow in A*), as well as a narrow cochlear aperture and internal auditory canal. In addition, the vestibular aqueduct is enlarged (*caliper in B*). There is partial tympanomastoid opacification.

schwannomas, meningiomas, ependymomas, and (less commonly) gliomas. In particular, vestibular schwannomas are present in 95% of individuals with neurofibromatosis type 2, often bilaterally.[37] High-resolution MR imaging is the modality of choice for screening and monitoring vestibular schwannomas.[38] The tumors are typically centered in the internal auditory canal and demonstrate enhancement on MR imaging (Fig. 15). Furthermore, MR imaging can also potentially

help identify patients with vestibular schwannomas who are at risk for developing hearing loss due to cochlear aperture obstruction and accumulation of intralabyrinthine protein,[39] which can appear as reduced fluid signal on heavily T2-weighted 3-dimensional gradient echo sequences.

SUMMARY

This article demonstrates that there is a wide spectrum of temporal bone imaging findings associated with congenital syndromes. Many syndromes that involve the temporal bone share common developmental aberrations but are distinguished from each other by particular combinations of anomalies and underlying gene mutations. Even among individuals affected by the same syndrome, the severity and scope of the temporal bone anomalies can vary considerably and thus influence patient management. Consequently, temporal bone imaging plays an important role in the treatment planning for patients with congenital syndromes and hearing loss, with particular attention to the anomalies listed in each syndrome section and common patterns that they may form.

REFERENCES

1. Kadakia S, Helman SN, Badhey AK, et al. Treacher Collins Syndrome: the genetics of a craniofacial disease. Int J Pediatr Otorhinolaryngol 2014;78(6): 893–8.

Fig. 15. Neurofibromatosis type 2. Coronal fat-suppressed postcontrast T1-weighted MR image shows enhancing tumors in bilateral internal auditory canals (*arrows*), compatible with vestibular schwannomas.

2. Taylor DJ, Phelps PD. Imaging of ear deformities in Treacher Collins syndrome. Clin Otolaryngol Allied Sci 1993;18(4):263–7.

3. van Vierzen PB, Joosten FB, Marres HA, et al. Mandibulofacial dysostosis: CT findings of the temporal bones. Eur J Radiol 1995;21(1):53–7.

4. Takegoshi H, Kaga K, Kikuchi S, et al. Mandibulofacial dysostosis: CT evaluation of the temporal bones for surgical risk assessment in patients of bilateral aural atresia. Int J Pediatr Otorhinolaryngol 2000; 54(1):33–40.

5. Rosa F, Coutinho MB, Ferreira JP, et al. Ear malformations, hearing loss and hearing rehabilitation in children with Treacher Collins syndrome. Acta Otorrinolaringol Esp 2016;67(3):142–7.

6. Gougoutas AJ, Singh DJ, Low DW, et al. Hemifacial microsomia: clinical features and pictographic representations of the OMENS classification system. Plast Reconstr Surg 2007 Dec;120(7): 112e–20e.

7. Davide B, Renzo M, Sara G, et al. Oculo-auriculo-vertebral spectrum: going beyond the first and second pharyngeal arch involvement. Neuroradiology 2017;59(3):305–16.

8. Bisdas S, Lenarz M, Lenarz T, et al. Inner ear abnormalities in patients with Goldenhar syndrome. Otol Neurotol 2005;26(3):398–404.

9. Hennersdorf F, Friese N, Löwenheim H, et al. Temporal bone changes in patients with Goldenhar syndrome with special emphasis on inner ear abnormalities. Otol Neurotol 2014;35(5):826–30.

10. McGaughran JM, Kuna P, Das V. Audiological abnormalities in the Klippel-Feil syndrome. Arch Dis Child 1998;79(4):352–5.

11. Yildirim N, Arslanoğlu A, Mahiroğullari M, et al. Klippel-Feil syndrome and associated ear anomalies. Am J Otolaryngol 2008;29(5):319–25.

12. Kochhar A, Fischer SM, Kimberling WJ, et al. Branchio-oto-renal syndrome. Am J Med Genet A 2007; 143A:1671–8.

13. Ginat DT, Ferro L, Gluth MB. Anatomic and quantitative temporal bone CT for preoperative assessment of branchio-oto-renal syndrome. Clin Neuroradiol 2016;26(4):481–3.

14. Propst EJ, Blaser S, Gordon KA, et al. Temporal bone findings on computed tomography imaging in branchio-oto-renal syndrome. Laryngoscope 2005;115:1855–62.

15. Ceruti S, Stinckens C, Cremers CW, et al. Temporal bone anomalies in the branchio-oto-renal syndrome: detailed computed tomographic and magnetic resonance imaging findings. Otol Neurotol 2002;23: 200–7.

16. Evans KN, Sie KC, Hopper RA, et al. Robin sequence: from diagnosis to development of an effective management plan. Pediatrics 2011;127: 936–48.

17. Igarashi M, Filippone MV, Alford BR. Temporal bone findings in Pierre Robin syndrome. Laryngoscope 1976;86:1679–87.

18. Gruen PM, Carranza A, Karmody CS, et al. Anomalies of the ear in the Pierre Robin triad. Ann Otol Rhinol Laryngol 2005;114:605–13.

19. Bergman JE, Janssen N, Hoefsloot LH, et al. CHD7 mutations and CHARGE syndrome: the clinical implications of an expanding phenotype. J Med Genet 2011;48(5):334–42.

20. Ha J, Ong F, Wood B, et al. Radiologic and audiologic findings in the temporal bone of patients with CHARGE syndrome. Ochsner J 2016;16(2):125–9.

21. Morimoto AK, Wiggins RH 3rd, Hudgins PA, et al. Absent semicircular canals in CHARGE syndrome: radiologic spectrum of findings. AJNR Am J Neuroradiol 2006;27(8):1663–71.

22. Bizhanova A, Kopp P. Genetics and phenomics of Pendred syndrome. Mol Cell Endocrinol 2010; 322(1–2):83–90.

23. Wémeau JL, Kopp P. Pendred syndrome. Best Pract Res Clin Endocrinol Metab 2017;31(2):213–24.

24. Phelps PD, Coffey RA, Trembath RC, et al. Radiological malformations of the ear in Pendred syndrome. Clin Radiol 1998;53(4):268–73.

25. Shott SR. Down syndrome: common otolaryngologic manifestations. Am J Med Genet C Semin Med Genet 2006;142C(3):131–40.

26. Clark CM, Patel HH, Kanekar SG, et al. Enlarged vestibular aqueducts and other inner-ear abnormalities in patients with Down syndrome. J Laryngol Otol 2017;131(4):298–302.

27. Ginat DT. Anomalous stapes in Down syndrome. Ear Nose Throat J 2017;96(1):15–9.

28. Blaser S, Propst EJ, Martin D, et al. Inner ear dysplasia is common in children with Down syndrome (trisomy 21). Laryngoscope 2006;116(12): 2113–9.

29. Intrapiromkul J, Aygun N, Tunkel DE, et al. Inner ear anomalies seen on CT images in people with Down syndrome. Pediatr Radiol 2012;42(12):1449–55.

30. Roberts W, Zurada A, Zurada-ZieliŃSka A, et al. Anatomy of trisomy 18. Clin Anat 2016;29(5):628–32.

31. Tadaki T, Kamiyama R, Okamura HO, et al. Anomalies of the auditory organ in trisomy 18 syndrome: human temporal bone histopathological study. J Laryngol Otol 2003;117(7):580–3.

32. Saito R, Jurado AB, Inokuchi I, et al. Temporal bone histopathology in trisomy 18 syndrome: a report of two cases. Acta Med Okayama 1987;41(3):125–31.

33. Makishima T, King K, Brewer CC, et al. Otolaryngologic markers for the early diagnosis of Turner syndrome. Int J Pediatr Otorhinolaryngol 2009;73(11): 1564–7.

34. Serra A, Cocuzza S, Caruso E, et al. Audiological range in Turner's syndrome. Int J Pediatr Otorhinolaryngol 2003;67(8):841–5.

35. Dhooge IJ, De Vel E, Verhoye C, et al. Otologic disease in turner syndrome. Otol Neurotol 2005;26(2):145–50.

36. Fish JH 3rd, Schwenter I, Schmutzhard J, et al. Morphology studies of the human fetal cochlea in turner syndrome. Ear Hear 2009;30(1):143–6.

37. Ardern-Holmes S, Fisher G, North K. Neurofibromatosis type 2. J Child Neurol 2017;32(1):9–22.

38. Slattery WH. Neurofibromatosis type 2. Otolaryngol Clin North Am 2015;48(3):443–60.

39. Asthagiri AR, Vasquez RA, Butman JA, et al. Mechanisms of hearing loss in neurofibromatosis type 2. PLoS One 2012;7(9):e46132.

Imaging of Temporal Bone Trauma

A Clinicoradiologic Perspective

Joshua E. Lantos, MD[a],[*], Kristen Leeman, MD[a],
Elizabeth K. Weidman, MD[a], Kathryn E. Dean, MD[a],
Tiffany Peng, MD[b], Aaron N. Pearlman, MD[b]

KEYWORDS

- Temporal bone fracture • Facial nerve injury • Cerebrospinal fluid leak • Hearing loss • Vertigo
- Perilymphatic fistula • Ossicular injury • Temporal bone surgery

KEY POINTS

- When there is clinical suspicion for temporal bone trauma, imaging is typically performed with high-resolution computed tomography. Other imaging modalities occasionally provide complementary information and may be indicated based on clinical or radiologic suspicion.
- Certain imaging findings can indicate a specific treatment or alter clinical and surgical management, including the type of surgery performed.
- Knowledge of clinical findings as well as medical and surgical management can aid in the detection of key findings.
- Radiologists should be familiar with the clinical scenarios of temporal bone trauma complicated by hearing loss, vertigo, perilymphatic fistula, cerebrospinal fluid leak, facial nerve injury, and vascular injury.

INTRODUCTION

The temporal bones are paired structures that form the inferior portion of the lateral skull and contribute to the skull base. In addition to protecting intracranial contents, the temporal bones house structures critical for hearing, balance, and facial expression. Injury to the temporal bone requires a substantial force, and patients often have concomitant neurologic or orthopedic injuries that require more immediate attention. Clinical evidence of temporal bone injury includes hemorrhagic otorrhea, hemotympanum, tympanic membrane perforation, vertigo, hearing loss, facial nerve paresis, nystagmus, and postauricular ecchymosis (Battle sign).[1,2] These clinical findings

will prompt imaging, and radiologic findings can guide or alter clinical management (Boxes 1 and 2). This article discusses the imaging findings of temporal bone injuries and potential impact on clinical decision-making.

IMAGING MODALITIES

High-resolution computed tomography (HRCT) of the temporal bone is the imaging modality of choice for evaluating temporal bone trauma.[1] Axial images should be acquired at less than 1-mm thickness, and can be reconstructed in the coronal or sagittal plane. Additional reconstructions parallel (Stenvers view) or perpendicular (Poschl view) to the petrous pyramid may also be useful for

Disclosure Statement: n/a.
[a] Department of Radiology, Weill Cornell Medicine, New York Presbyterian Hospital, 1305 York Avenue, 3rd Floor, New York, NY 1002, USA; [b] Department of Otolaryngology–Head and Neck Surgery, Weill Cornell Medicine, New York Presbyterian Hospital, 1305 York Avenue, 5th Floor, New York, NY 10021, USA
* Corresponding author.
E-mail address: jol9057@med.cornell.edu

Neuroimag Clin N Am 29 (2019) 129–143
https://doi.org/10.1016/j.nic.2018.08.005
1052-5149/19/Published by Elsevier Inc.

Box 1

Indications for surgery in temporal bone trauma (Ramsey[17])

- Persistent conductive hearing loss
- Persistent tympanic membrane perforation
- Severe facial nerve injury
- Persistent cerebrospinal fluid leak
- Severe comminuted fracture
- External auditory canal fracture causing stenosis

Box 2

Surgical approaches (Ramsey[17])

- Transcanal approach
  - Tympanoplasty for small posterior perforations
  - Ossicular chain reconstruction
  - External auditory canal (EAC) canalplasty
  - Perilymphatic fistula repair without concurrent mastoid pathology
- Postauricular approach
  - EAC canalplasty
  - Tympanoplasty for large anterior perforations (greater access than transcanal)
- Mastoidectomy approach
  - Mastoid and distal tympanic facial nerve repair/decompression
  - Tympanoplasty with concurrent mastoid pathology (eg, CSF leak)
  - CSF leak from tegmen mastoideum
- Translabyrinthine approach
  - Facial nerve repair when there is irreversible hearing loss
  - CSF leak repair when there is irreversible hearing loss
- Middle cranial fossa approach
  - Proximal facial nerve repair (geniculate, labyrinthine, internal auditory canal) when patient has serviceable hearing
  - CSF leak from tegmen tympani, petrous apex
  - Encephalocele repair
- Transmastoid/supralabyrinthine approach
  - Facial nerve decompression for lesions distal to the geniculate ganglion when patient has serviceable hearing

---

evaluation.[3] Computed tomography (CT) is the best modality for delineating bony anatomy and is therefore best for depicting fracture lines, the facial canal, ossicular chain, otic capsule, carotid canal, jugular fossa, and sigmoid plate. Dedicated arterial imaging with CT angiography (CTA), magnetic resonance (MR) angiography, or catheter angiography may be indicated in the case of suspected arterial injury, including when there is violation of the carotid canal on HRCT. CT or MR venogram should be considered for fractures that extend to the sigmoid plate or jugular foramen. Cisternography with CT, radionuclide, or MR imaging may assist in diagnosing and localizing cerebrospinal fluid (CSF) leaks. MR imaging is the best modality for diagnosing traumatic encephalocele.

FRACTURE CLASSIFICATION

Beginning with Ulrich[4] in 1926, fractures of the temporal bone have been classified as either longitudinal or transverse based on the orientation of the fracture line relative to the long axis of the petrous pyramid. Subsequent studies showed that most temporal bone fractures, approximately 80%, could be classified as longitudinal, whereas the remaining 20% were transverse.[5,6] Longitudinal fractures are more likely to involve the ossicular chain and result in conductive hearing loss (CHL), whereas transverse fractures are more likely to involve the otic capsule and result in sensorineural hearing loss (SNHL). However, subsequent studies found that most fractures were oblique relative to the long axis of the petrous pyramid, crossing the petrotympanic fissure laterally and then running anteromedially parallel to the long axis of the petrous ridge, whereas only a minority truly longitudinal.[7] Additionally, the classic longitudinal and transverse descriptors correlated poorly with patient outcome.[7–9]

To date, the best classification system correlating with patient outcomes is the otic capsule sparing (OCS) versus optic capsule violating (OCV) descriptor.[2,9–11] OCS fractures are usually caused by a temporoparietal blow involving the squamous portion of the temporal bone and extend through the posterosuperior external auditory canal, mastoid air cells, and middle ear to the tegmen.[12] OCS fractures typically result in a conductive or mixed hearing loss due to this tendency to involve the middle ear.[8] OCV fractures typically result from an occipital blow and extend from the foramen magnum up through the petrous pyramid and into the otic capsule.[11,12] OCV fractures often involve the jugular foramen, foramen lacerum, and internal auditory canal.[12] They are also associated with increased rates of facial nerve injury, SNHL, CSF leak, and intracranial complications.[8–10,12] For example, Little and Kesser[10] found a 5-fold increase in facial nerve injury, a 25-fold increase in SNHL, and an 8-fold increase in CSF otorrhea in OCV relative to OCS fractures. Kennedy and colleagues[3] provide an excellent summary of recent studies showing the improved predictive value of patient outcomes using the OCV versus OCS classification system.

CONDUCTIVE HEARING LOSS

The most common complication following temporal bone trauma is hearing loss, with a reported incidence ranging from 24% to 81%.[3,9,11] Bedside examination with a 512-Hz tuning fork in an alert patient is a reliable way to screen for hearing loss and help to distinguish between SNHL and CHL. When the combination of the Weber and Rinne examinations suggests CHL, physical examination should focus on the common causes of CHL, such as hemotympanum and tympanic membrane (TM) perforation.

Hemotympanum is the accumulation of blood within the middle ear cleft secondary to trauma and impaired drainage through the Eustachian tube, manifested clinically as discoloration of the TM. Hemotympanum is very common in temporal bone trauma, and when present, is an indication for temporal bone CT.[13] After approximately 6 to 8 weeks, hemotympanum should resolve, and an audiogram should be performed to evaluate for residual hearing loss, which may be an indication for imaging and surgical management.[2,17] CHL from TM perforation is managed similarly, because most patients regain hearing without intervention.[13] Patients with TM perforation should be reevaluated in 6 to 8 weeks, and patients with CHL from a persistent perforation referred to an otologist for tympanoplasty.[13]

Ossicular discontinuity occurs in approximately 20% of temporal bone fractures.[13] Dislocation is more common than fracture.[14] Ossicular injury is usually the result of longitudinal or OCS fractures, which typically involve the middle ear and mastoid air cells and have a higher incidence of CHL. In addition to direct trauma from fracture, indirect injury secondary to tetanic contraction of the stapedius or tensor tympani muscles may also cause ossicular dislocation.[1,3]

Five types of ossicular dislocation have been described: incudostapedial, incudomalleal, incus, stapediovestibular, and incudomalleal complex. Incudostapedial is the most common, followed by incudomallear.[1,2,15] The incus is the most commonly injured ossicle because it is the largest and has the fewest ligamentous attachments.[1,3,14] Ossicular joint injury may be suggested to be simply subluxed if there is minimal separation of the ossicles, or dislocated if there is frank separation.[3] Confirmation of the type of ossicular discontinuity can be confirmed with gentle intraoperative palpation.

Axial plane CT is optimal to visualize the incudomalleal joint within the epitympanum. The joint has a characteristic "ice-cream-cone" appearance on these images, with the body of the incus representing the cone, and the head of the malleus representing the ice cream. Disruption and widening of the incudomalleal joint is seen with traumatic subluxation and dislocation (Fig. 1). The integrity of the incudostapedial joint can be more challenging to discern, especially in the setting of hemotympanum, given the small size of the joint and subtle findings (Fig. 2).[3] Serial thin-slice axial and coronal CT images should be scrutinized to assess the articulation of the incus lenticular process with the head of the stapes. Even when the joint cannot be seen, an abnormal distance between the distal long process and the stapes can be a clue to dislocation.

Total incus dislocation is seen when both the incudomalleal and incudostapedial joints are disrupted. The incus can then freely move within the middle ear and may be extruded through a TM perforation (Fig. 3). The incudomalleal joint may remain intact and the incudomalleal complex itself may be displaced into the mesotympanum or hypotympanum when the ligamentous attachments of the malleus have been traumatically disrupted.[1,3] Malleus dislocation can occur when its ligamentous attachments have been disrupted with simultaneous incudomalleal dislocation (Fig. 4). Stapediovestibular dislocation results from disruption of the annular ligament of the stapes footplate to the oval window, resulting in a perilymphatic fistula (PLF) at the oval window. The stapes may be dislocated into the vestibule (internal) or into the middle ear (external).[1] Ossicular fracture is uncommon, and imaging findings can be subtle. These have been reported with incidence ranging from 2% to 11%, and most commonly involve the stapes.[6,14]

As with CHL related to hemotympanum and TM perforation, conservative management is often favored in the setting of minor ossicular disruption, because symptoms are often self-limiting.[3] A persistent CHL, defined as an air-bone gap of more than 20 dB on audiometry at 6 weeks,[16] raises suspicion for ossicular chain disruption.[2] Most otologists reserve exploratory tympanotomy with possible ossiculoplasty for a persistent CHL; however, if early surgical intervention is planned for

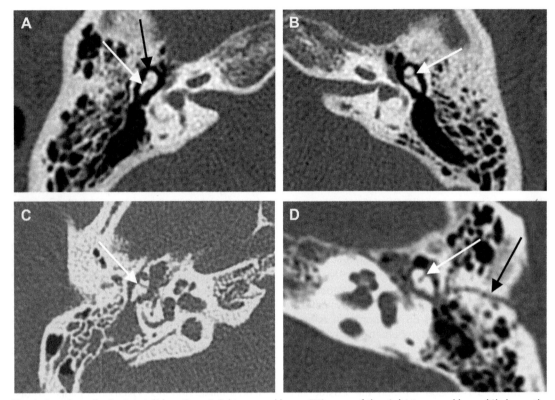

Fig. 1. Incudomalleolar joint dislocation. Axial temporal bone CT image of the right temporal bone (*A*) shows the normal appearance of the incudomalleal joint, with the head of the malleus (*A, black arrow*) articulating normally with the body of the incus (*A, white arrow*). There is nearly no perceptible gap between the 2 structures. There is abnormal widening of the joint (*B, white arrow*) on the contralateral side due to diving-related trauma with delayed CHL. Axial images of 2 other patients demonstrate traumatic incudomalleal dislocation (*C, D white arrows*). Incudomalleal dislocation is most often due to OCS fractures that extend through the middle ear (*D, black arrow*).

treatment of more emergent CSF leak or facial nerve decompression, early ossiculoplasty may be performed simultaneously.[2]

Surgical treatment for TM perforation may be performed with a fascial graft, usually temporalis, or a cartilage graft, such as tragal cartilage. Repair may be accomplished via a transcanal, postauricular, or endaural approach. The optimal approach for repair depends on the size and location of the perforation, with anteriorly based perforations typically requiring a postauricular approach due to limited anterior exposure with a transcanal approach. If CSF leak repair or facial nerve decompression will be performed, a postauricular approach is required due to the need for concurrent mastoidectomy. When required, ossicular

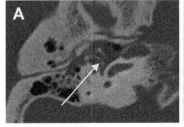
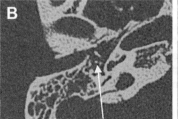
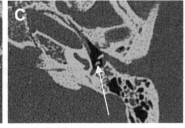

Fig. 2. Incudostapedial dislocation. Axial temporal bone CT images through 2 different patients (*A, B*) demonstrate widening between the lenticular process of the incus and the head of the stapes (*arrow*). Hemotympanum is present on both images and may obscure this subtle finding. Comparison with the contralateral normal side (*C* is the uninjured side of patient in *B*) shows the normal incudostapedial joint (*arrow*), which shows almost no separation between the incus lenticular process and stapes.

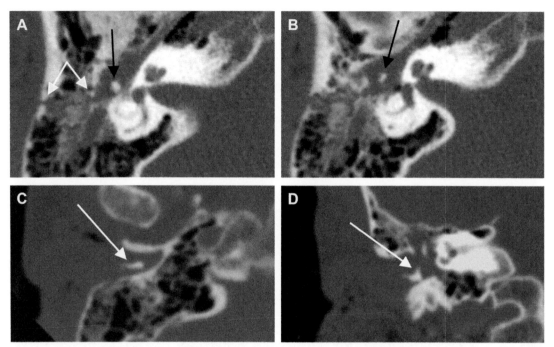

Fig. 3. Total incus dislocation. Axial (*A–C*) and coronal (*D*) images of the right temporal bone show an obliquely oriented fracture involving the middle ear (*A, white arrows*) and posterior displacement of the malleus head (*A, black arrow*) with absence of the incus body and short process in the epitympanum. Inferiorly, only the malleus handle is present (*B, arrow*) with absence of the incus long process. Further inferiorly within the external auditory canal, a dense bony structure (*C, arrow*) is identified resembling the incus, with coronal reconstruction confirming that this is the incus with the tip of the short process directed superiorly (*D, arrow*). A TM perforation can be inferred from external dislocation of the incus.

chain reconstruction is accomplished transcanal via tympanomeatal flap,[17] using either autologous (eg, incus interposition) or synthetic prosthesis to restore coupling of the TM with the stapes footplate and oval window.

SENSORINEURAL HEARING LOSS

SNHL may be the result of an OCV or OCS fracture, but is much more common with OCV. One study found a 25-fold increase in SNHL in OCV fractures as compared with OCS fractures.[10] OCV fractures typically result in severe or profound SNHL.[11] Potential mechanisms of SNHL include disruption of the membranous labyrinth, cochlear nerve injury, cochlear hemorrhage, or PLF.[12] Delayed and progressive SNHL after injury can be seen with both PLF and posttraumatic endolymphatic hydrops. SNHL can result from labyrinthine concussion in the absence of fracture.

Axial CT is the best way to evaluate OCV fractures, with fracture lines seen extending through the cochlea, vestibule, or semicircular canals (**Fig. 5**). Pneumolabyrinth can be a secondary sign of an OCV fracture and is important to recognize, as it may be the only indication of an OCV

injury. Hemorrhage within the labyrinth is not visible on CT, but can be appreciated by T1 shortening on MR imaging.[3]

One complication of an OCV fracture that may require surgical intervention is the development of labyrinthitis ossificans. Labyrinthitis ossificans is the pathologic replacement of the fluid-filled membranous labyrinth by fibrous tissue and then bone. High-resolution steady-state T2-weighted MR imaging is the imaging modality of choice to detect the earlier fibrous stage of labyrinthitis ossificans, because CT will show only end-stage bone formation (**Fig. 6**).[18] MR imaging findings have been well described in post-meningitic hearing loss.[19] The fibrous and bony disease states both show loss of normal T2 bright fluid signal within the membranous labyrinth on high-resolution T2-weighted steady-state sequences. CT can then be performed to distinguish fibrous tissue from bone. Enhancement within the labyrinth on post-gadolinium MR imaging precedes the fibrous stage,[19] reflecting inflammation before the deposition of fibrous tissue. Standard treatment to preserve hearing in labyrinthitis ossificans is cochlear implantation, and patients benefit from urgent surgical referral before obstructive

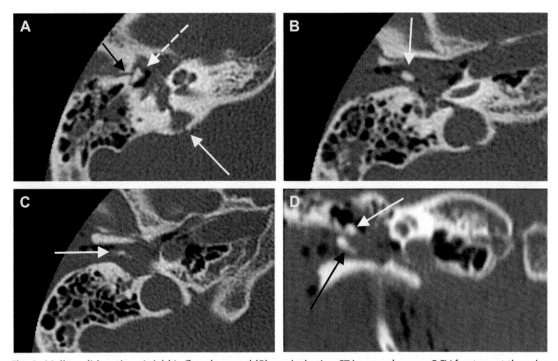

Fig. 4. Malleus dislocation. Axial (*A–C*) and coronal (*D*) cervical spine CT images show an OCV fracture at the edge of the film with a transverse component involving the jugular foramen and vestibule (*A, white arrow*) and an oblique component (*A, black arrow*) entering the middle ear. The malleus head is absent (*A, dashed arrow*) with only the incus body and short process seen within the epitympanum. More inferiorly, the malleus is seen in the external auditory canal, with head (*B, arrow*) and manubrium (*C, arrow*) seen on sequential images. Coronal image confirms the externally dislocated malleus (*D, black arrow*) and the incus still seen within the middle ear (*D, white arrow*). Like external incus dislocation, TM perforation can also be inferred in this case.

ossification of the cochlea makes implantation more technically challenging or impossible (**Fig. 7**).[18,20] Therefore, detecting labyrinthitis ossificans in its earliest stages is imperative to seize on a limited window of opportunity to restore hearing with cochlear implantation.

VERTIGO

Vertigo in temporal bone trauma may be the result of vestibular concussion or direct OCV injury to the vestibule, semicircular canals, vestibular aqueduct, or vestibular nerve.[2,3] Axial CT images are best for evaluating OCV fractures (see **Fig. 5**).[3] Careful evaluation of the vestibule and vestibular aqueduct should be performed. Stenvers and Poschl reconstructions aide in evaluation of the posterior and superior semicircular canals, allowing for easier detection of fracture lines extending into these structures.[3]

Many cases of posttraumatic vertigo may not have associated radiological findings and are managed conservatively because the condition is usually self-limiting, resolving in 6 to 12 months through central adaptation.[2] Benign paroxysmal positional vertigo, presumably caused by traumatic displacement of otoconia from the vestibule, is the most common cause of dizziness in the posttraumatic setting.[13] It may develop days to weeks after injury and is treated with standard rehabilitation, including repositioning maneuvers.[2] Delayed development of endolymphatic hydrops is a rare entity in the setting of temporal bone trauma. When it occurs, it is treated similar to Meniere disease, with a low-salt diet, diuretics, and steroids[2] Severe, persistent symptoms of vertigo and the presence or later development of auditory symptoms should warrant evaluation for possible PLF.

PERILYMPHATIC FISTULA

PLF is an abnormal communication between the inner and middle ear through a bony dehiscence in the otic capsule or, more frequently, disruption of the oval or round windows.[21] This can result in cochlear (SNHL) or vestibular (vertigo, tinnitus) symptoms. Patients often present in a delayed and progressive fashion following traumatic temporal bone injury. Before the widespread use of CT, exploratory surgery, including direct visualization of the oval and round windows, was

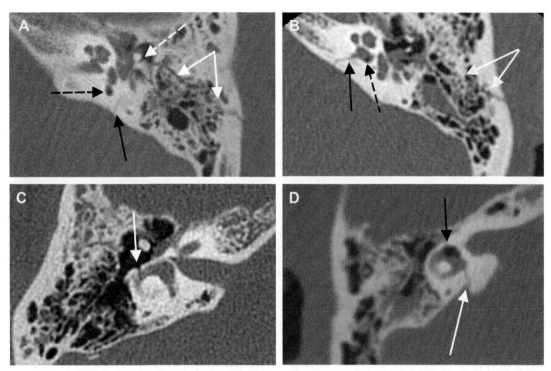

Fig. 5. OCV fractures. Axial temporal bone CT images in 4 different patients show a variety of otic capsule injuries. Mixed longitudinal (A, white arrows) and transverse (A, black arrow) components result in incudomalleal dislocation (A, dashed white arrow) and pneumolabyrinth within the ampulla of the posterior semicircular canal (A, dashed black arrow). Another mixed longitudinal (B, white arrows) and transverse (B, black arrow) fracture results in violation of the cochlea with pneumolabyrinth (B, dashed arrow). A third patient has an OCV injury to the lateral semicircular canal (C, white arrow). Final patient has a transversely oriented fracture through the vestibule (D, white arrow) with resultant pneumolabyrinth (D, black arrow).

performed to localize the source of clinically evident PLF.[22] First described by Mafee and colleagues[23] in 1984, pneumolabyrinth, or air within the otic capsule, can confirm the diagnosis of PLF on CT without the need for exploratory surgery.

Surgical repair and exploration for PLF is generally reserved for patients with persistent or progressive sensorineural hearing loss and vestibular symptoms.[22] Any bony defect in the otic capsule or injury in the location of the oval or round windows is a potential surgical target to treat

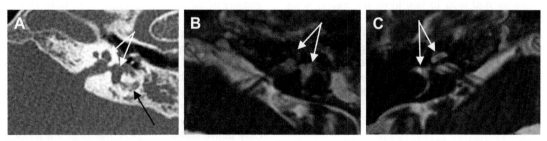

Fig. 6. Early labyrinthitis ossificans. Axial temporal bone CT demonstrates subtle labyrinthitis ossificans involving the lateral semicircular canal (A, black arrow) with no abnormality detected within the cochlea or vestibule (A, white arrows). Same-day MR image with high-resolution axial T2-weighted steady-state sequence demonstrates more significant replacement of normal T2 bright endolymphatic fluid in the IAC, cochlea, vestibule, and semicircular canals (B, arrows). Findings are therefore predominantly the earlier fibrous stage of labyrinthitis ossificans, with the bony stage seen only in the lateral semicircular canal. This patient may benefit from urgent cochlear implantation before significant ossification makes for a more challenging and potentially less successful procedure. Normal contralateral side showing expected T2-bright signal in these structures (C, arrows) is included for comparison.

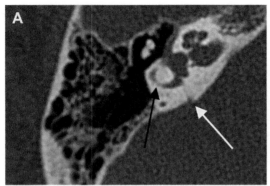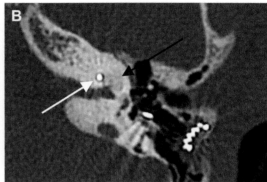

Fig. 7. Labyrinthitis ossificans. Axial temporal bone CT images in 2 different patients show labyrinthitis ossificans (LO). The first has LO in the lateral semicircular canal (*A, black arrow*). This patient presented for imaging in the subacute setting after an OCV fracture (*A, white arrow*). Like the patient in **Fig. 6**, this patient may benefit from relatively urgent cochlear implantation if there is significant SNHL. The second patient has significant LO, only some of which could be drilled out for cochlear implantation. Electrodes were placed as far as the middle turn (*B, white arrow*), with more distal cochlea completely ossified (*B, black arrow*), resulting in a suboptimal hearing result.

perilymphatic fistula, and should be localized preoperatively by CT. PLF fistula is typically repaired via a transcanal approach using a tympanotomy and a graft to close the leak. Any concurrent or alternate pathology that may present with similar findings, such as semicircular canal dehiscence, would be critical knowledge before surgical intervention, as all sources of perilymphatic fluid leak should be addressed concurrently.

One relatively rare and complicated clinical scenario in which the radiologist can add value is the setting of traumatic stapes dislocation into the vestibule as a cause of PLF, often the result of penetrating trauma.[24,25] There is no standard of care for when to perform surgery or whether to remove the dislocated stapes from the vestibule; those that advocate for early removal are concerned about scar tissue that may develop in the vestibule and lead to late inner ear injury, while those that caution against removal are concerned about the risk of sensorineural hearing loss.[24] Nonetheless, factors that can weigh in the decision to remove the stapes include the depth of extrusion into the vestibule and whether or not the stapes is fractured,[24] and should be described by the radiologist.

CEREBROSPINAL FLUID LEAK

Temporal bone trauma can result in violation of the dura, usually from direct tear by bony fracture, allowing CSF to leak extracranially. CSF leaks are seen associated with 13% to 45% of temporal bone fractures.[1,12,16,26] Disruption of the dura with temporal bone fractures has been described at the internal auditory canal (IAC), petrous apex,

posterior fossa, and along the tegmen tympani and tegmen mastoideum. CSF leak is suspected clinically when there is clear watery drainage from the ear canal though a TM defect or from the nose via the Eustachian tube when the TM is intact. On physical examination, otorhinorrhea in the posterior pharynx increases in flow with Valsalva when the TM is intact. CSF leaks are often subtle and may be positional in nature.[1] Fluid testing for the presence of ß −2 transferrin, an isoform of transferrin found only in the CSF, perilymph, and aqueous humor, or even more sensitive and specific ß-trace protein can help confirm clinically suspected leak.[12] Although patient history, patient signs and symptoms, and laboratory testing can lead to the diagnosis of CSF leak, it can be difficult to precisely locate the source of the leak clinically. Laboratory testing is sometimes limited by an inability to obtain a critical volume of fluid needed to confirm CSF leak.[13] Imaging plays an important role in CSF leak diagnosis, and can help surgeons decide on an appropriate surgical approach. HRCT of the temporal bones acquired in the axial plane should include both coronal and sagittal reformats to improve sensitivity in assessing for defects along the tegmen tympani and mastoideum.[1,27] HRCT has a sensitivity of 60% to 93% in detecting clinically active leaks.[27–29] OCV fractures are associated with a fourfold to eightfold increase in incidence of CSF leak.[9,30] OCV fractures typically result in dural injury to the IAC or posterior fossa, with CSF flowing from the posterior fossa through the otic capsule defect into the middle ear. OCS fractures are associated with CSF leaks arising from fractures through the tegmen tympani or tegmen mastoideum, with fluid accumulating in the epitympanum, mastoid antrum, and mastoid air cells.[9,12,31]

In the absence of gross fracture but continued high clinical suspicion, HRCT with intrathecal contrast (CT cisternogram) adds physiologic information and may unmask a subtle leak site by demonstrating contrast extravasation from the subarachnoid space into the middle ear or mastoids.[27] CT cisternogram may also help localize a leak when there are multiple bony defects on CT that are potential candidates for the site of leak, and it is uncertain where the dural tear resides. Radionuclide cisternography using either Tc-99m DTPA (diethylenetriaminepentaacetic acid) or indium-111 DTPA may unmask CSF leaks that are occult on traditional cross-sectional imaging studies[27]; however, anatomic detail is limited.

MR cisternography can be performed without intrathecal contrast or with intrathecal contrast. A benefit of MR imaging over CT cisternography and radionuclide cisternography is the absence of ionizing radiation. Noncontrast MR cisternography uses high-resolution T2-weighted steady-state images to morphologically depict the site of CSF leak. Contrast-enhanced MR cisternography offers similar physiologic information as CT cisternography and radionuclide cisternography because contrast can be seen exiting the subarachnoid space and into the middle ear or mastoids.[32] MR imaging may be indicated if symptoms of CSF leak persist beyond 7 to 10 days, and is the best imaging test to diagnose posttraumatic encephalocele and meningitis. MR imaging and CT are complementary, with CT best for depicting the bony defect and MR imaging distinguishing nonspecific opacification on CT as fluid, hemorrhage, or meningoencephalocele (Fig. 8).

Most CSF leaks will resolve spontaneously within 7 to 10 days,[2,11,16,26] with one large series reporting 78% resolution in this time frame.[11] Those that persist beyond 7 days are less likely to resolve without intervention and portend a higher risk of meningitis.[8,11] Initial management often includes conservative therapies of bed rest with reverse Trendelenburg positioning, avoidance of Valsalva maneuvers, and lumbar drain placement to minimize the CSF pressure gradient to below that of the tensile strength of the newly forming fibrous layer covering the dural defect.[3,12] The role of prophylactic antibiotics is controversial,[13,16] with multiple studies in the literature showing a decreased risk of meningitis in patients who receive prophylactic antibiotics, although with 2 meta-analyses showing no benefit.[12]

Aside from prolonged CSF leak (>7–10 days) and suspicion for meningitis, several factors visible on imaging can indicate the need for surgical intervention. The presence of a complex fracture on CT, including distracted fracture or rotated and angulated fracture fragments are important to describe. Fracture fragments can contribute to further dural tear as well as act like a wick guiding CSF flow extracranially if oriented perpendicular to the dura.[3] The presence of an encephalocele will also favor more urgent surgical management and may alter surgical approach.

For OCV fractures with profound SNHL and CSF leak, mastoidectomy with resection of the external auditory canal, TM, incus, and malleus is the surgical procedure of choice.[12,33] In OCS fractures, surgical management may depend on the location of the fracture and the presence of an encephalocele. Small defects that are located laterally through the tegmen mastoideum without encephalocele or those that involve the posterior fossa

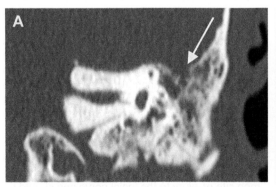
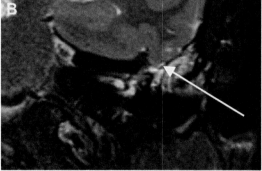

Fig. 8. Encephalocele. Coronal temporal bone CT image shows a defect in the tegmen mastoideum (A, arrow) in a patient with prior trauma. CT does not distinguish fluid within the mastoid air cells from encephalocele, but a suspicious defect such as this one should warrant further imaging with MR. MR image in the same patient demonstrates a temporal lobe encephalocele extending through a dural defect (B, arrow). Uncomplicated small tegmen mastoideum defects can be repaired through a mastoidectomy approach, but the presence of an encephalocele requires a middle cranial fossa approach.

may be repaired by a transmastoid approach. This requires a mastoidectomy followed by placement of a fascial graft or synthetic material over the dural defect.[12,34,35] For medial fractures through the tegmen tympani, petrous apex, large defects, multiple defects, or lateral fractures with an associated encephalocele, a middle cranial fossa approach to repair is necessary.[12]

FACIAL NERVE INJURY

Facial nerve injury occurs in 7% of temporal bone fractures and results in generalized hemifacial weakness.[11] Facial nerve function can be assessed in alert, cooperative patients by evaluating symmetry in the muscles of facial expression. Facial nerve paresis is graded using House-Brackmann system, ranging from normal (House-Brackmann I) to total (House-Brackmann VI) facial nerve palsy (Table 1). The time course and severity of facial nerve dysfunction provide clues to the degree of nerve injury. Complete hemifacial paralysis immediately following injury is less common and may indicate nerve transection, whereas delayed (1–16 days) onset of paralysis or partial paresis is more common and usually indicates injury to an intact nerve. One large series of temporal bone fractures found that 73% of patients with facial nerve injury had delayed onset of facial nerve dysfunction, and 27% had immediate onset of facial nerve dysfunction identified at admission.[11] Most patients with delayed onset of facial nerve dysfunction have good outcomes with conservative treatment, so it is essential to evaluate and document facial nerve function at the time of initial presentation.

Facial nerve injury in temporal bone fracture may occur secondary to nerve transection, stretching, or contusion. Contusion is the most common

cause of facial nerve injury in temporal bone fracture, and can be due to mass effect on the facial nerve from hematoma or edema exerting mass effect on the nerve within a rigid bony canal. In a study of facial nerve injuries treated surgically, 86% were due to contusion and 14% due to partial or complete transection.[36] High-impact trauma is typically implicated in cases of facial nerve injury, with most (63%) cases of facial nerve paralysis in temporal bone fractures due to motor vehicle accident, followed by industrial (7%) and sports-related (3%) injuries.[36]

The frequency and severity of facial nerve injury varies with type of temporal bone fracture. Using the traditional fracture classification scheme, 25% to 50% of transverse fractures are associated with facial nerve injury, compared with 20% to 25% of longitudinal fracture.[6,10] An autopsy study of 100 temporal bone fractures found that transverse fractures usually resulted in injury to the labyrinthine segment of the facial nerve canal and the facial nerve was frequently severed, whereas longitudinal fractures resulted in facial nerve injury in the region of the genu, usually without nerve transection.[15] Thus, facial nerve injury is more frequent and more severe in transverse compared with longitudinal fractures. OCV fracture is highly associated with facial nerve injury, with a fivefold increase in facial nerve injury compared with OCS fracture.[10] However, because OCS fractures are much more common than OCV fractures, most fracture-associated facial nerve palsies are caused by OCS fractures.[11]

High-resolution temporal bone CT is the preferred imaging modality to evaluate for injury to the facial nerve canal. One must search for fracture lines extending through the facial canal and bone fragments, ossicles, or hematoma impinging on the facial canal. Most injuries to the facial nerve occur in the region of the geniculate ganglion, with nerve injury identified intraoperatively in the geniculate ganglion in 66% of cases, second genu in 20%, and less commonly in the tympanic (8%) and mastoid (6%) segments.[36] High-resolution MR may reveal perineural hematomas, although CT is preferred in the acute setting because the course of the facial nerve is often obscured by hemorrhage and edema.[3,37]

It is essential for radiologists to report whether temporal bone fractures involve the facial canal (Fig. 9). The perigeniculate region is the most common site of injury to the facial nerve and should be carefully scrutinized.[3,15,38] A second fracture in the mastoid segment has been reported in 19% of fractures involving the perigeniculate region, so it is important to carefully examine the entire facial canal even after the detection of one site of injury

Table 1		
House-Brackmann scale		
Grade	**Description**	**Gross Function**
I	Normal	Normal
II	Mild dysfunction	Slight weakness with effort
III	Moderate dysfunction	Obvious asymmetry with movement
IV	Moderately severe dysfunction	Obvious disfiguring asymmetry
V	Severe dysfunction	Barely perceptible movement
VI	Total paralysis	None

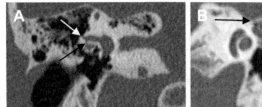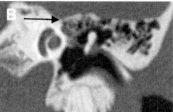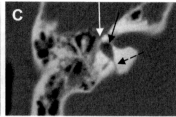

Fig. 9. Facial nerve injury. Coronal (*A, B*) and axial (*C*) temporal bone CT images in 3 different patients with facial canal fractures. Patient in (*A*) had an OCV fracture through the lateral semicircular canal (*A, white arrow*) that extended inferiorly into the facial canal injuring the tympanic segment (*A, black arrow*). Second patient has an OCV fracture extending to the genu (*B, black arrow*). Third patient has an OCV fracture (*C, dashed arrow*) extending into the vestibule where there is pneumolabyrinth (*C, black arrow*). The fracture line continues to the proximal facial canal injuring the tympanic segment (*C, white arrow*).

(Fig. 10).[38] It is also important to note whether there is disruption or displacement of the facial canal, as this may be an indication for early surgical decompression.[33] Imaging indicators of poor prognosis for facial nerve function include bony fragments disrupting the facial canal and displaced facial canal margins.[3]

It is also important to report fracture involvement of the otic capsule, as this correlates with the severity of injury, prognosis, and treatment planning. Case series have reported that 48% to 67% of OCV fractures result in facial nerve injury, whereas only 6% to 13% of patients with OCS fractures had facial nerve dysfunction.[10,11] Recovery of facial nerve function has been reported in 93% of OCV fractures and 100% of OCS fractures.[11]

Most patients with incomplete facial paralysis or delayed-onset paralysis can be managed conservatively. These patients are typically treated with

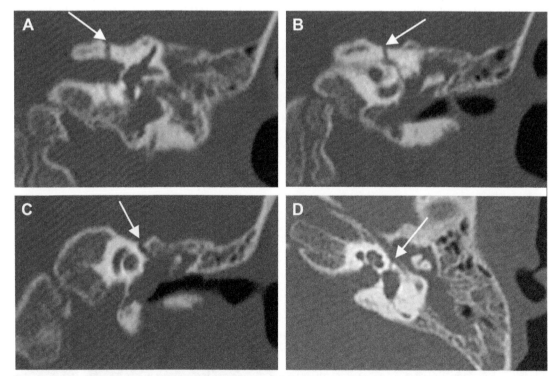

Fig. 10. Facial nerve injury, proximal and distal. Coronal (*A–C*) and axial (*D*) temporal bone CT images show an OCV injury involving the IAC (*A, arrow*), labyrinthine segment (*B, arrow*) and genu (*C, arrow*), as well as more distal injury involving the tympanic portion (*D, arrow*). Many patients with a proximal facial nerve injury have a second distal site of injury. Detecting injury proximal to the genu may change surgical management to require a middle cranial fossa approach.

observation or systemic corticosteroids.[39] Patients with delayed-onset facial paralysis or incomplete paralysis (<90% on electroneurography) have an excellent prognosis, with nearly all patients recovering facial nerve function with conservative management.[11,16] Most patients with facial nerve injury who recover spontaneously do so within the first few months after injury; Brodie and Thompson[11] reported 59% of these patients recover within 1 month, and 88% recover within 3 months.

Surgical management of facial nerve injuries is controversial, and is typically considered for patients with immediate complete facial nerve paralysis. Some investigators have advocated consideration of surgery based on severity and timing of facial nerve injury alone, whereas others have proposed a combination of electromyography and CT findings or electroneurography, showing degeneration of greater than 90% as indications for surgical intervention, regardless of timing of paralysis onset.[2,6,11,36] The goals of surgery are to explore, decompress, and repair the facial nerve. In cases of a disrupted facial nerve, rerouting the nerve, reanastomosis, or nerve grafting may be performed. Cable grafting is necessary when tension-free primary repair is not possible; it is usually performed with the greater auricular, sural, or peroneal nerves.[40] Patients who undergo surgical decompression of the facial nerve for immediate, complete facial paralysis usually have at least some return of function. A recent systemic review by Nash and colleagues[39] reported complete (House Brackman grade I) return of function in 16% of patients, partial return in 71% of patients, and persistent complete palsy (House Brackman grade VI) in 6% of patients who underwent surgery for immediate complete facial nerve paralysis.

Surgical approach depends on radiological and clinical features. For OCV fractures with unrecoverable hearing loss, translabyrinthine decompression of the nerve is preferred because it provides access to all segments of the facial nerve and does not have the morbidity associated with a middle cranial fossa approach requiring temporal lobe retraction. In patients with OCS fractures, a transmastoid, extended transmastoid (supralabyrinthine) or middle cranial fossa approach can be used for facial nerve decompression.[11,17] A transmastoid approach alone, however, allows access only to the tympanic and mastoid segments of the facial nerve.[40] The addition of the supralabyrinthine approach extends the mastoidectomy by extensively dissecting the epitympanum, removing additional bone to access the geniculate ganglion and allowing for bony decompression of the labyrinthine segment.[12,17] Some investigators advocate for labyrinthine segment decompression even in the absence of injury to this segment due to the possibility of retrograde degeneration in this narrowest portion of the facial canal.[17] One disadvantage of this approach is that it generally requires incus dislocation and ossiculoplasty.[12] When repair of the labyrinthine segment, rather than just decompression, or access to the IAC is required, a transmastoid/supralabyrinthine approach does not provide sufficient access, and a middle cranial fossa approach is necessary.[17,33,40]

VASCULAR INJURY

Vascular structures at risk for injury in temporal bone trauma include the internal carotid artery, transverse and sigmoid sinus, and internal jugular vein. Resnick and colleagues[41] found that 11% of patients with skull base fractures involving the

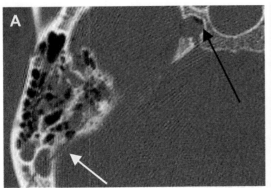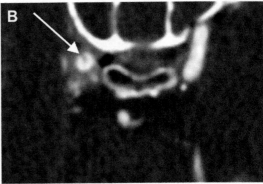

Fig. 11. Carotid canal injury. Axial temporal bone CT image shows a longitudinal fracture (A, *white arrow*) extending to the carotid canal, with resultant air within the canal (A, *black arrow*). Some advocate that this finding should prompt arterial imaging with CTA or catheter angiography. Same-day CTA showed a linear filling defect within the petrous internal carotid (B, *arrow*) consistent with traumatic dissection.

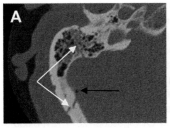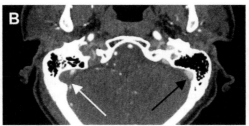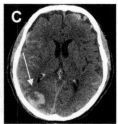

Fig. 12. Venous sinus injury. Axial temporal bone CT image shows an OCS fracture through the mastoid segment temporal bone extending to the occipitomastoid suture (*A, white arrows*). There is punctate air within the region of the proximal sigmoid sinus (*A, black arrow*) raising suspicion for venous sinus injury. This finding should prompt request for CT venogram. Axial image from same-day CTA shows an asymmetric filling defect in the right sigmoid sinus (*B, white arrow*), with normal filling of the left sigmoid sinus (*B, black arrow*), consistent with venous sinus thrombosis. Axial noncontrast head CT image shows patient went on to develop a venous hemorrhagic infarction (*C, arrow*).

carotid canal had evidence of vascular injury, and such injury is more common to occur to the petrous segment, despite higher incidence of fracture at the lacerum-cavernous junction. However, autopsy of 100 patients by Wysocki[15] found that although fractures of the carotid canal were common (50%), vessel injury was rare (only 1 patient of 100). With mixed results in the literature, some investigators advocate arterial imaging (CT angiography or catheter angiography) in all patients with fracture through the carotid canal.[42] Complications of carotid injury include transection, occlusion, dissection, pseudoaneurysm, and arteriovenous fistula (**Fig. 11**). In many of these clinical scenarios, anticoagulation, antiplatelet therapy, or aspirin may be indicated.[42] Antithrombotic therapies reduce the risk of stroke in the setting of blunt cerebrovascular injury.[43]

Fracture involvement of venous structures is common, with Wysocki[15] finding involvement of the sigmoid groove or jugular fossa in 40 of 100 autopsy subjects. These were more common in transverse-oriented fractures. This same review found that violation of the vessel wall occurred in all of these cases.[15] On temporal bone CT, it is important to review soft tissue algorithm reconstructions to assess for hyperdense venous thrombosis, venous epidural hematoma, and associated brain parenchymal hematoma (**Fig. 12**).[3] CT venogram should be performed when fractures extend to a dural venous sinus or the jugular bulb,[44] as filling defects within the sinus or jugular foramen are highly suggestive of thrombosis.[1] Rischall and colleagues[45] found that in 66 patients with fracture through the transverse-sigmoid sinus complex, more than one-third had extrinsic compression of the sinus from extra-axial hematoma, whereas a significant number (range: 8–15 patients, depending on observer) had dural venous sinus thrombosis. Petrous

temporal bone fractures are more likely than occipital fractures to result in dural venous sinus thrombosis.[44] There is concern over the use of anticoagulants in patients with head trauma, therefore first-line therapy for traumatic dural venous sinus thrombosis is aimed at lowering intracranial pressure with intravenous hyperosmolar agents, such as mannitol or hypertonic saline.[46] Second-line therapies may include systemic anticoagulation, endovascular treatment (thrombolysis, mechanical thrombectomy), or surgical decompression.[46,47]

SUMMARY

Imaging plays an important role in the evaluation of temporal bone trauma. Certain imaging findings can significantly change patient management or change surgical approach. Precise knowledge of clinical or surgical management can guide the interpretation of imaging to detect these key findings. This article reviewed the clinical and imaging findings as well as management of complications from temporal bone trauma, including hearing loss, vertigo, perilymphatic fistula, CSF leak, facial nerve injury, and vascular injury.

REFERENCES

1. Juliano AF, Ginat DT, Moonis G. Imaging review of the temporal bone: part II. Traumatic, postoperative, and noninflammatory nonneoplastic conditions. Radiology 2015;276(3):655–72.
2. Johnson F, Semaan MT, Megerian CA. Temporal bone fracture: evaluation and management in the modern era. Otolaryngol Clin North Am 2008;41(3): 597–618, x.
3. Kennedy TA, Avey GD, Gentry LR. Imaging of temporal bone trauma. Neuroimaging Clin N Am 2014; 24(3):467–86, viii.

4. Ulrich K. Verletzungen des Gehörorganes bei Schädelbasisfrakturen. Acta Otolaryngol Stockh 1926; Suppl VI:1–50.

5. Canalis R, Abemayor E, Shulman J, et al. Blunt and penetrating injuries to the ear and temporal bone. The ear: comprehensive otology. Philadelphia: Lippincott Williams & Wilkins; 2000. p. 785–800.

6. Nosan DK, Benecke JE Jr, Murr AH. Current perspective on temporal bone trauma. Otolaryngol Head Neck Surg 1997;117(1):67–71.

7. Ghorayeb BY, Yeakley JW. Temporal bone fractures: longitudinal or oblique? The case for oblique temporal bone fractures. Laryngoscope 1992;102(2): 129–34.

8. Ishman SL, Friedland DR. Temporal bone fractures: traditional classification and clinical relevance. Laryngoscope 2004;114(10):1734–41.

9. Dahiya R, Keller JD, Litofsky NS, et al. Temporal bone fractures: otic capsule sparing versus otic capsule violating clinical and radiographic considerations. J Trauma 1999;47(6):1079–83.

10. Little SC, Kesser BW. Radiographic classification of temporal bone fractures: clinical predictability using a new system. Arch Otolaryngol Head Neck Surg 2006;132(12):1300–4.

11. Brodie HA, Thompson TC. Management of complications from 820 temporal bone fractures. Am J Otol 1997;18(2):188–97.

12. Diaz RC, Cervenka B, Brodie HA. Treatment of temporal bone fractures. J Neurol Surg B Skull Base 2016;77(5):419–29.

13. Erbele ID, Sorensen MP, Rivera A. Otologic and temporal bone injuries, triage, and management. Atlas Oral Maxillofac Surg Clin North Am 2013;21(1): 117–25.

14. Meriot P, Veillon F, Garcia JF, et al. CT appearances of ossicular injuries. Radiographics 1997;17(6): 1445–54.

15. Wysocki J. Cadaveric dissections based on observations of injuries to the temporal bone structures following head trauma. Skull Base 2005;15(2): 99–106 [discussion: 106–7].

16. Cvorovic L, Jovanovic MB, Markovic M, et al. Management of complication from temporal bone fractures. Eur Arch Otorhinolaryngol 2012;269(2): 399–403.

17. Ramsey MJ. Temporal bone fractures. In: Resident manual of trauma to the face, head, and neck. Alexandria (VA): AAO-HNS Foundation; 2012. p. 140–63.

18. Young JY, Ryan ME, Young NM. Preoperative imaging of sensorineural hearing loss in pediatric candidates for cochlear implantation. Radiographics 2014;34(5):E133–49.

19. Kopelovich JC, Germiller JA, Laury AM, et al. Early prediction of postmeningitic hearing loss in children using magnetic resonance imaging. Arch Otolaryngol Head Neck Surg 2011;137(5):441–7.

20. Young NM, Tan TQ. Current techniques in management of postmeningitic deafness in children. Arch Otolaryngol Head Neck Surg 2010;136(10):993–8.

21. Gladwell M, Viozzi C. Temporal bone fractures: a review for the oral and maxillofacial surgeon. J Oral Maxillofac Surg 2008;66(3):513–22.

22. Prisman E, Ramsden JD, Blaser S, et al. Traumatic perilymphatic fistula with pneumolabyrinth: diagnosis and management. Laryngoscope 2011;121(4):856–9.

23. Mafee MF, Valvassori GE, Kumar A, et al. Pneumolabyrinth: a new radiologic sign for fracture of the stapes footplate. Am J Otol 1984;5(5):374–5.

24. Hatano A, Rikitake M, Komori M, et al. Traumatic perilymphatic fistula with the luxation of the stapes into the vestibule. Auris Nasus Larynx 2009;36(4):474–8.

25. Khoo LS, Tan TY. Traumatic perilymphatic fistula secondary to stapes luxation into the vestibule: a case report. Ear Nose Throat J 2011;90(5):E28–31.

26. Yilmazlar S, Arslan E, Kocaeli H, et al. Cerebrospinal fluid leakage complicating skull base fractures: analysis of 81 cases. Neurosurg Rev 2006;29(1):64–71.

27. Stone JA, Castillo M, Neelon B, et al. Evaluation of CSF leaks: high-resolution CT compared with contrast-enhanced CT and radionuclide cisternography. AJNR Am J Neuroradiol 1999;20(4):706–12.

28. Shetty PG, Shroff MM, Sahani DV, et al. Evaluation of high-resolution CT and MR cisternography in the diagnosis of cerebrospinal fluid fistula. AJNR Am J Neuroradiol 1998;19(4):633–9.

29. La Fata V, McLean N, Wise SK, et al. CSF leaks: correlation of high-resolution CT and multiplanar reformations with intraoperative endoscopic findings. AJNR Am J Neuroradiol 2008;29(3):536–41.

30. Rafferty MA, Mc Conn Walsh R, Walsh MA. A comparison of temporal bone fracture classification systems. Clin Otolaryngol 2006;31(4):287–91.

31. Oh JW, Kim SH, Whang K. Traumatic cerebrospinal fluid leak: diagnosis and management. Korean J Neurotrauma 2017;13(2):63–7.

32. Algin O, Turkbey B. Intrathecal gadolinium-enhanced MR cisternography: a comprehensive review. AJNR Am J Neuroradiol 2013;34(1):14–22.

33. Patel A, Groppo E. Management of temporal bone trauma. Craniomaxillofac Trauma Reconstr 2010; 3(2):105–13.

34. Sanna M, Fois P, Russo A, et al. Management of meningoencephalic herniation of the temporal bone: personal experience and literature review. The Laryngoscope 2009;119(8):1579–85.

35. Savva A, Taylor MJ, Beatty CW. Management of cerebrospinal fluid leaks involving the temporal bone: report on 92 patients. Laryngoscope 2003;113(1): 50–6.

36. Darrouzet V, Duclos JY, Liguoro D, et al. Management of facial paralysis resulting from temporal bone fractures: our experience in 115 cases. Otolaryngol Head Neck Surg 2001;125(1):77–84.

37. Jones RM, Rothman MI, Gray WC, et al. Temporal lobe injury in temporal bone fractures. Arch Otolaryngol Head Neck Surg 2000;126(2):131–5.

38. Lambert PR, Brackmann DE. Facial paralysis in longitudinal temporal bone fractures: a review of 26 cases. Laryngoscope 1984;94(8):1022–6.

39. Nash JJ, Friedland DR, Boorsma KJ, et al. Management and outcomes of facial paralysis from intratemporal blunt trauma: a systematic review. Laryngoscope 2010;120(7):1397–404.

40. Kong K. Temporal bone fracture requiring facial nerve decompression or repair. Operat Tech Otolaryngol Head Neck Surg 2017;28(4):277–84.

41. Resnick DK, Subach BR, Marion DW. The significance of carotid canal involvement in basilar cranial fracture. Neurosurgery 1997;40(6):1177–81.

42. McKinney A, Ott F, Short J, et al. Angiographic frequency of blunt cerebrovascular injury in patients with carotid canal or vertebral foramen fractures on multidetector CT. Eur J Radiol 2007;62(3):385–93.

43. Burlew CC, Biffl WL. Imaging for blunt carotid and vertebral artery injuries. Surg Clin North Am 2011; 91(1):217–31.

44. Delgado Almandoz JE, Kelly HR, Schaefer PW, et al. Prevalence of traumatic dural venous sinus thrombosis in high-risk acute blunt head trauma patients evaluated with multidetector CT venography. Radiology 2010;255(2):570–7.

45. Rischall MA, Boegel KH, Palmer CS, et al. MDCT venographic patterns of dural venous sinus compromise after acute skull fracture. AJR Am J Roentgenol 2016;207(4):1–7.

46. Ghuman MS, Salunke P, Sahoo SK, et al. Cerebral venous sinus thrombosis in closed head trauma: a call to look beyond fractures and hematomas! J Emerg Trauma Shock 2016;9:37–8.

47. Hsu PJ, Lee CW, Tang SC, et al. Pearls & Oysters: delayed traumatic intracerebral hemorrhage caused by cerebral venous sinus thrombosis. Neurology 2014;83(14):e135–7.

Temporal Bone Tumors
An Imaging Update

Philip Touska, MBBS, FRCR[a],*, Amy Fan-Yee Juliano, MD[b]

KEYWORDS

- Temporal bone tumors • Imaging • Vestibular schwannoma • Paraganglioma • Skull base

KEY POINTS

- Diagnostic imaging is invaluable in the assessment of temporal bone tumors and can reduce patient morbidity by reducing the need for invasive clinical interventions.
- Temporal bone tumors should be considered according to the site of their origin. For example, the differential diagnosis for a lesion originating in the internal auditory meatus will differ considerably from one arising in the middle ear, petrous apex, or posterior petrous ridge.
- Not all enhancing internal auditory canal lesions are vestibular schwannomas; consider nonvestibular schwannomas, meningiomas, and metastases.
- Temporal bone tumors in children should prompt the reader to consider differentials such as Langerhans cell histiocytosis, sarcomas (including rhabdomyosarcoma), and neurofibromatosis type 2 (in the setting of vestibular schwannomas).
- Masses arising in the temporomandibular joint may involve the temporal bone causing diagnostic uncertainty. Benign diseases, such as synovial chondromatosis and pigmented villonodular synovitis, have characteristic imaging features. It is important to be aware that sarcomas, such as synovial sarcomas, may also arise at this location.

INTRODUCTION

Tumors of the temporal bone are protean and typically inaccessible without surgical intervention; therefore, imaging is an indispensable part of their evaluation. The following review addresses key points in the imaging evaluation of common temporal bone tumors and highlights features of some rarer tumors to help avoid misdiagnosis. Tumors involving the temporomandibular joint (TMJ) are discussed because they may involve the temporal bone. Pediatric patients are considered separately, given the difference in diagnostic considerations compared with adults.

CEREBELLOPONTINE ANGLE, INTERNAL AUDITORY CANAL, AND FACIAL NERVE CANAL
Imaging Approach

MR imaging is the modality of choice for assessing the internal auditory canal (IAC) and cerebellopontine angle (CPA) cistern for a mass lesion. One of the most common indications for imaging is to exclude retrocochlear pathology in patients with asymmetrical sensorineural hearing loss (SNHL), although only 1% to 7.5% of these patients are ultimately diagnosed with a vestibular schwannoma (VS).[1]

Disclosures: None.
[a] Department of Radiology, Guy's and St. Thomas' Hospitals NHS Foundation Trust, Great Maze Pond, London SE1 9RT, UK; [b] Department of Radiology, Massachusetts Eye and Ear Infirmary, Harvard Medical School, 243 Charles Street, Boston, MA 02114, USA
* Corresponding author.
E-mail address: p.touska@nhs.net

Neuroimag Clin N Am 29 (2019) 145–172
https://doi.org/10.1016/j.nic.2018.09.007

The high-resolution, <1-mm, unenhanced, fluid-sensitive and heavily T2-weighted magnetic resonance (MR) sequence is a useful screening tool, with a sensitivity reaching 96% to 100% for the detection of small (≥2 mm) VS[1,2] (Fig. 1A). This sequence is also promising for monitoring known VS,[1,3–6] obviating the need for repeated contrast injections. Many 3-dimensional (3D) "cisternographic" sequences are available, using either steady-state gradient echo (GRE) or fast-recovery fast spin-echo (FRFSE) techniques. GRE-based techniques (eg, constructive interference steady state [CISS]) offer higher contrast-to-noise ratios (CNR), but are prone to susceptibility effects (eg, banding), which can cause artifacts in the IAC and labyrinth that are accentuated at higher field strengths. FRFSE-based techniques (eg, driven equilibrium [DRIVE]) are less prone to susceptibility effects, although the CNR is typically lower.[7]

Pregadolinium and postgadolinium high-resolution, 2-mm, T1-weighted sequences can be used to confirm a VS suspected on heavily T2-weighted imaging (Fig. 1B, C), or can help determine an alternate diagnosis, for example, neuritis, metastatic disease, or a neoplastic cause of facial paresis. In the case of facial nerve palsy, it is important to include sequences through the parotid gland. Fat-saturation sequences can help accentuate abnormal enhancement at the stylomastoid foramen.[8]

High-resolution, 3D, fluid-attenuated inversion recovery (FLAIR) sequences can detect abnormal signal within the labyrinth reflecting elevated protein content (see Fig. 1). A similar, but reciprocal, effect (with decreased labyrinthine fluid signal) can be seen on high-resolution T2-weighted sequences, although FLAIR demonstrates greater sensitivity.[9] Such intralabyrinthine signal changes have been seen in patients with VS and are associated with

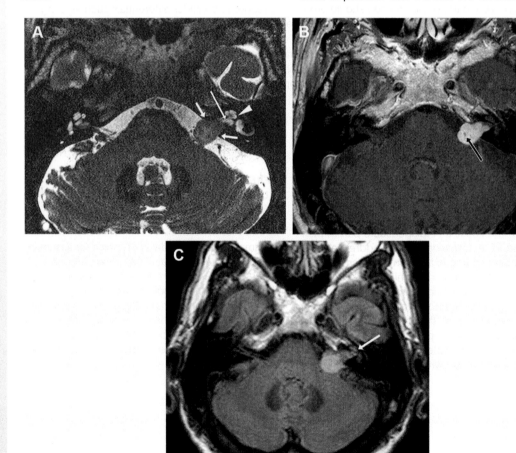

Fig. 1. VS on MR imaging. (*A*) Axial high-resolution 1-mm heavily T2-weighted MR image (3D DRIVE) demonstrates a space-occupying mass that effaces CSF in the IAC and CPA. Note expansion of the porus acusticus (*short arrows*) by the schwannoma. There is diminished fluid signal in the inner ear structures on the ipsilateral left side (*arrowhead*) compared with the normal right side. A "fundal fluid cap" is present (*long thin arrow*). (*B*) Postcontrast 2-mm T1-weighted MR image shows homogeneous enhancement of the schwannoma, except for a few tiny cystic areas within (*arrow*). (*C*) Axial FLAIR image shows abnormal increased signal in the inner ear structures on the left, presumably reflecting elevated protein content (*arrow*).

an increased preoperative severity of hearing loss and reduced hearing preservation rates following surgery for VS[10–13] (see **Fig. 1A**). Notably, similar intralabyrinthine signal changes are associated with a poor prognosis and greater severity in sudden SNHL.[9,14]

Diffusion-weighted imaging (DWI) is helpful for differentiating epidermoid cysts from other CPA lesions. A coronal non–echo planar imaging (EPI) technique is preferred due to decreased artifact from adjacent air when compared with an axial EPI technique (**Fig. 2**).[15]

There is increasing interest in the use of tractography to delineate the course of the facial nerve before surgery for VS with promising results, and this technique may become a useful adjunct to CPA/IAC imaging in the future.[16]

Computed tomography (CT) has a limited role in imaging evaluation of IAC pathology, but may be used to assess bone margins (eg, smooth expansion in VS) and osseous changes such as hyperostosis and sclerosis with a meningioma (**Fig. 3**). At times, CT is performed as an alternative in patients unable to undergo MR imaging, although its sensitivity is much lower particularly for intracanalicular VS. Dual-energy CT may be helpful for artifact reduction, and "bone removal" algorithms may aid visualization of CPA lesions.[17,18]

Common Lesions

Vestibular schwannoma

The vast majority (80%–90%) of CPA neoplasms are VS.[19] VS are typically T1-isointense, T2-hyperintense, homogeneously enhancing IAC lesions with variable CPA components (see **Fig. 1**). Cystic changes occur in up to 48% and are secondary to myxomatous material characteristic of Antoni B areas.[20,21] VS with cystic elements are associated with more rapid enlargement, greater degrees of hearing loss, unfavorable surgical outcomes and

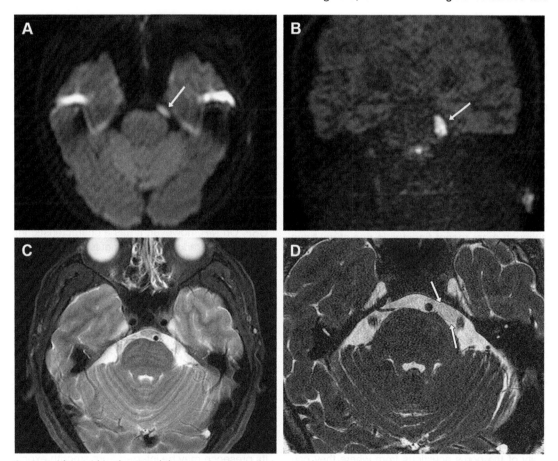

Fig. 2. Epidermoid in the CPA. (*A*) DWI using EPI technique in the axial plane. There is a focus of diffusion reduction in the left CPA that is discernible (*arrow*), although similar to artifact at bone/air-brain interface. In a subtler case, this could be missed. (*B*) DWI using non-EPI technique in the coronal plane shows unequivocal diffusion reduction in the lesion (*arrow*). (*C*) Axial T2-weighted spin-echo image; the lesion is not well appreciated and is isointense to CSF. (*D*) Axial high-resolution heavily T2-weighted image offers slightly better visibility of the lesion, which demonstrates subtle hypointensity relative to CSF (*arrows*).

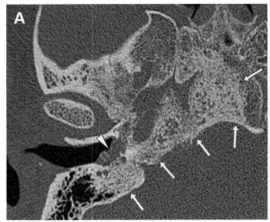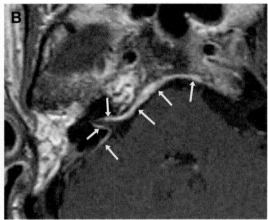

Fig. 3. Posterior fossa meningioma. (A) Axial CT image in bone algorithm shows bony sclerosis along the mastoid and petrous portions of the right temporal bone, extending to the clivus (*arrows*). The meningioma extends into the middle ear, which can be seen on this CT outlined by air (*arrowhead*). (B) Axial postcontrast T1-weighted MR image shows the "en plaque" meningioma extending along the dural surface of the posterior fossa, including into the IAC (*arrows*).

responses to stereotactic radiosurgery (SRS).[20,22,23] Some VS show minimal growth, whereas others (18%–73%) enlarge at rates of 0.5 to 4 mm per year, with faster growth observed in larger (>2 cm) lesions and those with CPA components.[4,24–26] Up to 22% demonstrate spontaneous regression[25] and there are recent studies suggesting that aspirin intake may inhibit VS growth.[27]

Imaging findings that may have prognostic relevance in VS cases include intralabyrinthine fluid signal abnormality and the presence of cerebrospinal fluid (CSF) at the fundus of the IAC ("fundal fluid cap") (see Fig. 1A). An absent fluid cap has been thought to be associated with reduced postoperative hearing preservation,[28,29] although more recent findings in one study have cast doubt on this.[30] Achieving successful hearing preservation after surgical resection may ultimately be more dependent on whether the tumor adheres to the cochlear nerve.[30]

Management of VS includes watchful waiting by serial MR surveillance imaging, surgical resection, and radiation therapy. Of note, there may be transient expansion of the lesion following SRS, which is not indicative of treatment failure unless there is progressive growth at 3 years.[31]

Meningioma

Meningiomas represent the second most common (10%–15%) CPA lesions and typically arise in the vicinity of the porus acusticus from where they can extend into the IAC.[32] Unlike VS, they only rarely cause canalicular expansion[33,34] (see Fig. 3; Fig. 4), may calcify (in ~20% of cases), can be associated with adjacent hyperostosis (see Fig. 3A), typically form an obtuse angle with the adjacent bone (see

Fig. 4), and may demonstrate transtentorial extension into the middle cranial fossa (see Fig. 4).[33,35,36] In addition, meningiomas with IAC extension are not typically associated with decreased T2 fluid signal in the labyrinth, unlike VS.[37] The presence of a "dural tail" is helpful but not pathognomonic, being present in other conditions as well such as lymphoma, chloroma, and metastasis.[38] Meningiomas involving the fundal region of the IAC may spread to infiltrate the labyrinth.[39]

Epidermoid cyst

Epidermoid cysts are the third most common CPA mass (although not a true neoplasm). On CT, an epidermoid cyst typically appears isodense to CSF. On MR, however, it has a characteristic imaging appearance that distinguishes it from an arachnoid cyst: nonenhancing, T1-hypointense, T2-hyperintense, and with reduced diffusivity on DWI (see Fig. 2).

Less Common Lesions

Facial nerve schwannoma

Facial nerve schwannoma (FNS) represents less than 1% of temporal bone tumors.[40] It appears as an enhancing, expansile mass on MR imaging (Fig. 5) but may have skipped segments, necessitating examination of the entire course of the nerve through the parotid gland.[41] On CT, an intratemporal FNS cannot be directly visualized, but if bulky, its presence may be inferred from smooth expansion of the facial nerve canal.[42]

At the IAC, FNS may be indistinguishable from VS on MR imaging; an anterosuperior location in the canal is suggestive but unreliable.[40] Symptoms of IAC FNS are often related to the

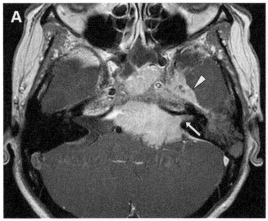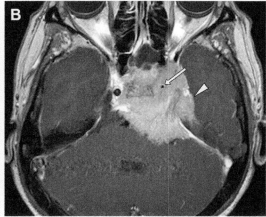

Fig. 4. CPA/IAC meningioma. Axial postcontrast T1-weighted MR images show a large bulky enhancing mass in the CPA extending into the IAC without expanding its lumen (*arrow* in *A*). There is extension over the petrous apex to the middle cranial fossa (*arrowheads* in *A, B*), and involvement of the clivus, sella, Meckel cave, and cavernous sinus, with severe narrowing of the encased left cavernous carotid (*arrow* in *B*). Note also the obtuse angles the meningioma forms with adjacent bone.

vestibulocochlear nerve (eg, hearing loss, dysequilibrium, vertigo, tinnitus) rather than the facial nerve.[43] In one large series, patients presented with asymmetrical hearing loss in 54%, facial paresis in 41%, and facial spasm in 26%.[44] Complete facial nerve paralysis is uncommon owing to the slow growing nature of the lesion.[40]

Bulbous extension of FNS to the geniculate fossa and greater superficial petrosal nerve may result in a middle cranial fossa mass.[42] FNS affecting the tympanic segment can present as a lobulated middle ear mass (see Fig. 5A), resulting in ossicular displacement or erosion leading to conductive hearing loss.[42] FNS within the mastoid segment often has irregular bone margins due to tumor "breaking through" into mastoid air cells (see Fig. 5B)[42] and may simulate an aggressive lesion.

An intraparotid FNS can be indistinguishable from a primary parotid neoplasm or abnormal node. Features such as peripherally elevated signal ("target sign") on T2-weighted imaging[45,46] and cystic change when large (see Fig. 5C) are helpful. If the mass continues through the stylomastoid foramen, a schwannoma is likely, but with the important differential diagnosis of perineural spread of tumor, usually from a primary skin or salivary gland malignancy.

Other schwannomas

A large schwannoma involving the cisternal portion of cranial nerves V, IX, X, or XI can bulge toward the CPA; when large, the structure of origin can be difficult to discern (Fig. 6).[47] Of note, the presence of multiple schwannomas is pathognomonic of neurofibromatosis type 2 (NF2) and should prompt imaging of the entire neuraxis.

Intralabyrinthine schwannoma is rare but possibly underrecognized.[48,49] It is suspected on MR imaging when there is focal loss of labyrinthine fluid signal on heavily T2-weighted images with corresponding enhancement. Intracochlear schwannoma is the most common form and may demonstrate transmodiolar extension into the IAC (Fig. 7). An intravestibular schwannoma may demonstrate transmacular extension into the IAC via the lamina/macula cribrosa. A transotic schwannoma is rarest, located in the labyrinth with extension to the IAC and middle ear.[49] Differential diagnosis includes inflammation, which demonstrates enhancement but no space-occupying mass; labyrinthitis ossificans, which shows mineralization on CT in the late stage; and intralabyrinthine lipoma or hemorrhage, which demonstrates intrinsic T1 hyperintense signal.[49]

Venous malformation ("facial nerve hemangioma")

The so-called facial nerve hemangioma is in fact a venous malformation rather than a neoplasm, arising from the perineural venous plexus. It occurs most often in the region of the geniculate ganglion due to its rich capillary plexus.[50,51] This lesion is associated with a more rapid onset of SNHL (for IAC lesions) and facial nerve paresis (for geniculate ganglion lesions) compared to VS. Earlier intervention is associated with more favorable outcomes following surgery.[52,53] In contrast to FNS, the bony margins of the lesion are typically irregular and enhancement is avid but heterogeneous. Intratumoral bone spicules may be identified on CT and MR imaging (leading to the previous term "ossifying hemangioma")[54] (Fig. 8).

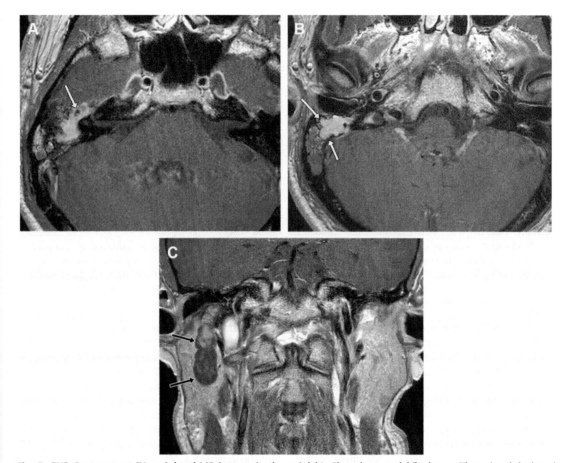

Fig. 5. FNS. Postcontrast T1-weighted MR images in the axial (*A, B*) and coronal (*C*) planes. There is a lobulated enhancing mass involving the tympanic segment of the facial nerve, protruding into the middle ear surrounding the ossicles (*arrow* in *A*). It continues into the mastoid segment, where there are irregular bone margins due to tumor expanding and filling the adjacent mastoid air cells (*arrows* in *B*). Coronal image shows continuation of the schwannoma into the parotid segment, where it has a bilobed segmented appearance and is cystic (*arrows* in *C*).

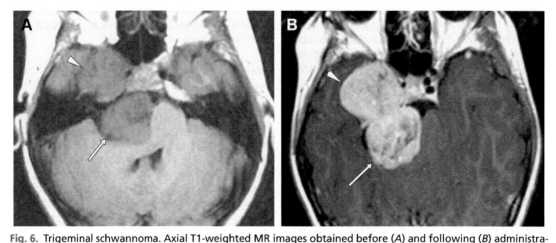

Fig. 6. Trigeminal schwannoma. Axial T1-weighted MR images obtained before (*A*) and following (*B*) administration of contrast. There is a bilobed mass, with one component adjacent to and compressing the brainstem (*arrows* in *A, B*), extending anteriorly to the region of Meckel cave and cavernous sinus, where it bulges laterally in a second lobulated component (*arrowheads* in *A, B*). There is avid enhancement with small internal cystic areas. The component around the brainstem protrudes toward the CPA (*arrow* in *A*), and viewed in isolation could be misinterpreted as a CPA mass, such as a meningioma or VS.

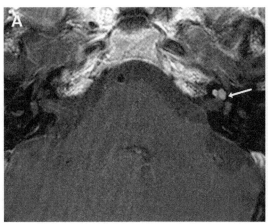
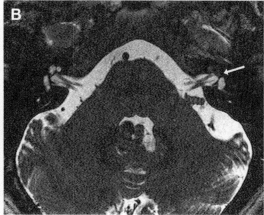

Fig. 7. Intracochlear labyrinthine schwannoma. (*A*) Axial 2-mm postcontrast T1-weighted MR image shows enhancement in the left cochlea (distal basal and middle turns shown on this image, *arrow*). (*B*) Axial 1-mm heavily T2-weighted MR image shows a space-occupying mass in the corresponding location (*arrow*).

Lipoma

Lipoma accounts for only 0.1% of CPA and IAC lesions. It has a characteristic appearance on MR imaging, following fat signal on all sequences[55,56] (Fig. 9). It may be asymptomatic or cause symptoms related to the vestibulocochlear and facial nerves. Removal is reserved only for severely symptomatic cases, because it tends to be infiltrative leading to an increased risk of neural injury during surgery.[55,57] Lipomas may occur in the inner ear vestibule, with an apparent propensity for an associated CPA lipoma.[56] Lipoma at the CPA may be differentiated from a dermoid by the absence of other ectodermal derivatives, such as calcifications.

PETROUS APEX
Imaging Approach

Petrous apex lesions are often noted as an incidental finding on imaging. When petrous apex

pathology is suspected at the outset (eg, due to cranial neuropathies localizing to the Gasserian ganglion and/or Dorello canal), MR imaging is usually the modality of choice. Sequences include high-resolution 2- to 3-mm axial and coronal T1-weighted pregadolinium and postgadolinium sequences, 2- to 3-mm axial T2-weighted fat-suppressed sequences, and a ≤1-mm axial heavily T2-weighted sequence through the skull base. Axial T2-weighted and postcontrast T1-weighted sequences through the whole brain can be included as well. Fat suppression is helpful in differentiating the boundaries of enhancing lesions from fatty marrow in the petrous apex and clivus. DWI is helpful in the diagnosis of epidermoid cysts and identification of cellular tumors; EPI-based DWI is suboptimal for small lesions and when there is substantial susceptibility artifact, a coronal non-EPI technique would be preferred. A heavily T2-weighted 3D sequence (eg, CISS or DRIVE) is

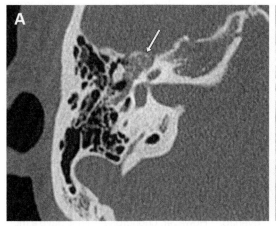
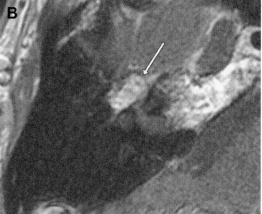

Fig. 8. Geniculate ganglion region venous malformation. (*A*) Axial CT image through the right temporal bone in bone algorithm shows an expansile mass with internal bone spicules centered at the geniculate ganglion (*arrow*). (*B*) Axial postcontrast T1-weighted MR image shows avid and slightly heterogeneous enhancement (*arrow*).

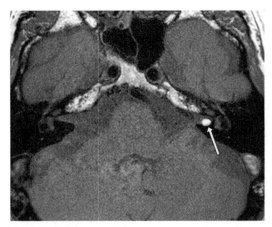

Fig. 9. IAC lipoma. Axial non-contrast-enhanced non-fat-suppressed T1-weighted MR image shows an intrinsically T1-hyperintense nodule in the left IAC (*arrow*). It follows fat signal on all sequences, compatible with a lipoma.

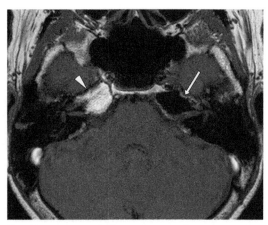

Fig. 10. Asymmetrically pneumatized petrous apices. Axial non-contrast-enhanced T1-weighted MR image shows hypointense signal in the left petrous apex representing air in pneumatized petrous apex air cells (*arrow*), and hyperintense signal in the right petrous apex representing fatty marrow in nonpneumatized bone (*arrowhead*). This asymmetry could be mistaken for a T1-hyperintense lesion on the right, such as a cholesterol granuloma.

useful when evaluation of the cisternal space and Meckel caves is required.[58] CT is helpful for assessment of lesion margins and identifying intralesional calcification (eg, in the case of chondrosarcoma).[59]

Common Lesions

Benign nonneoplastic lesions
It is more common to encounter normal variants and benign processes than true neoplasms in the petrous apex. For example, asymmetric pneumatization results in T1-hypointensity on the pneumatized side (reflecting air) and T1-hyperintensity on the nonpneumatized side (reflecting fatty marrow), which may be mistaken for a T1-hyperintense mass on the nonpneumatized side (Fig. 10). Benign cystic lesions, such as a petrous apex air cell effusion, mucocele, cholesterol granuloma, cholesteatoma, and meningocele, demonstrate characteristic imaging findings that enable straightforward diagnosis. Imaging assessment is more challenging with aggressive but nonneoplastic conditions, such as infection, in which case clinical features may be helpful (eg, a history of otitis media in petrous apicitis or a history of otitis externa, older age, and immunocompromised state in skull-base osteomyelitis).

Metastasis and local tumor involvement
Although rare, metastasis to the temporal bone is an important consideration when there is a history of malignancy (incidence of ~22% in one large autopsy series).[60] Breast, lung, prostate, and head and neck cancers are the most frequent primaries[60] and the petrous apex is the most common subsite, possibly as a result of slow blood flow through the petrous apex marrow.[61]

Imaging appearances are nonspecific, often revealing destructive, enhancing soft tissue.

The petrous apex may also be involved through direct invasion from an adjacent malignancy. For example, nasopharyngeal carcinoma can extend superiorly through foramen lacerum without traversing the pharyngobasilar fascia[62]; thus soft tissue expanding the foramen lacerum should prompt evaluation of the nasopharynx (Fig. 11). Meningiomas can abut the petrous apex causing hyperostosis and sclerosis (see Fig. 3A), simulating a sclerotic metastasis.[63]

Chondrosarcoma
Chondrosarcomas classically arise off-midline in the region of the petroclival synchondrosis, from where they can extend into the petrous apex. Hyaline components often undergo mineralization, leading to the classic "rings and arcs" pattern of calcification seen on CT.[64] On MR imaging, chondrosarcomas are characteristically T2-hyperintense with variable enhancement (Fig. 12). Of note, chondrosarcomas can occur in the setting of Ollier disease and Maffucci syndrome, which are nonhereditary chondrodysplasias characterized by enchondromatosis.[65]

Both the notochord-derived chordoma and the mesenchyme-derived chondrosarcoma may affect the petrous apex as a result of local extension, and there is some radiological and histopathological overlap.[66] However, chondrosarcomas have a more indolent course, whereas chordomas are more aggressive with higher rates of local recurrence.[67]

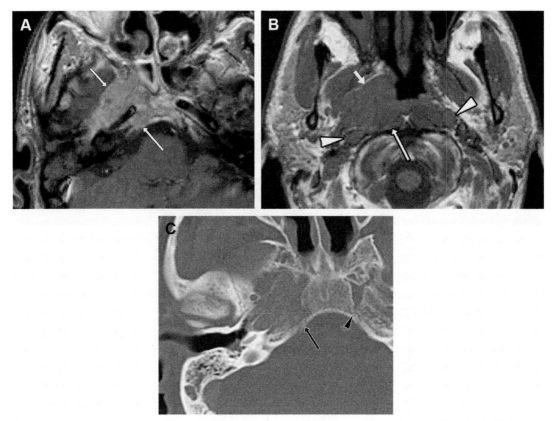

Fig. 11. Petrous apex invasion by nasopharyngeal carcinoma. (A) Axial contrast-enhanced T1-weighted MR image shows an enhancing mass invading the petrous apex (*arrows*), surrounding the petrous segment of the internal carotid artery. (B) Axial precontrast T1-weighted MR image at a slightly more caudal level reveals the lesion of origin: a bulky nasopharyngeal carcinoma (*short arrow*), which effaces the right fossa of Rosenmüller and invades the right longus colli muscle (*long arrow*). There are enlarged nodes of Rouvière bilaterally (*arrowheads*). (C) Axial CT image in bone algorithm shows lytic changes around the right foramen of lacerum (*arrow*), which is widened by tumor invading superiorly. Note the normal left foramen of lacerum (*arrowhead*).

Skull-base chordomas typically arise in the midline in the region of the spheno-occipital synchondrosis, but can affect any portion of the clivus along the course of the notochord. Involvement of the petrous apex is due to lateral extension, but these lesions can rarely arise within the petrous temporal bone, possibly secondary to embryonic notochordal branches.[67,68] Chordomas have a more heterogeneous appearance described as "honeycomb," (where mucinous or hemorrhagic components can lead to T1-shortening and nonenhancement)[68] and demonstrate lower ADC values on DWI compared with chondrosarcomas.[65,69]

Endolymphatic sac tumor
Endolymphatic sac tumors are thought to arise from the middle third (originally termed the "rugose" portion, or pars rugosa, and now called the "tubular" portion, or pars canalicularis) of the endolymphatic sac[70] and are therefore centered at the posterior (retrocanalicular and retrolabyrinthine) portion of the petrous apex.[71] Although some are sporadic, others are seen with von Hippel–Lindau disease (vHL) (11%–16% of vHL patients) where they may be bilateral (in approximately 30%).[72] Typical features on CT include retrolabyrinthine bone erosion in the region of the endolymphatic sac and duct, with intratumoral calcifications (Fig. 13A).[73] On MR imaging, foci of intrinsic T1-shortening are typical, reflecting hemorrhagic, proteinaceous, or cholesterol contents (Fig. 13B).[73]

The differential diagnosis for an erosive lesion seen on CT at the posterior face of the petrous apex also includes arachnoid granulations, metastases, and lymphoma. MR imaging is therefore very helpful for further characterization, because arachnoid granulations contain fluid isointense to adjacent cerebrospinal fluid, without enhancement. Clinical history is helpful when considering metastasis or lymphoma. Jugular foramen paragangliomas should be centered at the jugular

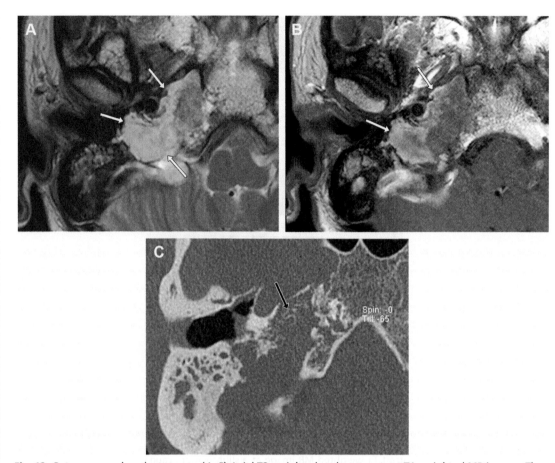

Fig. 12. Petrous apex chondrosarcoma. (*A, B*) Axial T2-weighted and postcontrast T1-weighted MR images. There is a petrous apex mass that is predominantly T2-hyperintense (*arrows* in *A*) with heterogeneous enhancement (*arrows* in *B*). (*C*) Axial CT image in bone algorithm shows lytic erosion of the petrous apex, with some internal "rings and arcs" calcifications (*arrow*). This patient has Maffucci syndrome, and the original enchondroma underwent malignant transformation to a chondrosarcoma.

foramen, and associated bony changes are typically characterized by an ill-defined, permeative, moth-eaten, "smudged" appearance rather than well-defined erosions (**Fig. 14**).[73,74]

Less Common Lesions

Rarer tumors involving the petrous apex include plasmacytoma and giant cell tumor, both of which cause lytic bone changes and appear relatively dense on CT and intermediate to hyperintense on T1-weighted MR imaging.[75–81] Xanthoma classically is of low density on CT and elevated signal on T1-weighted MR imaging, reflecting lipid content; it is more common in patients with hyperlipidemia.[82]

JUGULAR FORAMEN
Imaging Approach

CT and MR imaging are complementary modalities. On MR imaging, a heavily T2-weighted sequence can help delineate the cisternal portions

of cranial nerves X and XI, which enter pars vascularis, and the cisternal and foraminal portions of cranial nerve IX, which enters pars nervosa. MR angiography is useful for assessing the patency of the internal jugular vein[83] due to extrinsic mass effect or luminal invasion by tumor and can be performed without or with the use of intravenous contrast. High-resolution thin-slice CT is capable of detecting subtle erosions of the margins of the foramen that may be a clue to a mass. Conventional angiography is sometimes used preembolization for paragangliomas.[84]

Common Lesions

Paraganglioma
Paraganglioma is the second most common tumor of the temporal bone after VS, and the most common tumor at the jugular foramen.[74,84] Paragangliomas arise from neural crest-derived paraganglia, found along nerves in the autonomic

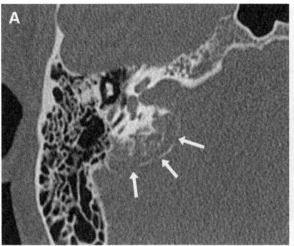
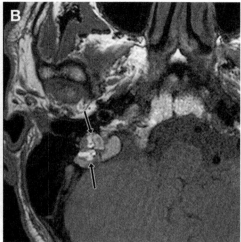

Fig. 13. Endolymphatic sac tumor. (A) Axial CT image in bone algorithm shows bone erosion in the retrolabyrinthine portion of the petrous apex (arrows), in the location of the endolymphatic sac and duct (vestibular aqueduct). (B) Axial non-contrast-enhanced T1-weighted MR image demonstrates foci of intrinsic T1-hyperintense signal (arrows), typical of endolymphatic sac tumors.

nervous system and cranial nerves. Those that occur in the region of the jugular foramen are referred to as glomus jugulare, or glomus jugulotympanicum if there is extension into the middle ear (see Fig. 14). The paraganglia that give rise to glomus jugulare and jugulotympanicum are located in the adventitia of the jugular bulb, in relation to the vagus nerve, tympanic branch of cranial nerve IX, and auricular branch of cranial nerve X.[85]

Forty percent of paragangliomas are associated with germline mutations in the succinate dehydrogenase complex subunits A–D, and genetic testing upon identification of a paraganglioma is now a

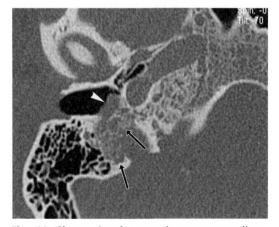

Fig. 14. Glomus jugulotympanicum paraganglioma on CT. Axial CT image in bone algorithm shows an ill-defined, permeative, "smudged" appearance to the jugular foramen margin (arrows), characteristic of bone changes related to a paraganglioma. The "tympanicum" portion of the tumor is well seen, outlined by air (arrowhead).

widespread practice.[86,87] Patients with multiple endocrine neoplasia type 2, vHL, and neurofibromatosis type 1 are also at increased risk.

Clinical presentation is dependent on the location of the lesion, with dysfunction of cranial nerves IX–XII in the case of jugular lesions and pulsatile tinnitus with conductive hearing loss in the case of tympanic lesions.[87] Only around 1% to 3% are endocrinologically functional.[88] Imaging features are dependent on lesion location. With jugular paragangliomas, CT demonstrates permeative erosion of the jugular foramen margin, most commonly at the caroticojugular spine, with variable extension superolaterally to the tympanic cavity where it may result in ossicular or facial nerve canal erosion.[74] On MR imaging, lesions are classically described to have a "salt-and-pepper" appearance: "salt"-like areas of T1 shortening reflecting hemorrhagic material or slow intravascular flow, and "pepper"-like flow voids due to the highly vascular nature of these tumors (Fig. 15A). On T2-weighted sequences, lesions are typically hyperintense with multiple flow voids (Fig. 15B).[74] Avid enhancement may be seen on MR imaging or CT. MR angiography can help delineate feeding vessels, with the ascending pharyngeal and occipital arteries most common.[89] With the genetic associations of paragangliomas, systemic imaging is often warranted to assess for additional tumors, for example, with ^{18}F-FDOPA (3,4-dihydroxy-6-[18F]-fluoro-L-phenylalanine) or ^{68}Ga-DOTA ([68Ga] tetraazacyclododecanetetraacetic acid–DPhe1-Tyr3-octreotate) PET-CT.[90] ^{18}F-FDG ([18F]-fluorodeoxyglucose) PET/CT may helpful, but is less specific and skull base lesions can be obscured by uptake from adjacent cerebral tissue.[91,92]

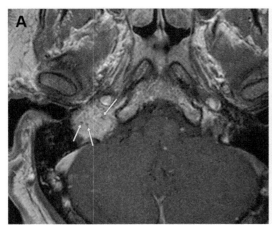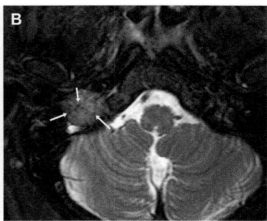

Fig. 15. Glomus jugulotympanicum paraganglioma on MR imaging. (*A*) Axial contrast-enhanced T1-weighted MR image shows an expansile enhancing mass centered at the jugular foramen with a "salt-and-pepper" appearance. The small hypointense areas (*arrows*) represent flow voids. (*B*) Axial T2-weighted MR image shows the flow voids as well (*arrows*), on a background of hyperintense signal.

Jugular foramen schwannomas

Schwannomas of the cranial nerves that traverse the jugular foramen may present with cranial neuropathy, or may only be discovered when large, with components extending into the posterior fossa or post–styloid parapharyngeal space. The majority arise from cranial nerves IX or X, possibly due to their ganglions located in the jugular foramen.[93]

On CT, schwannomas are typically of low attenuation and result in smooth expansile scalloping of the jugular foramen with a sclerotic rim.[94] On MR imaging, they appear as fusiform masses extending along the line of the cranial nerves with moderate to intense enhancement, but without the flow voids that typify paragangliomas (**Fig. 16**).[94] Cystic degeneration is more frequently seen in larger schwannomas and presents a greater surgical challenge.[95] Of note, patients with large jugular foramen schwannomas may occasionally present with asymmetric hearing loss, mimicking VS.[94]

Less Common Lesions

Meningioma

A meningioma arising primarily at the jugular foramen has a distinctive appearance. On CT, it is characterized by diffuse centrifugal infiltration of the bone surrounding the jugular foramen, including the jugular tubercle, hypoglossal canal, and clivus. Hence, the trajectory of spread of a meningioma differs from the superolateral trajectory of a paraganglioma.[96] In addition, the bony erosion appears mixed sclerotic and lytic, termed "permeative-sclerotic" (**Fig. 17**).[96] On MR imaging, an enhancing dural tail may be seen, and flow

voids are absent. These features enable differentiation of primary jugular foramen meningioma from schwannoma and paraganglioma.

Metastases

The jugular foramen can be a site of metastatic disease that can mimic a paraganglioma. Metastatic spread may occur hematogenously from distant tumors (eg, breast, lung, or prostate carcinoma), local invasion (eg, from nasopharyngeal carcinoma and chondrosarcoma),[97] or perineural spread from regional tumors (eg, lymphoma, melanoma, and squamous cell carcinoma [SCC] of the face and oral cavity).[98] Therefore, if an enhancing, erosive lesion is seen at the jugular foramen, metastasis should be considered and a search for a potential head and neck primary should be conducted in the absence of a history of known malignancy.

MIDDLE EAR AND MASTOID
Imaging Approach

High-resolution CT is the usual initial modality for assessment of the middle ear and mastoid. MR imaging is used for problem solving, to confirm lesional enhancement that is difficult to appreciate on CT, and may also be helpful if CT is unrevealing and/or no otoscopic abnormality is identifiable in the setting of pulsatile tinnitus.[99]

Common Lesions

Tympanic paraganglioma (glomus tympanicum)

The most common benign middle ear tumor is a tympanic paraganglioma (glomus tympanicum), which arises from paraganglia located along the tympanic plexus overlying the cochlear promontory

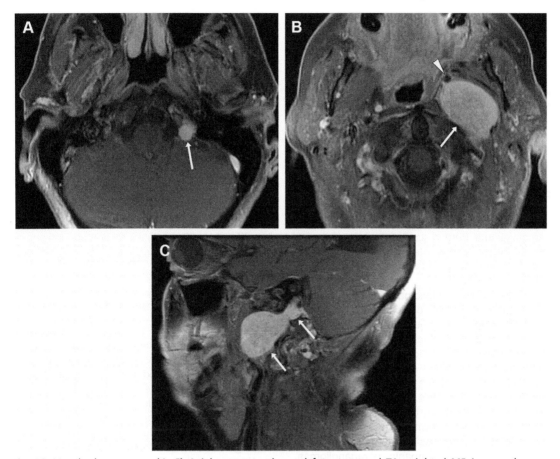

Fig. 16. Vagal schwannoma. (*A, B*) Axial contrast-enhanced fat-suppressed T1-weighted MR images show an enhancing mass in the left jugular foramen (*arrow* in *A*) that continues caudally exiting the skull base to the post-styloid parapharyngeal space (*arrow* in *B*). The internal carotid artery is displaced medially (*arrowhead* in *B*), because the vagus nerve resides lateral to it. (*C*) Sagittal contrast-enhanced T1-weighted MR image shows the mass following the course of the vagus nerve (*arrows*). Note the uniform homogeneous enhancement without flow voids.

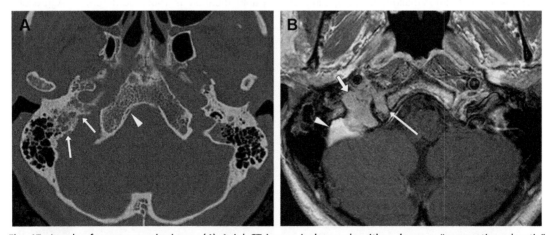

Fig. 17. Jugular foramen meningioma. (*A*) Axial CT image in bone algorithm shows a "permeative-sclerotic" appearance to the right skull base, including the right aspect of the clivus (*arrowhead*) and the bone around the right jugular foramen (*arrows*). (*B*) Axial contrast-enhanced T1-weighted image shows the enhancing tumor in the jugular foramen (*short arrow*), with intraluminal involvement of the internal jugular vein (*arrowhead*); the vein demonstrates higher signal intensity than the meningioma due to slow flow. There is also tumor through the hypoglossal canal (*long thin arrow*). Note the absence of flow voids within the tumor.

(Fig. 18).[100] The genetic aspects and clinical features common to paragangliomas have been discussed previously. In addition to conductive hearing loss and pulsatile tinnitus, otoscopic examination of patients with tympanic paragangliomas reveals an erythematous retrotympanic mass that may blanche with pneumatic pressure (Brown's sign).[100]

CT is the ideal modality for imaging assessment, showing the mass in the middle ear cavity outlined by air and demarcated from adjacent bone. CT can differentiate a glomus tympanicum from a persistent stapedial artery or aberrant carotid artery. CT can also differentiate a purely tympanic paraganglioma from a jugulotympanic paraganglioma, which demonstrates involvement of the jugular foramen and lytic changes to the floor of the middle ear cavity.

A tympanic paraganglioma typically manifests as a focal mass at the cochlear promontory (see Fig. 18A), which may engulf but not erode the ossicles; mastoid and eustachian tube involvement is also possible.[74] Once identified, MR imaging may be used to confirm avid enhancement (see Fig. 18B), distinguishing it from congenital cholesteatoma or chronic otitis media. The "salt-and-pepper" appearance may be difficult to appreciate if the lesion is small.[74] Tumor extent can be classified according to the Fisch system, used for both tympanic and jugulotympanic paragangliomas, grading them from A (confined to the middle ear space) to D (intracranial extension).[92]

Squamous cell carcinoma

Although rare overall, SCC of the middle ear represents the most common malignant cell type in that location.[101] There is an association between middle ear SCC and chronic otitis media, supporting the role of squamous metaplasia and chronic inflammation in carcinogenesis. Prior radiation is another important predisposing factor.[101] Patients are typically older and present with otorrhea, at times bloody. SCC is aggressive and locally infiltrative, with the potential to extend intracranially, to the jugular or carotid vessels, eustachian tube and TMJ.[102] CT is helpful for delineating the extent of bone destruction, but soft tissue extent is better assessed by MR imaging, which also allows for differentiation between tumor tissue and effusion. Nevertheless, imaging is nonspecific, and it may be difficult to differentiate infection and inflammation from malignancy; tissue sampling is ultimately required for diagnosis.[102]

Less Common Lesions

Adenomatous tumors

Adenomatous tumors are a rare cause of a tympanic cavity mass, and there has been controversy over their classification, given variable degrees of glandular and neuroendocrine differentiation as well as whether carcinoid tumors should be included. This has led to the use of the term "neuroendocrine adenoma of the middle ear."[103] On CT, adenomatous tumors may be embedded among the ossicles without erosion (akin to tympanic paragangliomas) (Fig. 19A); on MR imaging, they are T1 hypointense to isointense, T2 hyperintense, and enhance following contrast administration (Fig. 19B and C).[104] Adenomatous tumors may occur in the mastoid, eustachian tube, facial nerve canal, and jugular foramen, but a mesotympanic location is most common.[105] Aggressive

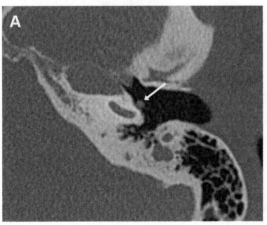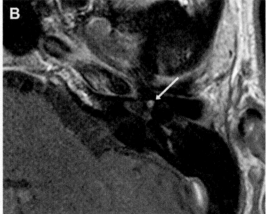

Fig. 18. Glomus tympanicum paraganglioma. (A) Axial CT image in bone algorithm demonstrates a focal round mass against the cochlear promontory (arrow). (B) Axial contrast-enhanced T1-weighted MR image shows enhancement of this mass (arrow). When the lesion is small, the classic "salt-and-pepper" MR appearance cannot be appreciated.

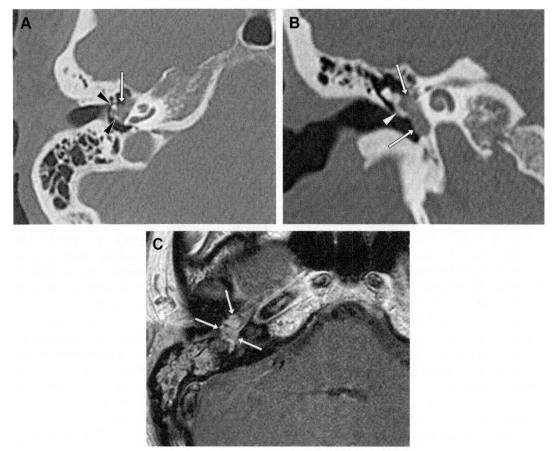

Fig. 19. Middle ear adenomatous tumor. (*A, B*) Axial and coronal CT images in bone algorithm demonstrate a soft tissue mass in the middle ear outlined by air (*arrows*). It is embedded within the ossicles (*arrowheads*) without eroding them. (*C*) Axial contrast-enhanced T1-weighted MR image shows enhancement of the tumor (*arrows*). (There is also proteinaceous fluid in the mastoid air cells on this follow-up study.) This mass was surgically resected.

varieties are similar histologically to endolymphatic sac tumors; they are locally invasive and more common in young women.[106]

Schneiderian papilloma
Schneiderian papillomas of the middle ear are extremely rare and may occur at this location as a primary lesion, possibly arising from ectopic foci of Schneiderian mucosa within middle ear mucosa.[107] Alternatively, they may occur in patients with prior sinonasal papillomas[108] as metastases. Presenting symptoms include hearing loss, otorrhea, and otalgia; facial nerve palsy is occasionally seen.[101,107] The risk of malignant transformation is at least as high as its sinonasal counterpart if not greater (up to 41%).[101,107] Postresection surveillance MR imaging is prudent to exclude recurrence.[107] There is little literature on the imaging appearance of middle ear Schneiderian papillomas, but they typically appear as enhancing, lobulated masses filling the middle ear and may involve the eustachian tube especially in the setting of a primary sinonasal Schneiderian papilloma.

Schwannoma
FNS is the most common schwannoma found in the middle ear and has been discussed previously (see **Fig. 5**). Rarely, schwannomas may arise from the chorda tympani, tympanic branch of cranial nerve IX (Jacobson nerve), and auricular branch of cranial nerve X (Arnold nerve), and present as a middle ear mass.[109,110] On imaging, they enhance and can scallop adjacent bone (eg, the cochlear promontory for lesions arising at the tympanic plexus).[109]

Choristoma
The middle ear can rarely be the site of heterotopic salivary and glial tissue, in which case it is considered a choristoma. Appearances are nonspecific on CT, manifesting as a focal opacity within the

middle ear.[111,112] Salivary gland choristomas tend to occur in the posterosuperior aspect of the tympanic cavity and may be associated with developmental anomalies of the ossicles, middle ear musculature, oval and round windows, as well as the facial nerve.[112]

Osteoma

In the temporal bone, osteomas most often occur in the external auditory canal (EAC), but can arise off of the mastoid process, cochlear promontory, or ossicles where they may result in conductive hearing loss.[101,113] Multiple osteomas are occasionally encountered.[114]

EXTERNAL AUDITORY CANAL
Imaging Approach

The choice of initial imaging modality is guided by the suspected clinical diagnosis. CT can identify bone erosion, calcifications, or expansion of the EAC margins. MR imaging is better able to assess soft tissue extent, differentiating enhancing from nonenhancing soft tissue, fluid, and CSF. Fat-suppression techniques can accentuate differences between enhancing tumor and fat planes around the EAC.[115]

Lesions

Squamous cell carcinoma

SCC is the most common primary malignant tumor of this area and typically presents with otalgia, otorrhea (which may be bloody), and soft tissue thickening within the EAC, mimicking otitis externa, albeit refractory to antimicrobial treatment.[116–118] Both chronic ear infection and prior radiation (for nasopharyngeal carcinoma in particular) are risk factors.[106]

Tumor spread is multidirectional and may exploit existing anatomic defects, such as the fissures of Santorini, petrosquamous suture, and foramen of Huschke (foramen tympanicum), resulting in extension to the TMJ and parotid gland without associated bony erosion.[115,117,119] Medial extension can lead to middle ear, otic capsule, or eustachian tube involvement. Posterior extension results in mastoid invasion. Craniocaudal extension leads to intracranial, facial nerve, and jugular foramen involvement, which are poor prognostic factors.[117,120] Nodal metastasis occurs in 10% to 20% of cases, beginning with parotid and periauricular nodes.[115,121]

On imaging, EAC SCC is heterogeneously enhancing on MR imaging; CT helps to identify bone erosion (Fig. 20).[115] Staging can be via the modified Pittsburgh staging system[118] or the recently released *American Joint Committee on*

Cancer (eighth edition) TNM system. Differential considerations include necrotizing otitis externa (although this is typified by greater inflammatory change and a higher incidence amongst older patients and diabetics) and radiation necrosis (which occurs within a previous radiation field and is usually associated with bony change that outweighs the accompanying soft tissue component). Ultimately, biopsy is almost certainly required.[115]

Osteoma

EAC osteomas are distinct from exostoses because they represent true tumors, rather than reactive osseous thickening. They are typically solitary, pedunculated, and associated with the tympanosquamous and tympanomastoid sutures,[122] readily appreciable on CT (Fig. 21). When large, EAC osteomas may obstruct normal epithelial migration, resulting in impaction of debris within the EAC medial to the lesion and predispose cholesteatoma formation.[122,123]

Other tumors

Other tumors may affect the EAC, including basal cell carcinoma (typically arising in the lateral EAC or pinna), ceruminous adenoma (benign, but may be locally destructive), ceruminous adenocarcinoma (the malignant counterpart to ceruminous adenoma), and minor salivary gland tumors, such as pleomorphic adenoma and adenoid cystic carcinoma (which has a propensity for subperiosteal and perineural spread).[124,125]

TEMPOROMANDIBULAR JOINT
Imaging Approach

Imaging techniques for tumors of the TMJ differ from those used to investigate TMJ joint mechanics, although CT and MR imaging remain the main modalities. CT can assess the osseous components of the TMJ and reveal soft tissue calcifications, whereas MR imaging is superior in evaluating tumoral soft tissue components. Axial and coronal T2-weighted MR sequences and T1-weighted precontrast and postcontrast MR sequences with a field of view encompassing the skull base and mandibular ramus are routine.

Lesions

Synovial chondromatosis

Primary synovial chondromatosis (SC) is a rare benign condition characterized by metaplastic cartilaginous nodules forming within proliferating synovium, eventually detaching to become intraarticular loose bodies. Primary SC is a distinct entity from secondary SC, which is more common and associated with degenerative arthropathy or prior trauma.[126–128] SC most commonly occurs

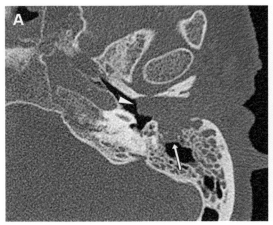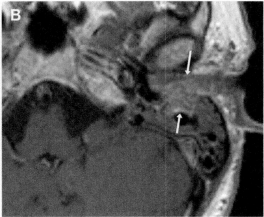

Fig. 20. EAC SCC. (*A*) Axial CT image in bone algorithm shows obliteration of the EAC lumen by a mass that continues into the mastoid region eroding the EAC posterior wall (*arrow*) and mastoid septations and protrudes medially toward the middle ear (*arrowhead*). (*B*) Axial contrast-enhanced T1-weighted MR image shows heterogeneous and intermediate enhancement of the tumor (*arrows*).

at large joints, such as the knee and hip, and only rarely occurs at the TMJ.[127,129] Malignant transformation to chondrosarcoma has been described.[128,130]

Patients with SC of the TMJ may present with pain, swelling, restricted mouth opening, joint clicking, crepitus, and joint displacement, most often in the third to fifth decades of life.[131–134]

On CT, multiple intra-articular calcifications of similar size and shape can be seen. They may become peripherally corticated or have a "target"-like appearance with central and peripheral calcifications. Occasionally, the calcified foci can coalesce to become a conglomerate mass[127] (**Fig. 22**A). The joint space may become widened, and erosive changes may affect the condyle and glenoid fossa.[132] On MR imaging, SC demonstrates variable signal characteristics.

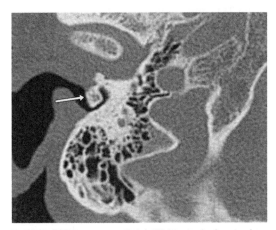

Fig. 21. EAC osteoma. Axial CT image in bone algorithm shows a solitary, pedunculated osseous growth off of the EAC margin (*arrow*).

The mineralized cartilaginous foci may appear as signal hypointensities on T1- and T2-weighted sequences (**Fig. 22**B), with central T1 signal hyperintensity if ossified. A T2 hyperintense joint effusion may be present, accompanied by thickening and enhancement of the joint capsule (see **Fig. 22**B).[127,135,136] SC can extend deep into the temporal bone, with involvement of the middle ear and carotid, and intracranially to the middle cranial fossa (5% of cases in one systematic review) (**Fig. 22**C).[131,137]

Pigmented villonodular synovitis

Pigmented villonodular synovitis (PVNS), also known as "diffuse-type giant cell tumor," is a rare, proliferative neoplastic disorder of the synovium typically seen in young to middle-aged adults,[138,139] usually affecting large joints, such as the knee, hip, and ankle; it occurs less commonly at the TMJ.[139–141] It is characterized histologically by the proliferation of epithelioid mononuclear cells interspersed with multinucleated giant cells; hemosiderin deposits and aggregates of foamy cells may also be present. PVNS at the TMJ often presents as a slowly enlarging preauricular mass with pain and trismus and can be mistaken for a parotid mass clinically.[142,143] It can be locally aggressive, infiltrating into the temporal bone and intracranially (approximately one-third of cases).[143–146] Recurrence rates following surgical resection are thought to be on the order of 9%, but data are limited. In large joints, the mean time to recurrence is 5 years.[143]

Imaging appearances are variable, depending on the extent of hemosiderin deposition and cystic components.[147,148] CT shows erosion of the joint and periarticular bone (**Fig. 23**A). Condylar

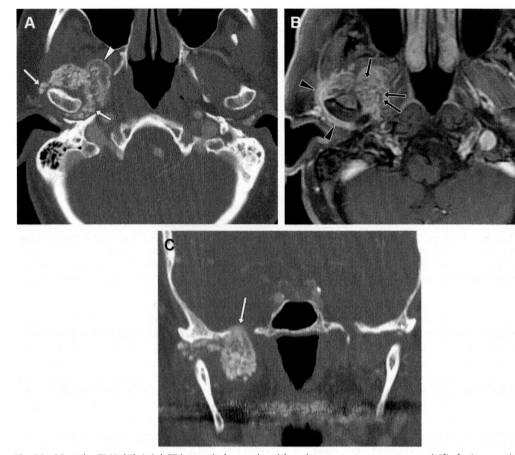

Fig. 22. SC at the TMJ. (*A*) Axial CT image in bone algorithm demonstrates numerous calcific foci around the TMJ (*arrows*), and portions that have coalesced into a conglomerate calcific mass (*arrowhead*). (*B*) Axial contrast-enhanced fat-suppressed T1-weighted MR image shows hypointense signal of the calcific foci (*arrows*), and thickening and enhancement of the joint capsule (*arrowheads*). (*C*) Coronal CT image in bone algorithm shows the lesion eroding through the floor of the middle cranial fossa (*arrow*) lateral to foramen ovale.

sclerosis and periosteal reaction may also occur. Lesions may be of higher density than surrounding soft tissue (**Fig. 23**B) and may demonstrate calcification.[2,145,148–150] On MR imaging, the presence of hemosiderin leads to variable levels of signal hypointensity on T1- and T2-weighted spin-echo sequences (**Fig. 23**C, D) and "blooming" on susceptibility-weighted sequences. This hypointensity may be diffuse, or predominantly peripheral (ringlike) or central (nodular).[147,148,150,151] T2-hyperintense cystic components may be seen within the lesion, potentially reflecting entrapped synovial fluid (see **Fig. 23**C), whereas areas of T1-hyperintensity may reflect lipid-laden macrophages.[147] Lesions may also be hypervascular, with enhancement of the soft tissue component (see **Fig. 23**).[147,151]

Malignancies

The TMJ can be a site of synovial malignancies, including synovial sarcoma and synovial

chondrosarcoma. Synovial sarcomas typically occur in adolescents or young adults, and 3% occur in the head and neck, including the region of the TMJ and infratemporal fossa, although the most common subsite in the head and neck is the hypopharynx.[152] Despite being synovial tumors, these lesions can occur in locations remote from joints, arising from mesenchymal stem cells affected by a chromosomal translocation (X;18), which leads to the formation of an oncogenic SS18-SSX fusion gene.[152,153]

Imaging appearances are variable: lesions may be well defined and homogenous (demonstrating isointense signal on T1-weighted MR sequence and high signal on T2-weighted MR sequence) or heterogenous and multiloculated, with cystic and hemorrhagic foci.[152,154–156] Enhancement may be homogenous or heterogenous. In addition, calcifications can occasionally be seen and are associated with better prognosis.[152] Metastasis may occur in up to 70% of cases, with nodal

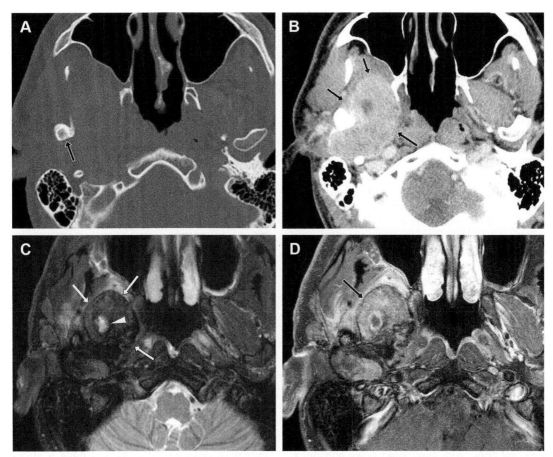

Fig. 23. PVNS at the TMJ. (*A*) Axial CT image in bone algorithm shows smooth erosion of the mandibular condyle (*arrow*). (*B*) Axial CT image in soft tissue algorithm; the mass is hyperdense to surrounding soft tissues (*arrows*). (*C*) Axial T2-weighted fat-suppressed MR image demonstrates substantial signal hypointensity of the lesion (*arrows*), except for a small cystic component (*arrowhead*). (*D*) Axial fat-suppressed postcontrast T1-weighted MR image; the mass demonstrates some enhancement on a background of hypointense components (*arrow*).

involvement being most common.[157] Lesions in the vicinity of the TMJ can occasionally involve the overlying skull base and extend intracranially.[158]

As discussed previously, synovial chondrosarcoma may occasionally complicate SC, but is extremely rare at the TMJ and can be difficult to differentiate from recurrent benign SC based on imaging alone.[127,159,160] Clinical features such as rapid growth and imaging features such as marrow invasion and suspected metastatic foci should alert the reader to potential malignant transformation.[127]

PEDIATRIC PATIENTS
Imaging Approach

In children, temporal bone pathology is more often related to benign or developmental lesions rather than malignant tumors.[161] Detailed clinical information is essential for selecting the appropriate imaging modality. Given the greater radiosensitivity of

pediatric patients, ionizing radiation should be used judiciously, and the need for and risks of general anesthesia required for MR imaging must also be considered.

Lesions

Tumors in the cerebellopontine angle cistern and internal auditory canal

As in adults, VS remains the most common extra-axial tumor at the IAC/CPA in children, but the association with NF2 is much higher (61% in one series) in the pediatric population; therefore, identification of a VS should prompt a search for additional schwannomas, meningiomas, and ependymomas.[162–165] By the same token, given the rarity of meningiomas among children especially at the CPA, identification of one should prompt a search for additional lesions, due to associations with conditions such as NF2 and Gorlin syndrome.[144]

In children, intra-axial lesions extending into the CPA and IAC can mimic a primary CPA/IAC mass, especially when large, and should be considered in the differential diagnosis, (eg, glioma, ependymoma, medulloblastoma, peripheral neuroectodermal tumor, and immature teratoma).[165,166] Indeed, determining the site of origin of a large mass can be challenging and there are reports of pedunculated glial tumors that can mimic VS.[167]

Langerhans cell histiocytosis

Langerhans cell histiocytosis (LCH) is a rare hematological disorder of uncertain pathophysiology that typically manifests in childhood.[168,169] LCH can be divided into 2 groups: single system and multisystem, with "risk organs" designated as the liver, spleen, and hematopoietic system, which confer a poorer prognosis if involved.[168] LCH can affect the skin, lymph nodes, lungs, central nervous system (including pituitary), thyroid, liver, spleen, and bone marrow, but bone lesions are most common, affecting around 75% of patients.[170]

The temporal bone is involved by LCH in 15% to 61% of cases and is the most commonly affected site in the skull base. Lesions may be bilateral and associated with multisystem disease.[171,172] Imaging features include well-defined osseous destruction usually centered at the mastoid portion of the temporal bone, with associated bulky enhancing soft tissue that is T2-hyperintense and of variable intensity on T1-weighted MR imaging (Fig. 24).[171,172] Ossicular destruction is uncommon. Clinical differential diagnoses include otitis externa, otitis media, and mastoiditis,[173,174] whereas the imaging differential includes coalescent mastoiditis, rhabdomyosarcoma, other granulomatous diseases, such as granulomatosis with polyangiitis, and metastatic disease, such as from neuroblastoma. LCH more commonly involves the mastoid than the middle ear and petrous apex,[175] so if a lesion noted on imaging relatively spares the mastoid, then LCH is probably less likely.

Rhabdomyosarcoma

Rhabdomyosarcoma is the most common pediatric soft tissue sarcoma and the most common malignancy of the temporal bone in children.[176,177] It occurs more frequently in male children, presenting usually around ages 4 to 6 years.[178] It is locally destructive and can infiltrate bone, including the facial nerve canal, resulting in facial palsy, and the tegmen to reach the intracranial compartment. When involving the middle ear and mastoid, rhabdomyosarcoma can mimic inflammatory middle ear disease clinically with otorrhea and middle ear polyposis, except with a failure to respond to therapy.[177,178] Thus, in that setting, imaging is warranted and biopsy is advised.[178] Metastasis is most frequently to the lungs and bones, with local nodal disease less frequent by comparison.[179]

On imaging, rhabdomyosarcoma manifests as osseous destruction by an enhancing mass (Fig. 25). CT assesses bone destruction, whereas MR imaging determines soft tissue extent, including regional spread, for example, along the eustachian tube, skull-base foramina, and intracranially and below the skull base. Tumor tissue can show variable MR signal characteristics and may be of intermediate signal on T1- and T2-weighted MR imaging sequences with intermediate to avid enhancement.[175,180]

Ewing sarcoma

Ewing sarcoma can rarely arise within the temporal bone, typically presenting with features of raised intracranial pressure and/or facial nerve palsy.[181] On CT, bony erosion and a periosteal reaction may be seen; MR imaging findings are nonspecific but can delineate tumor extent and relationships to vessels.[181,182]

Myeloid sarcoma

Myeloid sarcomas (synonymous with chloroma and granulocytic sarcoma) are composed of immature granulocytic cells and have a strong association with hematological disease, notably acute myeloid leukemia (AML); indeed, it is thought to represent an extramedullary manifestation of acute leukemia.[183] Myeloid sarcoma may precede AML or herald the blastic phase of myelodysplastic syndrome/chronic myeloid leukemia and may occur following allogenic bone marrow transplantation.[183–185] Myeloid sarcomas are seen in a wide age range (1 month to 89 years), and it is therefore important to consider the diagnosis in both children and adults, especially because rapid, aggressive treatment is needed to maximize survival prospects.[185–187]

Clinically, myeloid sarcoma can mimic otomastoiditis,[188] but, on imaging, its appearance is not typical of infection. On unenhanced CT, the lesion appears well defined and hyperdense (Fig. 26A). On MR imaging, it is of intermediate signal on T2-weighted sequences, and similar to that of bone marrow on precontrast T1-weighted sequences, with enhancement following contrast administration (see Fig. 26).[184] It may be difficult to differentiate myeloid sarcoma from meningioma or lymphoma, and clinical history is paramount.[184]

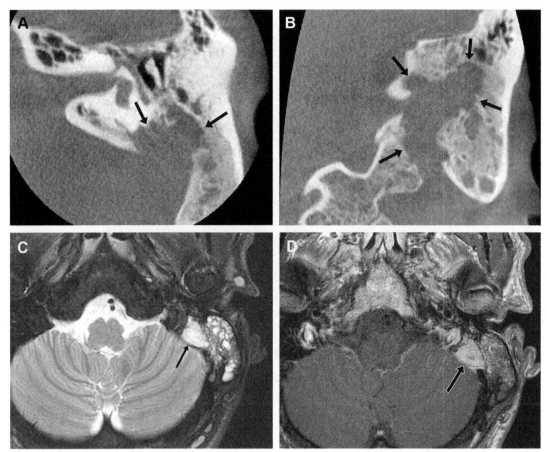

Fig. 24. LCH. (*A, B*), Axial and coronal CT images in bone algorithm show well-defined bone destruction centered at the mastoid portion of the temporal bone (*arrows*). (*C, D*) Axial T2-weighted and postcontrast T1-weighted images reveal the underlying soft tissue mass that is T2-hyperintense with avid enhancement (*arrows*).

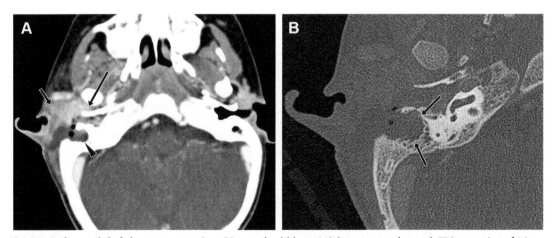

Fig. 25. Embryonal rhabdomyosarcoma in a 32-month-old boy. Axial contrast-enhanced CT images in soft tissue (*A*) and bone (*B*) algorithms. There is an avidly enhancing soft tissue mass underlying the right pinna infiltrating into the EAC (*short arrow* in *A*), invading the mastoid where there is associated bone erosion (*arrows* in *B*) and necrosis (*arrowhead* in *A*), and insinuating into the TMJ (*long arrow* in *A*).

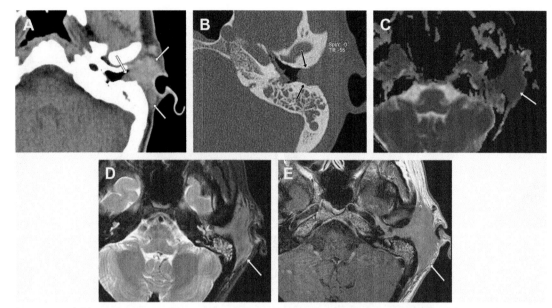

Fig. 26. Myeloid sarcoma in a patient with no known history of malignancy or lymphoproliferative disorder. (*A, B*) Axial CT images in soft tissue and bone algorithms show a dense and bulky soft tissue mass deep to the pinna infiltrating around the mastoid and into the EAC lumen (*arrows* in *A*) without aggressive bone erosion (*arrows* in *B*). (*C*) ADC map from an axial DWI MR sequence shows reduced diffusivity within this soft tissue mass (*arrow*), indicating high cellularity. (*D, E*) Axial T2-weighted and postcontrast T1-weighted images show a well-delineated mass that is intermediate in T2-signal intensity with homogeneous enhancement (*arrows*).

SUMMARY

The temporal bone may be affected by a wide variety of tumors. Although a definitive diagnosis by imaging alone is not always possible, it can help to narrow the differential diagnosis, differentiate malignancies from benign variants, and guide treatment planning.

REFERENCES

1. Fortnum H, O'Neill C, Taylor R, et al. The role of magnetic resonance imaging in the identification of suspected acoustic neuroma: a systematic review of clinical and cost-effectiveness and natural history. Health Technol Assess 2009;13(18). iii–iv, ix–xi.

2. Abele TA, Besachio DA, Quigley EP, et al. Diagnostic accuracy of screening MR imaging using unenhanced axial CISS and coronal T2WI for detection of small internal auditory canal lesions. AJNR Am J Neuroradiol 2014;35(12):2366–70.

3. Coelho DH, Tang Y, Suddarth B, et al. MRI surveillance of vestibular schwannomas without contrast enhancement: clinical and economic evaluation. Laryngoscope 2018;128(1):202–9.

4. Zou J, Hirvonen T. "Wait and scan" management of patients with vestibular schwannoma and the relevance of non-contrast MRI in the follow-up. J Otol 2017;12(4):174–84.

5. Buch K, Juliano A, Stankovic KM, et al. Noncontrast vestibular schwannoma surveillance imaging including an MR cisternographic sequence: is there a need for postcontrast imaging? J Neurosurg 2018. [Epub ahead of print].

6. Sharma A, Viets R, Parsons MS, et al. A two-tiered approach to MRI for hearing loss: incremental cost of a comprehensive MRI over high-resolution T2-weighted imaging. AJR Am J Roentgenol 2014; 202(1):136–44.

7. Lane JI, Ward H, Witte RJ, et al. 3-T imaging of the cochlear nerve and labyrinth in cochlear-implant candidates: 3D fast recovery fast spin-echo versus 3D constructive interference in the steady state techniques. AJNR Am J Neuroradiol 2004;25(4): 618–22.

8. Hudgins PA, Baugnon KL. Head and neck: skull base imaging. Neurosurgery 2018;82(3):255–67.

9. Yoshida T, Sugiura M, Naganawa S, et al. Three-dimensional fluid-attenuated inversion recovery magnetic resonance imaging findings and prognosis in sudden sensorineural hearing loss. Laryngoscope 2008;118(8):1433–7.

10. Bhadelia RA, Tedesco KL, Hwang S, et al. Increased cochlear fluid-attenuated inversion recovery signal in patients with vestibular schwannoma. AJNR Am J Neuroradiol 2008; 29(4):720–3.

11. Kim DY, Lee JH, Goh MJ, et al. Clinical significance of an increased cochlear 3D fluid-attenuated

inversion recovery signal intensity on an MR imaging examination in patients with acoustic neuroma. AJNR Am J Neuroradiol 2014;35(9):1825–9.

12. Miller ME, Mafee MF, Bykowski J, et al. Hearing preservation and vestibular schwannoma. Otol Neurotol 2014;35(2):348–52.

13. Somers T, Casselman J, de Ceulaer G, et al. Prognostic value of magnetic resonance imaging findings in hearing preservation surgery for vestibular schwannoma. Otol Neurotol 2001;22(1):87–94.

14. Lee JI, Yoon RG, Lee JH, et al. Prognostic value of labyrinthine 3D-FLAIR abnormalities in idiopathic sudden sensorineural hearing loss. AJNR Am J Neuroradiol 2016;37(12):2317–22.

15. Schwartz KM, Lane JI, Bolster BD Jr, et al. The utility of diffusion-weighted imaging for cholesteatoma evaluation. AJNR Am J Neuroradiol 2011;32(3):430–6.

16. Zolal A, Juratli TA, Podlesek D, et al. Probabilistic tractography of the cranial nerves in vestibular schwannoma. World Neurosurg 2017;107: 47–53.

17. Potter CA, Sodickson AD. Dual-energy CT in emergency neuroimaging: added value and novel applications. Radiographics 2016;36(7):2186–98.

18. Prevedello LM. Advances in computed tomography evaluation of skull base diseases. Int Arch Otorhinolaryngol 2014;18(Suppl 2):S123–6.

19. Frisch CD, Eckel LJ, Lane J, et al. Intralabyrinthine schwannomas. Otolaryngol Clin North Am 2015; 48(3):423–41.

20. Charabi S, Tos M, Thomsen J, et al. Cystic vestibular schwannoma - clinical and experimental studies. Acta Otolaryngol Suppl 2000;120(S543): 11–3.

21. Frisch CD, Jacob JT, Carlson ML, et al. Stereotactic radiosurgery for cystic vestibular schwannomas. Neurosurgery 2016;80(1):1.

22. Pendl G, Ganz JC, Kitz K, et al. Acoustic neurinomas with macrocysts treated with gamma knife radiosurgery. Stereotact Funct Neurosurg 1996; 66(1):103–11.

23. Thakur JD, Khan IS, Shorter CD, et al. Do cystic vestibular schwannomas have worse surgical outcomes? Systematic analysis of the literature. Neurosurg Focus 2012;33(3):E12.

24. Lin EP, Crane BT. The management and imaging of vestibular schwannomas. AJNR Am J Neuroradiol 2017;38(11):2034–43.

25. Nikolopoulos TP, Fortnum H, O'Donoghue G, et al. Acoustic neuroma growth: a systematic review of the evidence. Otol Neurotol 2010;31(3):478–85.

26. Dunn IF, Bi WL, Mukundan S, et al. Congress of neurological surgeons systematic review and evidence-based guidelines on the role of imaging in the diagnosis and management of patients with vestibular schwannomas. Neurosurgery 2018; 82(2):E32–4.

27. Kandathil CK, Cunnane ME, McKenna MJ, et al. Correlation between aspirin intake and reduced growth of human vestibular schwannoma: volumetric analysis. Otol Neurotol 2016;37(9): 1428–34.

28. Goddard JC, Schwartz MS, Friedman RA. Fundal fluid as a predictor of hearing preservation in the middle cranial fossa approach for vestibular schwannoma. Otol Neurotol 2010;31(7):1128–34.

29. Farid N. Imaging of vestibular schwannoma and other cerebellopontine angle tumors. Operat Tech Otolaryngol Head Neck Surg 2014;25:87–95.

30. Sun DQ, Kung RW, Hansen MR, et al. Does a "fundal fluid cap" predict successful hearing preservation in vestibular schwannoma resections via the middle cranial fossa approach? Otol Neurotol 2018;39(6):772–7.

31. Delsanti C, Roche PH, Thomassin JM, et al. Morphological changes of vestibular schwannomas after radiosurgical treatment: pitfalls and diagnosis of failure. Prog Neurol Surg 2008;21:93–7.

32. Tahara A, de Santana PA Jr, Calfat Maldaun MV, et al. Petroclival meningiomas: surgical management and common complications. J Clin Neurosci 2009;16(5):655–9.

33. Bonneville F, Savatovsky J, Chiras J. Imaging of cerebellopontine angle lesions: an update. Part 1: enhancing extra-axial lesions. Eur Radiol 2007; 17(10):2472–82.

34. Roser F, Nakamura M, Dormiani M, et al. Meningiomas of the cerebellopontine angle with extension into the internal auditory canal. J Neurosurg 2005; 102(1):17–23.

35. Atlas MD, Fagan PA, Turner J. Calcification of internal auditory canal tumors. Ann Otol Rhinol Laryngol 1992;101(7):620–2.

36. Nakamura M, Roser F, Mirzai S, et al. Meningiomas of the internal auditory canal. Neurosurgery 2004; 55(1):119–27. discussion 127-8.

37. Ishikawa K, Haneda J, Okamoto K. Decreased vestibular signal intensity on 3D-FIESTA in vestibular schwannomas differentiating from meningiomas. Neuroradiology 2013;55(3):261–70.

38. Sotoudeh H, Yazdi HR. A review on dural tail sign. World J Radiol 2010;2(5):188–92.

39. Hamilton BE, Salzman KL, Patel N, et al. Imaging and clinical characteristics of temporal bone meningioma. AJNR Am J Neuroradiol 2006;27(10):2204–9.

40. Mundada P, Purohit BS, Kumar TS, et al. Imaging of facial nerve schwannomas: diagnostic pearls and potential pitfalls. Diagn Interv Radiol 2016;22(1):40–6.

41. Chiang CW, Chang YL, Lou PJ. Multicentricity of intraparotid facial nerve schwannomas. Ann Otol Rhinol Laryngol 2001;110(9):871–4.

42. Wiggins RH, Harnsberger HR, Salzman KL, et al. The many faces of facial nerve schwannoma. AJNR Am J Neuroradiol 2006;27(3):694–9.

43. Dort J, Fisch U. Facial nerve schwannomas. Skull Base Surg 1991;1:51–7.

44. Carlson ML, Deep NL, Patel NS, et al. Facial nerve schwannomas: review of 80 cases over 25 years at Mayo Clinic. Mayo Clin Proc 2016; 91(11):1563–76.

45. Shimizu K, Iwai H, Ikeda K, et al. Intraparotid facial nerve schwannoma: a report of five cases and an analysis of MR imaging results. AJNR Am J Neuroradiol 2005;26(6):1328–30.

46. Singh AK, Bathla G, Altmeyer W, et al. Imaging spectrum of facial nerve lesions. Curr Probl Diagn Radiol 2015;44(1):60–75.

47. Al-Mefty O, Ayoubi S, Gaber E. Trigeminal schwannomas: removal of dumbbell-shaped tumors through the expanded Meckel cave and outcomes of cranial nerve function. J Neurosurg 2002;96(3): 453–63.

48. Jacob A, Robinson LL Jr, Bortman JS, et al. Nerve of origin, tumor size, hearing preservation, and facial nerve outcomes in 359 vestibular schwannoma resections at a tertiary care academic center. Laryngoscope 2007;117(12):2087–92.

49. Salzman K, LChilds AM, Davidson HC, et al. Intralabyrinthine schwannomas: imaging diagnosis and classification. AJNR Am J Neuroradiol 2012;33(1): 104–9.

50. Balkany T, Fradis M, Jafek BW, et al. Hemangioma of the facial nerve: role of the geniculate capillary plexus. Skull Base Surg 1991;1(1):59–63.

51. Benoit MM, North PE, McKenna MJ, et al. Facial nerve hemangiomas: vascular tumors or malformations? Otolaryngol Head Neck Surg 2010;142(1): 108–14.

52. Dufour JJ, Michaud LA, Mohr G, et al. Intratemporal vascular malformations (angiomas): particular clinical features. J Otolaryngol 1994;23(4): 250–3.

53. Oldenburg MS, Carlson ML, Van Abel KM, et al. Management of geniculate ganglion hemangiomas. Otol Neurotol 2015;36(10):1735–40.

54. Curtin HD, Jensen JE, Barnes L Jr, et al. "Ossifying" hemangiomas of the temporal bone: evaluation with CT. Radiology 1987;164(3):831–5.

55. Brodsky JR, Smith TW, Litofsky S, et al. Lipoma of the cerebellopontine angle. Am J Otolaryngol 2006;27(4):271–4.

56. Dahlen RT, Johnson CE, Harnsberger HR, et al. CT and MR imaging characteristics of intravestibular lipoma. AJNR Am J Neuroradiol 2002;23(8): 1413–7.

57. Bigelow DC, Di Lella F, Ventura E, et al. Lipomas of the internal auditory canal and cerebellopontine angle. Laryngoscope 1998;108(10):1459–69.

58. Bathla G, Hegde AN. The trigeminal nerve: an illustrated review of its imaging anatomy and pathology. Clin Radiol 2013;68(2):203–13.

59. Razek AA, Huang BY. Lesions of the petrous apex: classification and findings at CT and MR imaging. Radiographics 2012;32(1):151–73.

60. Gloria-Cruz TI, Schachern PA, Paparella MM, et al. Metastases to temporal bones from primary nonsystemic malignant neoplasms. Arch Otolaryngol 2000;126(2):209.

61. Isaacson B, Kutz JW, Roland PS. Lesions of the petrous apex: diagnosis and management. Otolaryngol Clin North Am 2007;40:479–519.

62. Chong VFH, Fan YF, Khoo JBK. Nasopharyngeal carcinoma with intracranial spread: CT and MR characteristics. J Comput Assist Tomogr 1996; 20(4):563–9.

63. Schmalfuss IM. Petrous apex. Neuroimaging Clin N Am 2009;367–91. https://doi.org/10.1016/j.nic. 2009.06.009.

64. Brown E, Hug EB, Weber JL. Chondrosarcoma of the skull base. Neuroimaging Clin N Am 1994; 4(3):529–41.

65. Noël G, Feuvret L, Calugaru V, et al. Chondrosarcomas of the base of the skull in Ollier's disease or Maffucci's syndrome three case reports and review of the literature. Acta Oncol 2004;43(8): 705–10.

66. Pamir MN, Özduman K. Analysis of radiological features relative to histopathology in 42 skull-base chordomas and chondrosarcomas. Eur J Radiol 2006;58(3):461–70.

67. Almefty K, Pravdenkova S, Colli BO, et al. Chordoma and chondrosarcoma: similar, but quite different, skull base tumors. Cancer 2007;110(11): 2467–77.

68. Erdem E, Angtuaco EC, Van Hemert R, et al. Comprehensive review of intracranial chordoma. Radiographics 2003;23(4):995–1009.

69. Yeom KW, Lober RM, Mobley BC, et al. Diffusion-weighted MRI: distinction of skull base chordoma from chondrosarcoma. AJNR Am J Neuroradiol 2013;34(5):1056–61.

70. Lo WW, Daniels DL, Chakeres DW, et al. The endolymphatic duct and sac. AJNR Am J Neuroradiol 1997;18:881–7.

71. Lo WW, Applegate LJ, Carberry JN, et al. Endolymphatic sac tumors: radiologic appearance. Radiology 1993;189(1):199–204.

72. Lonser RR, Kim HJ, Butman JA, et al. Tumors of the endolymphatic sac in von Hippel–Lindau disease. N Engl J Med 2004;350(24):2481–6.

73. Patel NP, Wiggins RH, Shelton C. The radiologic diagnosis of endolymphatic sac tumors. Laryngoscope 2006;116(1):40–6.

74. Rao AB, Koeller KK, Adair CF. From the archives of the AFIP. Paragangliomas of the head and neck: radiologic-pathologic correlation. Armed Forces Institute of Pathology. Radiographics 1999;19(6): 1605–32.

75. Cerase A, Tarantino A, Gozzetti A, et al. Intracranial involvement in plasmacytomas and multiple myeloma: a pictorial essay. Neuroradiology 2008; 50(8):665–74.

76. Connor SEJ. The skull base in the evaluation of sinonasal disease. Neuroimaging Clin N Am 2015; 25(4):619–51.

77. Freeman JL, Oushy S, Schowinsky J, et al. Invasive giant cell tumor of the lateral skull base: a systematic review, meta-analysis, and case illustration. World Neurosurg 2016;96:47–57.

78. Nofsinger YC, Mirza N, Rowan PT, et al. Head and neck manifestations of plasma cell neoplasms. Laryngoscope 1997;107(6):741–6.

79. Saleh EA, Taibah AK, Naguib M, et al. Giant cell tumor of the lateral skull base: a case report. Otolaryngol Head Neck Surg 1994;111(3P1): 314–8.

80. Tang J-Y, Wang CK, Su YC, et al. MRI appearance of giant cell tumor of the lateral skull base: a case report. Clin Imaging 2003;27(1):27–30.

81. Holland J, Trenkner DA, Wasserman TH, et al. Plasmacytoma. Treatment results and conversion to myeloma. Cancer 1992;69(6):1513–7.

82. Bonhomme GR, Loevner LA, Yen DM, et al. Extensive intracranial xanthoma associated with type II hyperlipidemia. AJNR Am J Neuroradiol 2000; 21(2):353–5.

83. van den Berg R, Verbist BM, Mertens BJ, et al. Head and neck paragangliomas: improved tumor detection using contrast-enhanced 3D time-of-flight MR angiography as compared with fat-suppressed MR imaging techniques. AJNR Am J Neuroradiol 2004;25(5):863–70.

84. Ong CK, Fook-Hin Chong V. Imaging of jugular foramen. Neuroimaging Clin N Am 2009;469–82. https://doi.org/10.1016/j.nic.2009.06.007.

85. Seth R, Ahmed M, Hoschar AP, et al. Cervical sympathetic chain paraganglioma: a report of 2 cases and a literature review. Ear Nose Throat J 2014; 93(3):E22–7.

86. Fishbein L. Pheochromocytoma and paraganglioma: genetics, diagnosis, and treatment. Hematol Oncol Clin North Am 2016;30(1):135–50.

87. Smith JD, Harvey RN, Darr OA, et al. Head and neck paragangliomas: a two-decade institutional experience and algorithm for management. Laryngoscope Investig Otolaryngol 2017;2(6):380–9.

88. Hornbeek H, Iyer NG, Carlson DL, et al. Functional vagal paraganglioma: a case report illustrating diagnosis and management. Skull Base 2010; 20(6):491–6.

89. van den Berg R, Wasser MN, van Gils AP, et al. Vascularization of head and neck paragangliomas: comparison of three MR angiographic techniques with digital subtraction angiography. AJNR Am J Neuroradiol 2000;21(1):162–70.

90. Castinetti F, Kroiss A, Kumar R, et al. Imaging and imaging-based treatment of pheochromocytoma and paraganglioma. Endocr Relat Cancer 2015; 22. T135–R145.

91. Chang CA, Pattison DA, Tothill RW, et al. (68)Ga-DOTATATE and (18)F-FDG PET/CT in paraganglioma and pheochromocytoma: utility, patterns and heterogeneity. Cancer Imaging 2016;16(1):22.

92. Gjuric M, Gleeson M. Consensus statement and guidelines on the management of paragangliomas of the head and neck. Skull Base 2009;19(1): 109–16.

93. Song MH, Lee HY, Jeon JS, et al. Jugular foramen schwannoma: analysis on its origin and location. Otol Neurotol 2008;387–91. https://doi.org/10.1097/MAO.0b013e318164cb83.

94. Eldevik OP, Gabrielsen TO, Jacobsen EA. Imaging findings in schwannomas of the jugular foramen. AJNR Am J Neuroradiol 2000;21(6):1139–44.

95. Brasilino de Carvalho M. Quantitative analysis of the extent of extracapsular invasion and its prognostic significance: a prospective study of 170 cases of carcinoma of the larynx and hypopharynx. Head Neck 1998;20(1):16–21.

96. Macdonald AJ, Salzman KL, Harnsberger HR, et al. Primary jugular foramen meningioma: imaging appearance and differentiating features. AJR Am J Roentgenol 2004;182(2):373–7.

97. Chong VFH, Fan YF. Jugular foramen involvement in nasopharyngeal carcinoma. J Laryngol Otol 1996;110(10):987–90. https://doi.org/10.1017/S0022215100135534.

98. Vogl TJ, Bisdas S. Differential diagnosis of jugular foramen lesions. Skull Base 2009;19(1):3–16.

99. Madani G, Connor SEJ. Imaging in pulsatile tinnitus. Clin Radiol 2009;319–28. https://doi.org/10.1016/j.crad.2008.08.014.

100. Sweeney AD, Carlson ML, Wanna GB, et al. Glomus tympanicum tumors. Otolaryngol Clin North Am 2015;293–304. https://doi.org/10.1016/j.otc.2014.12.004.

101. Wackym PA, Friedman I. Unusual tumors of the middle ear and mastoid. In: Jackler RK, Driscoll CLW, editors. Tumors of the ear and temporal bone. Philadelphia: Lippincott Williams & Wilkins; 2000. p. 128–43.

102. Friedman DP, Rao VM. MR and CT of squamous cell carcinoma of the middle ear and mastoid complex. AJNR Am J Neuroradiol 1991;12(5):872–4.

103. Cardoso FA, Monteiro EMR, Lopes LB, et al. Adenomatous tumors of the middle ear: a literature review. Int Arch Otorhinolaryngol 2017;21(3): 308–12.

104. Zan E, Yousem DM, Aygun N. Asymmetric mineralization of the arytenoid cartilages in patients without laryngeal cancer. AJNR Am J Neuroradiol 2011;32(6):1113–8.

105. Saliba I, Evrard A-S. Middle ear glandular neoplasms: adenoma, carcinoma or adenoma with neuroendocrine differentiation: a case series. Cases J 2009;2:6508.

106. Thompson LDR. Update from the 4th edition of the world health organization classification of head and neck tumours: tumours of the ear. Head Neck Pathol 2017;11(1):78–87.

107. Schaefer N, Chong J, Griffin A, et al. Schneiderian-type papilloma of the middle ear: a review of the literature. Int Surg 2015;100(6):989–93.

108. Shen J, Baik F, Mafee MF, et al. Inverting papilloma of the temporal bone: case report and meta-analysis of risk factors. Otol Neurotol 2011;32(7):1124–33.

109. Aydin K, Maya MM, Lo WW, et al. Jacobson's nerve schwannoma presenting as middle ear mass. AJNR Am J Neuroradiol 2000;21(7):1331–3.

110. Browning ST, Phillipps JJ, Williams N. Schwannoma of the chorda tympani nerve. J Laryngol Otol 2000;114(1):81–2.

111. Martinez-Peñuela A, Quer S, Beloqui R, et al. Glial choristoma of the middle ear: report of 2 cases. Otol Neurotol 2011;32(3):e26–7.

112. Vasama JP, Ramsay H, Markkola A. Choristoma of the middle ear. Otol Neurotol 2001;22(3):421–2.

113. Toro PC, Castillo AC, Moya Martínez R, et al. Middle ear promontory osteoma. Am J Otolaryngol 2014;35(5):626–7.

114. Kim CW, Oh SJ, Kang JM, et al. Multiple osteomas in the middle ear. Eur Arch Otorhinolaryngol 2006; 263(12):1151–4.

115. Ong CK, Pua U, Chong VFH. Imaging of carcinoma of the external auditory canal: a pictorial essay. Cancer Imaging 2008;8(1):191–8.

116. Chin RY, Nguyen TBV. Synchronous malignant otitis externa and squamous cell carcinoma of the external auditory canal. Case Rep Otolaryngol 2013;837169. https://doi.org/10.1155/2013/837169.

117. Moffat D, Chiossone-Kerdel J, Da Cruz M. Squamous cell carcinoma. In: Jackler RK, Driscoll CLW, editors. Tumors of the ear and temporal bone. Philadelphia: Lippincott Williams & Wilkins; 2000. p. 67–77.

118. Moody SA, Hirsch BE, Myers EN. Squamous cell carcinoma of the external auditory canal: an evaluation of a staging system. Am J Otol 2000;21(4):582–8.

119. Gillespie MB, Francis HW, Chee N, et al. Squamous cell carcinoma of the temporal bone: a radiographic-pathologic correlation. Arch Otolaryngol Head Neck Surg 2001;127(7):803–7.

120. Higgins TS, Moody Antonio SA. The role of facial palsy in staging squamous cell carcinoma of the temporal bone and external auditory canal. Otol Neurotol 2010;31(9):1.

121. Lobo D, Llorente JL, Suárez C. Squamous cell carcinoma of the external auditory canal. Skull Base 2008;18(3):167–72.

122. Hester T, Silverstein H. Osteoma and exostoses. In: Jackler RK, Driscoll CLW, editors. Tumors of the ear and temporal bone. Philadelphia: Lippincott Williams & Wilkins; 2000. p. 103–10.

123. Carbone PN, Nelson BL. External auditory osteoma. Head Neck Pathol 2012;6(2):244–6.

124. Chang J, Cheung S. Auditory canal: glandular tumors. In: Jackler RK, Driscoll CLW, editors. Tumors of the ear and temporal bone. Philadelphia: Lippincott Williams & Wilkins; 2000. p. 84–101.

125. Vandeweyer E, Thill MP, Deraemaecker R. Basal cell carcinoma of the external auditory canal. Acta Chir Belg 2002;102(2):137–40.

126. Maclean F, Bonar S, Bullough P. Joints: primary synovial chondromatosis. In: Mills SE, Greenson JK, Hornick JL, et al, editors. Sternberg's diagnostic surgical pathology. 6th edition. Philadelphia: Lippincott Williams & Wilkins; 2015. p. 248.

127. Murphey MD, Vidal JA, Fanburg-Smith JC, et al. Imaging of synovial chondromatosis with radiologic-pathologic correlation. Radiographics 2007;27(5):1465–88.

128. Neumann JA, Garrigues GE, Brigman BE, et al. Synovial chondromatosis. JBJS Rev 2016;4(5):1.

129. Wu C-W, Chen YK, Lin LM, et al. Primary synovial chondromatosis of the temporomandibular joint. J Otolaryngol 2004;33(2):114–9.

130. Evans S, Boffano M, Chaudhry S, et al. Synovial chondrosarcoma arising in synovial chondromatosis. Sarcoma 2014;2014:647939.

131. Guarda-Nardini L, Piccotti F, Ferronato G, et al. Synovial chondromatosis of the temporomandibular joint: a case description with systematic literature review. Int J Oral Maxillofac Surg 2010;39(8):745–55.

132. Liu X, Huang Z, Zhu W, et al. Clinical and imaging findings of temporomandibular joint synovial chondromatosis: an analysis of 10 cases and literature review. J Oral Maxillofac Surg 2016;74(11):2159–68.

133. Pinto AAC, Ferreira e Costa R, de Sousa SF, et al. Synovial chondromatosis of the temporomandibular joint successfully treated by surgery. Head Neck Pathol 2015;9(4):525–9.

134. Narváez JA, Narváez J, Ortega R, et al. Hypointense synovial lesions on T2-weighted images: differential diagnosis with pathologic correlation. AJR Am J Roentgenol 2003;181(3):761–9.

135. Kramer J, Recht M, Deely DM, et al. Mr appearance of idiopathic synovial osteochondromatosis. J Comput Assist Tomogr 1993;17(5):772–6.

136. Peyrot H, Montoriol PF, Beziat JL, et al. Synovial chondromatosis of the temporomandibular joint:

CT and MRI findings. Diagn Interv Imaging 2014; 95(6):613–4.

137. McCaffery C, Dodd M, Bekiroglu F, et al. Synovial chondromatosis of the temporomandibular joint with extension into the middle cranial fossa and internal carotid canal. Int J Oral Maxillofac Surg 2017;46(7):867–70.

138. van der Heijden L, Gibbons CL, Dijkstra PD, et al. The management of diffuse-type giant cell tumour (pigmented villonodular synovitis) and giant cell tumour of tendon sheath (nodular tenosynovitis). J Bone Joint Surg Br 2012;94–B(7):882–8.

139. Stephan SR, Shallop B, Lackman R, et al. Pigmented villonodular synovitis: a comprehensive review and proposed treatment algorithm. JBJS Rev 2016;1. https://doi.org/10.2106/JBJS.RVW.15.00086.

140. Mendenhall WM, Mendenhall CM, Reith JD, et al. Pigmented villonodular synovitis. Am J Clin Oncol 2006;29:548–50.

141. Palmerini E, Staals EL, Maki RG, et al. Tenosynovial giant cell tumour/pigmented villonodular synovitis: outcome of 294 patients before the era of kinase inhibitors. Eur J Cancer 2015;51(2):210–7.

142. Ren R, Mueller S, Kraft AO, et al. Giant cell tumor of temporomandibular joint presenting as a parotid tumor: challenges in the accurate subclassification of giant cell tumors in an unusual location. Diagn Cytopathol 2018;46(4):340–4.

143. Safaee M, Oh T, Sun MZ, et al. Pigmented villonodular synovitis of the temporomandibular joint with intracranial extension: a case series and systematic review. Head Neck 2015;37(8):1213–24.

144. Gump WC. Meningiomas of the pediatric skull base: a review. J Neurol Surg B Skull Base 2015; 76(1):66–73.

145. Pianosi K, Rigby M, Hart R, et al. Pigmented villonodular synovitis of the temporomandibular joint: a unique presentation. Plast Reconstr Surg Glob Open 2016;4(4):e674.

146. Vaca M, Polo R, Martínez-San-Millán J, et al. Pigmented villonodular synovitis of the temporomandibular joint with petrous bone invasion. Otol Neurotol 2017;e58–9. https://doi.org/10.1097/MAO.0000000000001390.

147. Bemporad JA, Chaloupka JC, Putman CM, et al. Pigmented villonodular synovitis of the temporomandibular joint: diagnostic imaging and endovascular therapeutic embolization of a rare head and neck tumor. AJNR Am J Neuroradiol 1999;20(1):159–62.

148. Kim I-K, Cho HY, Cho HW, et al. Pigmented villonodular synovitis of the temporomandibular joint - computed tomography and magnetic resonance findings: a case report. J Korean Assoc Oral Maxillofac Surg 2014;40(3):140–6.

149. Le W-J, Li MH, Yu Q, et al. Pigmented villonodular synovitis of the temporomandibular joint: CT imaging findings. Clin Imaging 2014;38(1):6–10.

150. Song MY, Heo MS, Lee SS, et al. Diagnostic imaging of pigmented villonodular synovitis of the temporomandibular joint associated with condylar expansion. Dentomaxillofac Radiol 1999;28(6):386–90.

151. Kim KW, Han MH, Park SW, et al. Pigmented villonodular synovitis of the temporomandibular joint: MR findings in four cases. Eur J Radiol 2004; 49(3):229–34.

152. Rangheard A-S, Vanel D, Viala J, et al. Synovial sarcomas of the head and neck: CT and MR imaging findings of eight patients. AJNR Am J Neuroradiol 2001;22(5):851–7.

153. Naka N, Takenaka S, Araki N, et al. Synovial sarcoma is a stem cell malignancy. Stem Cells 2010; 28(7):1119–31.

154. Blacksin MF, Siegel JR, Benevenia J, et al. Synovial sarcoma: frequency of nonaggressive MR characteristics. J Comput Assist Tomogr 1997;21(5):785–9.

155. Hirsch RJ, Yousem DM, Loevner LA, et al. Synovial sarcomas of the head and neck: MR findings. AJR Am J Roentgenol 1997;169(4):1185–8.

156. Valenzuela RF, Kim EE, Seo JG, et al. A revisit of MRI analysis for synovial sarcoma. Clin Imaging 2000;24(4):231–5.

157. Nomura F, Kishimoto S. Synovial sarcoma of the temporomandibular joint and infratemporal fossa. Auris Nasus Larynx 2014;41(6):572–5.

158. Ji T, Ma CY, Ow A, et al. Synovial sarcoma involving skull base – a retrospective analysis of diagnosis and treatment of 21 cases in one institution. Oral Oncol 2011;47(7):671–6.

159. Coleman MA, Matsumoto J, Carr CM, et al. Bilateral temporal bone langerhans cell histiocytosis: radiologic pearls. Open Neuroimag J 2013;7:53–7.

160. Ichikawa T, Miyauchi M, Nikai H, et al. Synovial chondrosarcoma arising in the temporomandibular joint. J Oral Maxillofac Surg 1998;56(7):890–4.

161. Chandra T, Maheshwari M, Kelly TG, et al. Imaging of pediatric skull base lesions. Neurographics 2015;5(2):72–84.

162. Cunningham CD, Friedman RA, Brackmann DE, et al. Neurotologic skull base surgery in pediatric patients. Otol Neurotol 2005;26(2):231–6.

163. Holman MA, Schmitt WR, Carlson ML, et al. Pediatric cerebellopontine angle and internal auditory canal tumors. J Neurosurg Pediatr 2013;12(4):317–24.

164. Tsai MH, Wong AM, Jaing TH, et al. Treatment of cerebellopontine angle tumors in children. J Pediatr Hematol Oncol 2009;31(11):832–4.

165. Zúccaro G, Sosa F. Cerebellopontine angle lesions in children. Childs Nerv Syst 2007;23(2):177–83.

166. Phi JH, Wang KC, Kim IO, et al. Tumors in the cerebellopontine angle in children: warning of a high probability of malignancy. J Neurooncol 2013; 112(3):383–91.

167. Bonneville F, Sarrazin JL, Marsot-Dupuch K, et al. Unusual lesions of the cerebellopontine angle: a segmental approach. Radiographics 2001;21(2): 419–38.

168. Hutter C, Minkov M. Insights into the pathogenesis of Langerhans cell histiocytosis: the development of targeted therapies. ImmunoTargets Ther 2016; 5:81–91.

169. Krooks J, Minkov M, Weatherall AG. Langerhans cell histiocytosis in children: history, classification, pathobiology, clinical manifestations, and prognosis. J Am Acad Dermatol 2018;78(6):1035–44.

170. Zinn DJ, Chakraborty R, Allen CE. Langerhans cell histiocytosis: emerging insights and clinical implications. Oncology (Williston Park) 2016; 30(2):122–32, 139.

171. D'Ambrosio N, Soohoo S, Warshall C, et al. Craniofacial and intracranial manifestations of langerhans cell histiocytosis: report of findings in 100 patients. AJR Am J Roentgenol 2008;191(2):589–97.

172. Fernández-Latorre F, Menor-Serrano F, Alonso-Charterina S, et al. Langerhans' cell histiocytosis of the temporal bone in pediatric patients. AJR Am J Roentgenol 2000;174(1):217–21.

173. Nelson BL. Langerhans cell histiocytosis of the temporal bone. Head Neck Pathol 2008;2(2):97–8.

174. Quraishi MS, Blayney AW, Breatnach F. Aural symptoms as primary presentation of Langerhan's cell histiocytosis. Clin Otolaryngol allied Sci 1993; 18(4):317–23.

175. Chevallier KM, Wiggins RH, Quinn NA, et al. Differentiating pediatric rhabdomyosarcoma and langerhans cell histiocytosis of the temporal bone by imaging appearance. AJNR Am J Neuroradiol 2016;37(6):1185–9.

176. Gluth MB. Rhabdomyosarcoma and other pediatric temporal bone malignancies. Otolaryngol Clin North Am 2015;48(2):375–90.

177. Sbeity S, Abella A, Arcand P, et al. Temporal bone rhabdomyosarcoma in children. Int J Pediatr Otorhinolaryngol 2007;71(5):807–14.

178. Durve DV, Kanegaonkar RG, Albert D, et al. Paediatric rhabdomyosarcoma of the ear and temporal bone. Clin Otolaryngol Allied Sci 2004;29(1): 32–7.

179. Kim JR, Yoon HM, Koh KN, et al. Rhabdomyosarcoma in children and adolescents: patterns and risk factors of distant metastasis. AJR Am J Roentgenol 2017;209(2):409–16.

180. Castillo M, Pillsbury HC 3rd. Rhabdomyosarcoma of the middle ear: imaging features in two children. AJNR Am J Neuroradiol 1993;14(3):730–3.

181. Kadar AA, Hearst MJ, Collins MH, et al. Ewing's sarcoma of the petrous temporal bone: case report and literature review. Skull Base 2010; 20(3):213–7.

182. Singh P, Jain M, Singh DP, et al. MR findings of primary Ewing's sarcoma of greater wing of sphenoid. Australas Radiol 2002;46(4):409–11.

183. Yilmaz AF, Saydam G, Sahin F, et al. Granulocytic sarcoma: a systematic review. Am J Blood Res 2013;3(4):265–70.

184. Lee B, Fatterpekar GM, Kim W, et al. Granulocytic sarcoma of the temporal bone. AJNR Am J Neuroradiol 2002;23(9):1497–9.

185. Pileri S, Orazi A, Falini B. Myeloid sarcoma. In: Swerdlow SH, World Health Organization, and International Agency for Research on Cancer, editors. WHO classification of tumours of haematopoietic and lymphoid tissues. Lyon (France): International Agency for Research on Cancer; 2017. p. 167.

186. Chandrasekhar S. Temporal bone tumors in children. In: Jackler RK, Driscoll CLW, editors. Tumors of the ear and temporal bone. Philadelphia: Lippincott Williams & Wilkins; 2000. p. 449.

187. Roby BB, Drehner D, Sidman JD. Granulocytic sarcoma of pediatric head and neck: an institutional experience. Int J Pediatr Otorhinolaryngol 2013; 77(8):1364–6.

188. Chang KH, Kim DK, Jun BC, et al. Temporal bone myeloid sarcoma. Clin Exp Otorhinolaryngol 2009; 2(4):198–202.

Management of Vestibular Schwannomas for the Radiologist

Apoorva T. Ramaswamy, MD, Justin S. Golub, MD, MS*

KEYWORDS

- Vestibular schwannoma • Skull base surgery • Lateral Skull Base • Radiosurgery • Hearing loss
- Cerebellopontine angle

KEY POINTS

- Vestibular schwannomas are the most common tumor of the cerebellopontine angle.
- The history of their management has driven advances in imaging, lateral skull base surgery, as well as radiosurgery.
- With these advances, a shift has occurred from life-saving treatment for late-stage disease to quality of life focused management of smaller tumors.
- The complicated treatment paradigms involving observation, stereotactic radiosurgery, and surgery require close communication between the treatment and neuroradiology teams.

BACKGROUND

Vestibular schwannomas (VSs) are benign neoplasms originating from the nerve sheath of the vestibular segment of cranial nerve VIII. The incidence of these lesions is more than 3300 per year in the United States, and they represent 90% of cerebellopontine angle tumors.[1] Although these tumors are relatively uncommon temporal bone pathologies, they have played an outsized historical influence on the development of lateral skull base surgery and neuroimaging. Today, in the era of high-resolution MR imaging and early diagnosis, death related to these lesions is exceedingly rare. However, case reports persist of mortality owing to severe hydrocephalus and brain herniation secondary to VSs.[2] Furthermore, morbidity owing to hearing loss and even facial weakness remains a stubborn reality. Although the previous management of these tumors was based on the oncologic model of complete resection and tolerance of significant subsequent morbidity, today management is driven primarily by the goals of functional preservation and symptom control. In light of this transition, there is significant variation of treatment patterns and philosophies. A knowledgeable neuroradiologist is a critical member of the multidisciplinary team required for the management of these patients. By understanding the important decisions ahead for each of these patients, a radiologist can anticipate questions affecting the appropriateness of observation, the feasibility of surgical versus stereotactic radiotherapy, and the potential for functional preservation.

HISTORY OF VESTIBULAR SCHWANNOMA IMAGING AND DIAGNOSIS

The history of diagnostics is integral to the history of VSs, and patient outcomes have improved in lockstep with improvements in imaging and audiologic testing. The first VSs, or acoustic neuromas as they were originally named, were localized solely based on symptomatology. Because they primarily presented with hearing loss, they were

Otolaryngology—Head and Neck Surgery, Vagelos College of Physicians & Surgeons, NewYork-Presbyterian/Columbia University Irving Medical Center, 180 Fort Washington Avenue, New York, NY 10032, USA
* Corresponding author.
E-mail address: justin.golub@columbia.edu

Neuroimag Clin N Am 29 (2019) 173–182
https://doi.org/10.1016/j.nic.2018.09.003
1052-5149/19/© 2018 Elsevier Inc. All rights reserved.

thought to originate in the auditory nerve, thus explaining the retrospectively incorrect moniker. Because of the difficult-to-access location, during this period from the 1890s to the early 1900s surgical mortality reached 80%. In 1910, the first images of the lateral skull base were obtained with the development of radiographs of the petrous pyramid.[3] However, it was not until 1918 when Walter Dandy developed ventriculography that surgeons could determine preoperatively the size and location of the lesion. Still, only large tumors could be visualized with this technology. It was not until the development of positive contrast cisternography around 1920 that moderately sized tumors could be seen. With the advent of Polytome Pantopaque technology in 1942 smaller intracanalicular (within the internal auditory canal [IAC]) tumors could be visualized.[4,5]

The development of MR imaging in the 1980s ushered in a golden age for early diagnosis of VSs with experienced neuroradiologists being able to diagnose these lesions with high sensitivity and specificity. With this advance, the number of tumors larger than 3 cm decreased from 48% to 7% over the span of 20 years. Similarly, the share of tumors less than 1 cm in diameter increased from 5% in 1978 to 24% in 1993.[3] With this increased sensitivity for smaller tumors and earlier diagnosis, the goals of intervention shifted from the prevention of catastrophic neurologic consequences to the finer tuned preservation of hearing and facial nerve function.

DIAGNOSIS

As discussed, the way patients are diagnosed with VS has changed significantly since the introduction of MR imaging. With the resulting earlier diagnosis, the presentation of patients with VSs has changed as well. Furthermore, with the increased use of MR imaging for other indications and the slow-growing nature of VSs, many are now being diagnosed incidentally while still in the asymptomatic stage. The presentation of patients with VS varies based on location of the lesion as well as its size. Because most VSs are unilateral, with the rare exception of neurofibromatosis type II, the symptoms lateralize to the side of the lesion. The most common presenting symptom is hearing loss. This loss is of the sensorineural pattern and usually is slowly progressive. Occasionally, the hearing loss will progress in spurts. The reason for this pattern is unclear, and it may be a vascular phenomenon. In the post-MR imaging era, approximately 8% of VSs present as sudden sensorineural hearing loss.[6] In fact, the primary route to the diagnosis of VSs is workup of

asymmetric hearing symptoms. Other reasons for presentation include unilateral tinnitus or, very rarely, subtle nonvertiginous vestibular symptoms. When tumors are large, facial weakness (cranial nerve VII), facial hypesthesia (cranial nerve V) or compression-related symptoms may present (Table 1).

Audiologic Evaluation

The primary presentation of patients with VS is asymmetric hearing loss. Other hearing-related causes for presentation include sudden hearing loss and unilateral tinnitus. The first step in workup of a patient with these symptoms is the comprehensive audiologic examination (CAE; often referred to as an audiogram). This battery of tests is commonly performed for hearing complaints, and it provides information regarding multiple aspects of hearing, ranging from the tympanic membrane integrity, to middle ear/Eustachian tube physiology, to the inner ear and cochlear nerve function. From the CAE, the diagnosis of conductive versus sensorineural hearing loss can be made easily. Sensorineural hearing loss is caused by dysfunction of the cochlea or auditory nerve. Conductive hearing loss is due to anatomic dysfunction of the external or middle ear structures that ultimately transmit mechanical sound waves to the cochlea where they are encoded as an electrochemical signal.

Hearing tests with atypical findings are often the primary reason for screening for VSs. These tests are extremely common, and the vast majority of abnormalities are symmetric sensorineural hearing losses owing to age-related hearing loss. Occasionally, an asymmetric sensorineural hearing loss will be found incidentally. In this situation, the current practice is to obtain an MR image to rule out a retrocochlear lesion (the most common of which is VS). Classically, 1% to 2% of patients who undergo MR imaging for asymmetric sensorineural hearing loss are found to have a VS.[7]

Other audiologic indications for MR imaging to rule out a retrocochlear lesion include unilateral sudden sensorineural hearing loss or significant and persistent unilateral tinnitus.[8] In a retrospective analysis of 291 patient in South Korea with sudden sensorineural hearing loss, 13 (4.5%) were found to have an abnormality on MR imaging and 9 (3.1% of original sample) were diagnosed with VS.[9] The rates of abnormal findings detected on MR imaging in patients will likely increase in patients with sudden sensorineural hearing loss as high-resolution and 3-dimensional fluid-attenuated inversion recovery technologies improve.[10] Thus, imaging should be recommended for the diagnosis of other etiologies

Table 1
Symptoms of patients with vestibular schwannoma at initial diagnosis

Class of Symptom	Symptom	Percentage of Patients at Presentation
Auditory	Asymmetric hearing loss	51%–88%
	Sudden sensorineural hearing loss	8%–18%
	Unilateral tinnitus	7.6%–88%
Vestibular	Disequilibrium	29%–55%
	Vertigo (illusion of frank movement)	Rare
Increased intracranial pressure	Headache	3%–17%
	Nausea/vomiting	Rare in modern era
	Decreased vision/diplopia/papilledema	Rare in modern era
	Anosmia	Rare in modern era
	Obtundation	Rare in modern era
Other neurologic symptoms	Facial nerve	3%–22%
	Trigeminal nerve	3%–24%
	Lower cranial nerve	Rare in modern era
	Long tract	Rare in modern era
	Ataxia/cerebellar	Rare in modern era
Asymptomatic (incidentally discovered)	—	11%–24%

Data from Stucken EZ, Brown K, Selesnick SH. Clinical and diagnostic evaluation of acoustic neuromas. Otolaryngol Clin North Am 2012;45:269–84, vii; and Marinelli JP, Lohse CM, Carlson ML. Incidence of vestibular schwannoma over the past half-century: a population-based study of Olmsted County, Minnesota. Otolaryngol Head Neck Surg 2018;159(4):717–23.

of sudden sensorineural hearing loss outside of VS. The CAE findings characteristic of VS are listed in **Table 2**. Importantly, CAE should be performed on all patients diagnosed with VS, even if the patient does not complain of hearing loss, to establish a baseline. The baseline CAE will also allow prognostication of hearing preservation with different treatment techniques. When observation is chosen, it will guide appropriate hearing rehabilitation, which can include a variety of devices depending on the level of hearing loss.

Historically and in resource-poor areas, the investigation of retrocochlear pathology includes auditory brainstem response audiometry. This test can be analogized to an electroencephalograph for hearing in which the patient's response to a small click or similar sound is recorded with scalp electrodes. It is based on the principle that evoked potentials from the cochlea are generated when it undergoes sound stimulus. The progression of these evoked potentials through the hearing pathway can be recorded as waves. An analysis of the morphology of these waves provides insight into the functionality of the component parts. However, with the advent of MR imaging with far greater sensitivity and specificity as well as widespread availability, auditory brainstem response audiometry is less commonly performed. A modification of the traditional auditory brainstem response audiometry, known as a stacked auditory brainstem response audiometry, has been found to have improved sensitivity, but it cannot surpass MR imaging in terms of localization and treatment planning.

Vestibular Testing

Disequilibrium can be a sensitive and early sign of pathology. For patients reporting these symptoms, vestibular testing can detect a unilateral weakness in the vestibular system. Lustig and colleagues[11] found that 5% of patients with VS present with symmetric hearing, and of these 41% have persistent complaints of disequilibrium that lead to MR imaging and ultimate diagnosis. Additionally, a more recent study found that 3.6% of patients were diagnosed with VS of 253 with suspicious findings on vestibular testing who underwent MR imaging.[12] Ataxia is a rare presentation, and indicates brainstem compression from a large VS. Vertigo (ie, spinning or the frank illusion of movement) is rare in VS. Vertigo results from an acute change in vestibular function, whereas VS tends to grow slowly over time. With slow progression

Table 2
Audiogram findings of patients with VS

Audiogram Finding	Patients with VS (%)
Profound hearing loss	14–16
Descending audiogram	51–65
Flat audiogram	22–28

Audiogram Finding	Score
Mean speech discrimination (word recognition) score	73 ± 34

Data from Kim SH, Lee SH, Choi SK, et al. Audiologic evaluation of vestibular schwannoma and other cerebellopontine angle tumors. Acta Otolaryngol 2016;136:149–53, and Hirsch A, Anderson H. Audiologic test results in 96 patients with tumors affecting the eighth nerve. A clinical study with emphasis on the early audiological diagnosis. Acta Otolaryngol Suppl 1980;369:1–26.

of vestibular nerve dysfunction, the brain is able to progressively compensate for the asymmetric input, preventing symptoms of vertigo.

Imaging

VSs are extraaxial, contrast-enhancing lesions of the cerebellopontine angle (CPA). They are typically centered on the IAC and lack stigmata of rarer lesions on the differential diagnosis (eg, the dural tails of meningiomas). Imaging is the gold standard for diagnosis. MR imaging allows localization and exceptional soft tissue delineation within the IAC. However, computed tomography (CT) scans with contrast can diagnose moderate to large VSs in patients unable to undergo MR imaging (eg, ferromagnetic implants, severe claustrophobia, or body habitus). Although less sensitive for smaller or intracanalicular tumors, CT scanning does provide excellent delineation

Table 3
Advantages and disadvantages of computed tomography scanning with contrast for the diagnosis and management of vestibular schwannoma

Advantages	Disadvantages
Good bony definition	Poor delineation of tumors <1 cm
Decreased cost	Poor visualization of intracanalicular tumors
Increased tolerance	
Speed	
No contraindications for ferromagnetic implants	Radiation

of bony erosion. The advantages and disadvantages of CT imaging for VSs are listed in Table 3. Often the first sign of a VS on CT scanning will be widening of the bony IAC. In addition, bone erosion may be important for prognostication of functional preservation of both the facial and cochlear nerves. Unsurprisingly, Matthies and colleagues[13] found that a larger IAC diameter on CT scanning (which probably correlates with a larger underlying tumor) was associated with increased likelihood of preoperative deafness.

The gold standard imaging modality for VS diagnosis is T1-weighted image MR imaging of the IAC with and without contrast. Without contrast, VSs are hyperintense relative to cerebrospinal fluid and are isointense to hypointense relative to gray matter on T1-weighted sequences. VSs avidly enhance with contrast. Cystic VSs can also occur with frequency of 11% to 48%. With the combination of T1 with and without contrast and T2-weighted imaging, VSs can be successfully diagnosed and largely differentiated from other lesions with 96% to 100% sensitivity and 88% to 93% specificity.[14] Fig. 1 lists the imaging characteristics of VSs in comparison with other lesions that may present similarly.

One of the disadvantages of this protocol is the need for gadolinium-based contrast. This requirement adds to duration of the test, increases cost, and has the potential for allergic reaction and nephrogenic systemic sclerosis. For this reason, several protocols using high-resolution T2-weighted imaging without contrast have been developed. These protocols go by many names given by the particular MR imaging manufacturers, including fast imaging employing steady-state acquisition (FIESTA), constructive interference in steady state (CISS), and gradient echo sequences. A recent retrospective analysis of 348 patients found that CPA lesions were detected with 90% sensitivity and 99.5% specificity on high-resolution T2-weighted MR imaging compared with T1-weighted MR imaging with contrast.[15]

TREATMENT

Because of improving imaging capabilities, more VSs are diagnosed at early stages with minimal symptoms. The goals of management have thus shifted from the prevention of catastrophic neurologic events (stroke, death) to functional preservation (avoiding facial nerve and hearing injury). Because of this shift, as well as the unique location of these tumors in the space adjoining the brain and temporal bone, the treatment team is necessarily multidisciplinary. Table 4 lists the team members vital for VS patient care. All of these

Differential Diagnosis of CPA Lesions

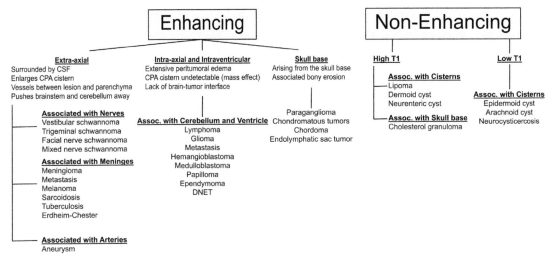

Fig. 1. Imaging characteristics of vestibular schwannomas in contrast with other lesions on the differential diagnosis. Assoc., associated; CPA, cerebellopontine angle; CSF, cerebrospinal fluid; DNET, dysembryoplastic neuroepithelial tumor. (*Data from* Hentschel MA, Kunst HPM, Rovers MM, et al. Diagnostic accuracy of high-resolution T2-weighted MR imaging vs contrast-enhanced T1-weighted MR imaging to screen for cerebellopontine angle lesions in symptomatic patients. Clin Otolaryngol 2018;43(3):805–11.)

members are essential because of the various modalities of VS management, including surgery, stereotactic radiation therapy, and serial imaging.

STAGING

After the initial diagnosis and workup of a patient with a VS, the treatment plan must be devised.

Table 4 Clinical team for patients with vestibular Schwannomas	
Treatment	Neurotologist
	Neurosurgeon
	Radiation oncologist
	Oncologist (for patients with neurofibromatosis type 2)
Diagnostic	Neuroradiologist
	Audiologist
	Neurologist
	Pathologist
	Neurotologist/ Otolaryngologist
	Neurosurgeon
	Geneticist (for patients with neurofibromatosis type 2)
Rehabilitation	Audiologist
	Neurotologist
	Speech and language therapist
	Vestibular therapist
	Neurophysiologist

As a first step, it is important to synthesize the patient's clinical and radiologic findings to understand their prognosis and potential for functional preservation with different treatment modalities. Several staging systems have been devised for VS with regard to both symptom score and radiologic findings (Table 5). These systems take into account the size of the VS and its effects on surrounding structures. The sizing is also controversial, with many staging systems using the maximum CPA diameter. However, this neglects IAC extension, which is important for functional preservation. It also ignores two of the other dimensions in 3-dimensional space. A volume-based system may be a better measure. However, this parameter is currently labor intensive to routinely assess.

One finding not taken into account by these systems is the presence of cystic degeneration in the VS. Cystic tumors are more likely to be large and rapidly growing. They also tend to be less responsive to stereotactic radiosurgery (SRS) and have higher rates of complication with surgical interventions, although this is controversial.[14,16]

Since the shift to functional and quality of life preservation, the objective measurement of symptoms is also critical for guiding serial imaging, as well as the postprocedural course after surgery or radiation. For this reason, functional grading systems for hearing, facial nerve function, tinnitus, and dizziness can be important clinical guides. A list of the quality-of-life measures relevant to

Table 5
Imaging-based staging systems for vestibular schwannoma

Tumor Size (mm)	Description	Sterkers	House	Koos	Samii
0	Confining to IAC	Tube type	Intracanalicular	Grade I	T1
≤10	Surpassing IAC	Small	Grade 1 (small)	Grade II	T2
≤15	Occupying CPA	Small	Grade 1 (small)	Grade II	T3a
≤20	Occupying CPA	Mild	Grade 2 (medium)	Grade II	T3a
≤30	Occupy CPA and contract the brainstem without compression	Mild	Grade 2 (medium)	Grade III	T3b
≤40	Compressing the brain stem	Large	Grade 4 (large)	Grade IV	T4a
>40	Severe brainstem displacement with deformation of the 4th ventricle	Huge	Grade 5 (giant)	Grade IV	T4b

Abbreviations: CPA, cerebellopontine angle; IAC, internal auditory canal.

Adapted from Wu H, Zhang L, Han D, et al. Summary and consensus in 7th International Conference on acoustic neuroma: an update for the management of sporadic acoustic neuromas. World J Otorhinolaryngol Head Neck Surg 2016;2:236; with permission.

patients with VS is provided in **Table 6**. It is important for the entire treatment team to be unified in their understanding of the staging so as to effectively use it to drive decision making. It also allows for standardized outcomes, a necessity for research and quality improvement.

Management of Small to Moderate Vestibular Schwannomas

Patients whose VSs are smaller than 2 cm have the greatest amount of flexibility for treatment options. Decisions regarding the management of these patients are likewise the most complex and nuanced. In these cases, hearing preservation is paramount, and prognostication of hearing preservation depends on the quality of hearing at diagnosis. Patients with good to excellent hearing have better prognoses, whereas those with only serviceable hearing (ie, impaired hearing but can still be serviced with a hearing aid) have poorer outcomes for all management modalities. **Fig. 2** presents a flowchart for hearing preservation prognosis. At this stage, serial imaging, SRS, and surgical intervention are all reasonable decisions. Patient preference and clinical status can be important factors in deciding on treatment at this stage. Younger patients with excellent hearing may prefer surgical intervention, whereas those with more tenuous but serviceable hearing or poorer surgical candidates may choose SRS. Observation with serial imaging remains a viable option, and methodologies for monitoring may become even more

advanced in the future. Although there is no consensus, a common practice is a 6-month T1-weighted MR imaging with/without contrast or high-resolution T2 (with FIESTA, CISS, or similar sequences) followed by yearly scans for the next 4 to 5 years, followed by increased intervals thereafter, depending on stability.[14] Observation may be particularly useful in patients with the following characteristics:

- Elderly or poor surgical candidate,
- Small tumor and excellent hearing,
- Strong patient preference, and
- Tumor on the side of an only hearing ear.

Management of Moderately Large to Large Vestibular schwannomas

For patients with a tumor greater than 3 cm, serial imaging is no longer an option. The majority of the data in this population suggest the management of these lesions with surgery, although some more recent research suggests that SRS can potentially be used safely in select circumstances.[17] The chief concern with SRS on larger tumors is postradiation edema with worsening of symptoms from mass effects. Accordingly, the presence of hydrocephalus is an absolute contraindication to SRS. The management of these tumors is more complicated because they tend to apply more pressure around surrounding structures, causing an increased risk of cranial nerve injury. The challenges particularly apply to facial nerve function,

Table 6
Quality-of-life and functional outcome measures

Symptom	Measure
Hearing	AAO-HNS Hearing Classification System Gardner–Robertson Hearing Classification
Dizziness	Dizziness Handicap Inventory
Tinnitus	Tinnitus Handicap Inventory
Facial Nerve	House-Brackmann Scale

Abbreviation: AAO-HNS, American Academy of Otolaryngology–Head and Neck Surgery.

Data from Wu H, Zhang L, Han D, et al. Summary and consensus in 7th International Conference on acoustic neuroma: an update for the management of sporadic acoustic neuromas. World J Otorhinolaryngol Head Neck Surg 2016;2:234–9.

which has been shown to be worse in patients who undergo complete tumor removal relative to a subtotal excision.[18,19] Improving outcomes in these patients without compromising tumor control is an area of active inquiry as the role of subtotal resection or near total resection is investigated as a replacement to the traditional goal of gross total resection. For regrowth after surgery, SRS is a good option.

Surgery

The surgical approach for VS depends on the size, location, and functions to be preserved (particularly hearing and the facial function). It is also highly dependent on individual surgeon preferences. The 3 main approaches are the middle cranial fossa (also sometimes called subtemporal), the retrosigmoid (also sometimes called suboccipital), and the translabyrinthine (Table 8). The middle cranial fossa and the retrosigmoid approaches both allow for hearing preservation, whereas the translabyrinthine approach necessitates obliteration of the cochlea and vestibular structures. However, the translabyrinthine approach provides the most direct visualization of the facial nerve, thus better enabling intraoperative preservation in patients who do not have serviceable hearing preoperatively. Between the middle cranial fossa and retrosigmoid approaches, the retrosigmoid approach provides a more extensive view of the CPA. However, the middle cranial fossa is superior for intracanalicular visualization, particularly in its lateral extent. Recent studies have explored the use of an endoscopic-assisted retrosigmoid approach to successfully address intracanalicular tumors.[20] The extent of lateral IAC extension of the VS is not only important for planning the approach, but also as a prognostic factor for facial nerve and hearing preservation. High-resolution T2-weighted imaging can

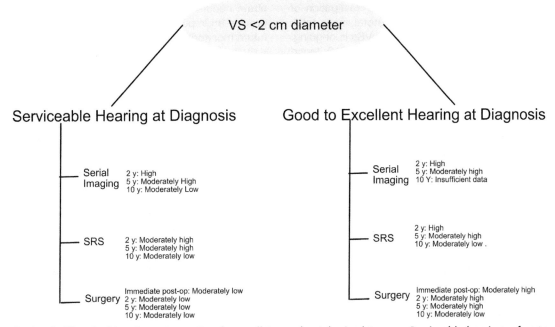

Fig. 2. Likelihood of hearing preservation for small to moderately sized tumors. Serviceable hearing refers to hearing sufficient enough to allow amplification with a hearing aid. SRS, stereotactic radiosurgery; VS, vestibular Schwannoma.

Table 7
Postoperative imaging in patient undergoing near total resection or subtotal resection

Type of Imaging	Frequency of Imaging	Relevant Measurements
• MR imaging of the posterior fossa and internal auditory canal with and without contrast and fat saturation • Continuous 1 mm-thick slices of the post contrast images with fat suppression • If the postcontrast images are <1 mm, or the patient was not administered contrast, then use fast imaging employing steady-state acquisition (FIESTA)/ constructive interference in steady state (CISS) thin slice sequences	• Preoperatively • Postoperatively (≤3 mo after surgery) • 6 mo • 1 y • Annually for 10 y	• Tumor diameter: longest dimension in the cerebello-pontine angle only excluding the intracanalicular portion (less accurate) versus the cerebellopontine angle plus the intracanalicular portion (more accurate) • Volumetric analysis: measuring the area of the tumor in each slice and multiplying it by the slice thickness • Imaging definitions: gross total resection = no tumor was visible; near total resection = only a very thin rim of tumor was visible on the brainstem and the facial nerve measuring no larger than 0.5 cm^3; and subtotal resection = any larger remnant

From Monfared A, Corrales CE, Theodosopoulos PV, et al. Facial nerve outcome and tumor control rate as a function of degree of resection in treatment of large acoustic neuromas: preliminary report of the Acoustic Neuroma Subtotal Resection Study (ANSRS). Neurosurgery 2016;79:196; with permission.

be particularly helpful in determining the position of the tumor within the IAC.

A multicenter, nonrandomized investigation of the long-term outcomes of subtotal, near total, and gross total resection of large VSs is ongoing. The preliminary results, published in 2016, found 21% regrowth in patients with remnant tumor. Regrowth was associated with larger remnant tumor. However, good facial nerve function was achieved in 67% of patients immediately postoperatively and in 81% at 1 year.[21] For these purposes, gross total resection was defined as the absence of visible tumor at the end of surgery; near total resection when the tumor remnant measured less than 5 × 5 × 2 mm over the brainstem and the facial nerve; and subtotal resection when the tumor was resected 80% to 90% by volume and 60% to 70% by surface area.[21] Because the radiologic postoperative monitoring for these procedures has not been fully established, the methods used for this trial are listed in Table 7.

As discussed in the case of subtotal resection and near total resection, monitoring for recurrence is also paramount in the context of gross total resection. The postoperative bed normally demonstrates thin linear enhancement. However, nodular enhancement in the postoperative bed raises

concern for regrowth. Because some of the postoperative materials used for packing may demonstrate nodularity, early postsurgical imaging can provide an important baseline for comparison for future monitoring.[14]

Radiation

The role for SRS is well-established in the treatment of VS, particularly in the management of small to medium sized tumors for patients with neurofibromatosis type II and for patients with spontaneous VS. The advantages of SRS relative to surgery include decreased length of stay, decreased cost, and lower periprocedural morbidity. The disadvantages of SRS relative to surgery include the need for prolonged surveillance with repeat MR imaging studies, subsequently increased technical difficulty of salvage surgery, radiation-induced hydrocephalus, functional compromise owing to postprocedural swelling, and incremental risk (albeit small) for a radiation-induced malignancy.[22] Multiple modalities for administration of SRS exist, including Gamma Knife (Elekta, Stockholm, Sweden), linear accelerator (LINAC [Elekta, Stockholm, Sweden], which includes Cyber Knife [Accuray, Sunnyvale,

Table 8
Summary of surgical approaches to the cerebellopontine angle

Approach	Indications	Advantages	Disadvantages
Translabyrinthine	• Nonserviceable hearing • Low likelihood of hearing preservation	• No cerebellar retraction • Any size tumor • Early identification and accessibility of facial nerve • Extradural drilling of IAC	• Sacrifice of residual hearing • Contraindications: otitis media, high-riding jugular bulb, anterior sigmoid sinus
Middle cranial fossa	• Small intracanalicular tumors • Hearing preservation	• Possibility of hearing preservation • Access to fundus (lateral internal auditory canal)	• Limited tumor size • Temporal lobe retraction • Decreased access to CPA
Retrosigmoid	• Broad	• Possibility of hearing preservation • Any size tumor	• Decreased access to fundus • Decreased access to facial nerve • Cerebellar retraction • Intradural drilling of IAC • Postoperative headache

Abbreviations: CPA, cerebellopontine angle; IAC, internal auditory canal.

CA]), and proton beam. The comparative efficacy of these technologies has not been studied rigorously, and the choice is generally made on an institution-by-institution basis, based on availability and experience. More recent changes to SRS techniques have involved modified dosage schemes that allow for better facial nerve, cochlear nerve, and cochlear preservation.[23]

SUMMARY

VSs are the most common tumor of the CPA. The history of their management has driven advances in imaging, lateral skull base surgery, as well as radiosurgery. With these advances, a shift has occurred from life-saving treatment for late-stage disease to quality-of-life focused management of smaller tumors. The complicated treatment paradigms involving observation, SRS, and surgery require close communication between the treatment and neuroradiology teams.

REFERENCES

1. Kshettry VR, Hsieh JK, Ostrom QT, et al. Incidence of vestibular schwannomas in the United States. J Neurooncol 2015;124:223–8.
2. Mohammadi A, Jufas N. Sudden death due to vestibular schwannoma: caution in emergent management. Otol Neurotol 2016;37:564–7.
3. Stucken EZ, Brown K, Selesnick SH. Clinical and diagnostic evaluation of acoustic neuromas. Otolaryngol Clin North Am 2012;45:269–84, vii.
4. McRackan TR, Brackmann DE. Historical perspective on evolution in management of lateral skull base tumors. Otolaryngol Clin North Am 2015;48: 397–405.
5. Siqueira EB, Bucy PC, Cannon AH. Positive contrast ventriculography, cisternography and myelography. Am J Roentgenol Radium Ther Nucl Med 1968; 104:132–8.
6. Marinelli JP, Lohse CM, Carlson ML. Incidence of vestibular schwannoma over the past half-century: a population-based study of Olmsted County, Minnesota. Otolaryngol Head Neck Surg 2018;159(4): 717–23.
7. Saliba I, Martineau G, Chagnon M. Asymmetric hearing loss: rule 3,000 for screening vestibular schwannoma. Otol Neurotol 2009;30:515–21.
8. Sweeney AD, Carlson ML, Shepard NT, et al. Congress of neurological surgeons systematic review and evidence-based guidelines on otologic and audiologic screening for patients with vestibular schwannomas. Neurosurgery 2018;82:E29–31.
9. Jeong KH, Choi JW, Shin JE, et al. Abnormal magnetic resonance imaging findings in patients with sudden sensorineural hearing loss: vestibular schwannoma as the most common cause of MRI abnormality. Medicine (Baltimore) 2016;95:e3557.

10. Conte G, Di Berardino F, Sina C, et al. MR imaging in sudden sensorineural hearing loss. Time to talk. AJNR Am J Neuroradiol 2017;38:1475–9.

11. Lustig LR, Rifkin S, Jackler RK, et al. Acoustic neuromas presenting with normal or symmetrical hearing: factors associated with diagnosis and outcome. Am J Otol 1998;19:212–8.

12. Gandolfi MM, Reilly EK, Galatioto J, et al. Cost-effective analysis of unilateral vestibular weakness investigation. Otol Neurotol 2015;36:277–81.

13. Matthies C, Samii M, Krebs S. Management of vestibular schwannomas (acoustic neuromas): radiological features in 202 cases–their value for diagnosis and their predictive importance. Neurosurgery 1997;40:469–81 [discussion: 481–2].

14. Dunn IF, Bi WL, Mukundan S, et al. Congress of neurological surgeons systematic review and evidence-based guidelines on the role of imaging in the diagnosis and management of patients with vestibular schwannomas. Neurosurgery 2018;82: E32–4.

15. Hentschel MA, Kunst HPM, Rovers MM, et al. Diagnostic accuracy of high-resolution T2-weighted MRI vs contrast-enhanced T1-weighted MRI to screen for cerebellopontine angle lesions in symptomatic patients. Clin Otolaryngol 2018;43(3):805–11.

16. Frisch CD, Jacob JT, Carlson ML, et al. Stereotactic radiosurgery for cystic vestibular schwannomas. Neurosurgery 2017;80:112–8.

17. Huang CW, Tu HT, Chuang CY, et al. Gamma Knife radiosurgery for large vestibular schwannomas greater than 3 cm in diameter. J Neurosurg 2018; 128(5):1380–7.

18. Gurgel RK, Dogru S, Amdur RL, et al. Facial nerve outcomes after surgery for large vestibular schwannomas: do surgical approach and extent of resection matter? Neurosurg Focus 2012;33:E16.

19. Gurgel RK, Theodosopoulos PV, Jackler RK. Subtotal/near-total treatment of vestibular schwannomas. Curr Opin Otolaryngol Head Neck Surg 2012;20:380–4.

20. Tatagiba MS, Roser F, Hirt B, et al. The retrosigmoid endoscopic approach for cerebellopontine-angle tumors and microvascular decompression. World Neurosurg 2014;82:S171–6.

21. Monfared A, Corrales CE, Theodosopoulos PV, et al. Facial nerve outcome and tumor control rate as a function of degree of resection in treatment of large acoustic neuromas: preliminary report of the Acoustic Neuroma Subtotal Resection Study (ANSRS). Neurosurgery 2016;79:194–203.

22. Glasscock ME, Gulya AJ. Glasscock-Shambaugh surgery of the ear. 5th edition. Hamilton (Canada): BC Decker; 2003.

23. Germano IM, Sheehan J, Parish J, et al. Congress of neurological surgeons systematic review and evidence-based guidelines on the role of radiosurgery and radiation therapy in the management of patients with vestibular schwannomas. Neurosurgery 2018;82:E49–51.

Common Otologic Surgical Procedures

Clinical Decision-Making Pearls and the Role of Imaging

Tiffany Peng, MD, Apoorva T. Ramaswamy, MD,
Ana H. Kim, MD*

KEYWORDS

- Temporal bone • Middle and posterior fossa • Otologic surgery • Neuroradiology

KEY POINTS

- Assessment of middle ear ossicles, facial nerve course, position of the sigmoid, and integrity of tegmen and semicircular canals are important roadmaps preoperatively.
- Identifying aberrancies in the course of facial nerve is a critical component to preoperative planning and counseling for any patient undergoing middle ear surgery.
- Every temporal bone is unique. As such, radiographic imaging provides the surgeon with a road map on what to expect intraoperatively.

INTRODUCTION: A SURGEON'S PERSPECTIVE

Neuro-otologists rely on the expertise and judgment of a skilled neuroradiologist to identify radiographic abnormalities in the complicated regional anatomy of the temporal bone and middle and posterior fossa, and more importantly, to alert the surgeon to potential operative pitfalls. This article highlights some of the common otologic surgical procedures that stress this important dynamic.

Operative decision-making in neuro-otology is based on a triad of the patient's history, physical examination, and imaging studies. For example, a finding of chronic otitis media on computed tomography (CT) temporal bone in an asymptomatic patient does not necessarily require surgery, but a superimposed radiographic or clinical suspicion for cholesteatoma would prompt surgical intervention. Similarly, a nondraining tympanic membrane (TM) perforation does not require surgery. However, a patient reporting chronic otorrhea or symptomatic hearing loss in the presence of pertinent radiographic findings will more likely find themselves in consultation for surgical options.

Surgeons face another branching point in surgical consultation when determining the appropriate approach to the middle ear and lateral skull base. A cholesteatoma may be addressed transcanal, endaural, postauricular, or transmastoid with or without leaving the external auditory canal (EAC) intact, and a cerebellopontine angle mass may be removed through a middle fossa, retrosigmoid, or translabyrinthine approach. In addition to delivering radiographic diagnoses, a skilled neuroradiologist offers important insight regarding patient anatomy that may change the operative approach when surgery is indicated.

This article offers the surgical perspective on quick and effective clinical decision-making pearls to keep in mind during a thorough radiographic analysis of the ear and lateral skull base (**Fig. 1**).

No commercial or financial conflict for all three authors.
Department of Otolaryngology–Head and Neck Surgery, Columbia University Medical Center, 180 Fort Washington Avenue, Harkness Pavilion, Room 864, New York, NY 10032, USA
* Corresponding author.
E-mail address: ahk2166@cumc.columbia.edu

Neuroimag Clin N Am 29 (2019) 183–196
https://doi.org/10.1016/j.nic.2018.09.008

neuroimaging.theclinics.com

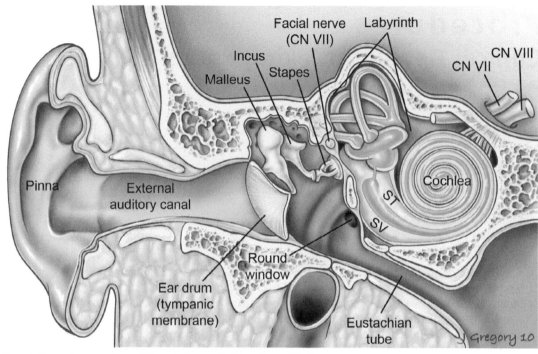

Fig. 1. Normal ear anatomy. ST, scala tympani; SV, scala vestibuli.

TYMPANIC MEMBRANE PERFORATION AND TYMPANOPLASTY

A TM perforation causes hearing loss by disrupting the conversion of acoustic sound energy entering the EAC into mechanical energy that normally occurs with the movement of the middle ear ossicles, which are connected to the TM. The goals of preoperative assessment and operative intervention are to address the perforation with a successful hearing outcome. CT of the temporal bone showing a poorly pneumatized mastoid or a mastoid cavity that is poorly aerated is reflective of underlying eustachian tube (ET) dysfunction and/or chronic otitis media. These ears have a higher risk of reperforation or development of middle ear disease (chronic otitis media, TM retraction, acquired cholesteatoma) compared with a well-pneumatized and aerated mastoid. In addition, status of the middle ear ossicles and patency of the oval and round window are predictors of postoperative hearing outcome.

Decision to Offer Tympanoplasty
- Patient has been infection free seeking improved hearing outcome.
- Chronic otorrhea unresponsive to conservative medical interventions caused by the presence of the TM perforation.
- Active patients for whom taking water precautions impacts quality of life.

Surgical Approaches

Transcanal approach is performed entirely within the EAC and is indicated for small (<30%) TM perforations, posterior or inferior pars tensa location, and demonstrates adequate EAC caliber (ideally >5 mm) to allow for adequate middle ear visualization. If the anterior rim of the TM is not well-visualized or there is concurrent disease to be addressed in the mastoid, alternate approaches to repair are favored.

Endaural approach involves extension of canal incision to the helical root. It is more commonly used in Europe, but may be used with all perforation sizes if there is no concurrent mastoid disease or indication for mastoidectomy.

Postauricular approach involves an incision in the postauricular sulcus for improved access to the anterior TM. It is performed most commonly in the United States and is warranted in the presence of perforations of all sizes and locations. This approach offers a higher success (>95%) of TM closure.

The patient's underlying disease state or clinical history may warrant concurrent mastoidectomy with tympanoplasty.[1] Examples of such clinical scenarios include concern or presence of chronic otitis media and cholesteatoma in the attic or mastoid. Concurrent mastoidectomy with tympanoplasty in uncomplicated TM perforations or sclerotic mastoid development suggestive of underlying ET dysfunction (**Fig. 2**) remains contro-versial. McGrew and colleagues[2] demonstrated that although mastoidectomy was not required for successful repair of TM perforations, concurrent mastoidectomy reduced the need for future procedures even in the absence of evidence of active infection, whereas a 2014 review reported no additional benefit to concurrent mastoidectomy in this population.[3]

Eustachian Tube Status

The ET is the only conduit for middle ear and mastoid aeration by way of the nasopharynx. The ET functions to equalize pressure across the TM, protect the middle ear from reflux of nasopharyngeal contents to the middle ear space, and clearance of middle ear secretions. When unilateral otitis media with effusion is seen, it is important to assess the posterior nasopharynx to rule out any type of mass obstructing the ET when reviewing imaging studies.

Take Home Points
- Subtotal/total TM perforation and anterior location favor postauricular approach.
- Concurrent mastoid pathology and recurrent perforation favor tympanoplasty with concurrent mastoidectomy.
- Sclerotic mastoid and symptomatic ET dysfunction (nasal congestion/obstruction, sinus disease) is a poor prognostic indicator for adequate functional outcome after tympanoplasty.

CHRONIC OTITIS MEDIA

Chronic otitis media is a common finding among patients presenting to an otolaryngologist. Radiographically, this condition may manifest as opacification or mucosal thickening of the middle ear or mastoid air cells without osseous erosion or coalescence. The scutum is typically not blunted, and the tegmen intact (**Fig. 3**). Radiographic finding of chronic otitis media is not a surgical indication in the absence of other clinical symptoms or findings.

Symptoms of Chronic Otitis Media
- Presence of a TM perforation with
  - Hearing Loss
  - Tinnitus
  - Aural fullness
  - Dizziness
  - Otalgia
  - Otorrhea

Neuro-otolologists base surgical intervention on active symptomology, clinical examination, hearing status, and radiographic findings. History of recurrent infections or chronic otorrhea refractory to medical treatment, or impaired hearing loss favor surgery over surveillance. A radiographic finding of cortical bone erosion in the setting of painless otorrhea with multiple TM perforations warrants consideration for tuberculosis otitis media, particularly if the patient also has significant granulation tissue in the middle ear and early severe hearing loss.[4] If on examination there is frank keratin debris visualized or posterior scutum erosion suspicious for acquired cholesteatoma, surgical intervention is warranted and CT is helpful in identifying disease extent. In the absence of this clinical suspicion, however, routine preoperative CT scanning is of questionable value because imaging alone cannot reliably distinguish between mucosal disease, fluid, and cholesteatoma.[5] This

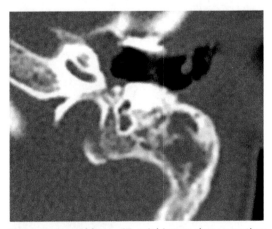

Fig. 3. Temporal bone CT, axial image demonstrating sclerotic mastoid that is opacified without septal coalescence, and tympanic membrane retraction with middle ear opacification. Note the high-riding jugular bulb and lateral sigmoid sinus, both critical information for surgical planning.

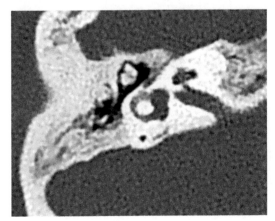

Fig. 2. Temporal bone CT, axial image demonstrating severely sclerotic mastoid.

is covered further in the cholesteatoma section of this article.

Take Home Points
- Chronic otitis media is a common radiographic finding manifesting as opacification or mucosal thickening of the middle ear and mastoid air cells, but operative intervention is based on patient symptoms, physical findings, and audiogram.
- Chronic otitis media with concurrent mastoid disease or cholesteatoma warrants tympanomastoidectomy surgery. In these cases, careful assessment of the middle ear ossicles, facial nerve course, position of the sigmoid (lateralized, dehiscence), and integrity of the tegmen and semicircular canals are important roadmaps preoperatively.

CHOLESTEATOMA

Cholesteatoma is a benign squamous epithelial proliferation that is locally destructive with the potential to erode delicate bony structures within the middle ear (ossicles, fallopian canal, scutum, tegmen epitympanum, otic bone), inner ear structures (cochlea and semicircular canals), and extend into the mastoid cavity or skull base (Fig. 4). It is congenital, primary acquired (typically found in the pars flaccida or the posterosuperior quadrant of the TM), or secondary acquired (located medial to the TM in association with a TM perforation).

The acquired cases are typically associated with either ET dysfunction or chronic ear disease. In the pediatric population, cholesteatomas are considered congenital in the presence of an intact TM and no history of ear surgery or myringotomy. There is a male predominance for this condition, and a predilection for occurrence in the anterosuperior quadrant.[6]

In addition, incomplete congenital EAC atresia on radiographic evaluation (Fig. 5) is associated with canal cholesteatoma caused by impaired clearance of squamous debris from the EAC and requires careful clinical surveillance, diffusion-weighted MR

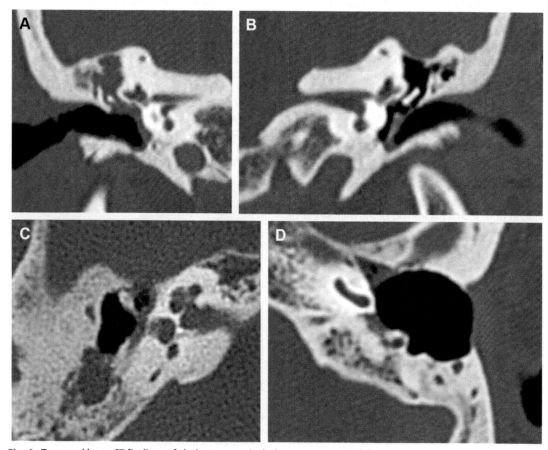

Fig. 4. Temporal bone CT findings of cholesteatoma include scutum erosion (*A*) compared with normal side (*B*), facial nerve dehiscence (*C*), and automastoidectomy whereby the posterior external bony canal and ossicles are eroded (*D*).

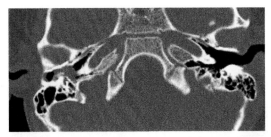

Fig. 5. Canal stenosis resulting in medial canal cholesteatoma formation on the right compared with the normal left canal.

imaging (Fig. 6), or surgical repair (canalplasty). Unlike other entities discussed in this article, cholesteatoma warrants surgery for removal even when the patient is asymptomatic to prevent further disease progression and complications.

Complications of Untreated Cholesteatoma
- Hearing loss
- Dizziness
- Facial paralysis
- Cerebrospinal fluid (CSF) leak

Surgical Approaches

Cholesteatoma may be managed transcanal if limited to the meso or hypotympanum with adequate EAC caliber for adequate visualization and room for instrumentation. Postauricular approach is favored with narrow EAC, disease involving the epitympanum/attic, and large TM perforations. Mastoidectomy is indicated if there is mastoid involvement.

There are two types of mastoidectomy: canal wall up or canal wall down depending on whether the bony EAC is left intact or drilled down to the level of the facial nerve course from the second genu and mastoid segment.

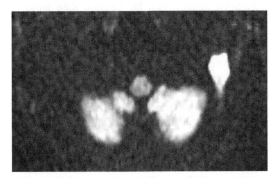

Fig. 6. Diffusion-weighted MR image demonstrating restricted diffusion on the left suggestive of cholesteatoma within the left mastoid cavity.

Radiographic Indications for Canal Wall Down Mastoidectomy
- Extensive mastoid cholesteatoma with semicircular canal dehiscence
  - Complete removal of the disease is not favorable without rupturing the membranous labyrinth, which can result in sensorineural hearing loss and dizziness.
- Erosion of the fallopian canal
  - The cholesteatoma matrix may not be able to be peeled off completely from the facial nerve epineurium.
- Automastoidectomy
  - The cholesteatoma has already partially eroded the posterior EAC.
- Epitympanic or supratubal cholesteatoma involvement with low-riding tegmen
  - Precludes adequate visualization and thus difficulty removing disease from these regions.
- Cholesteatoma within the sinus tympani
  - Carries the highest recidivism rate because of its blind location.
- Recurrent disease and prior canal wall up tympanomastoidectomy

Take Home Points
- Cholesteatoma in a pediatric patient with an intact TM and no history of ear surgery is congenital.
- Primary acquired cholesteatoma occurs in the pars flaccida, the weakest and nonvibratory portion of the TM. Hearing loss is a late finding as such.
- Radiographic identification of cholesteatoma with automastoids, extensive facial nerve involvement, semicircular canal dehiscence, low tegmen precluding adequate visualization and access to the epitympanum/attic, extensive disease in the sinus tympani, and recurrent cholesteatoma favor canal wall down tympanomastoidectomy.

HEARING LOSS

The radiographic evaluation of a patient with hearing loss is broad, with special distinction to be made between congenital versus acquired. Hearing loss is categorized into conductive, sensorineural, or mixed as determined by the patient's audiogram, and this information is critical to appropriate analysis of radiographic findings that may otherwise be nonspecific.

Congenital Causes of Hearing Loss (Fig. 7)
- Mondini malformation
- Absent or narrow IAC

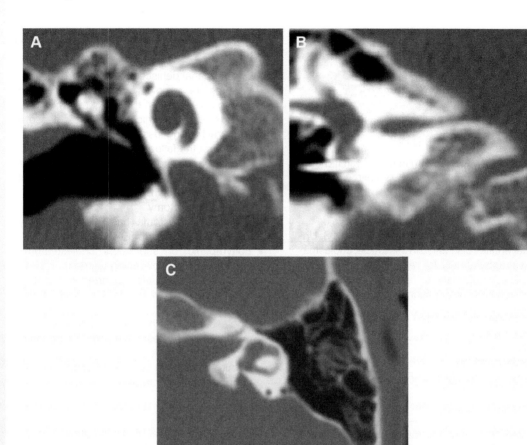

Fig. 7. Congenital causes of hearing loss include Mondini malformation (*A*), absent or narrow internal auditory canal (*B*), and enlarged vestibular aqueduct (*C*).

- Incomplete partition
- Enlarged vestibular aqueduct
- Congenital fixed stapes footplate
- Atresia
- Genetic

Acquired Causes of Hearing Loss (Fig. 8)
- Otitis media with effusion
- Tympanic membrane perforation
- Ossicular chain discontinuity (Fig. 9)
- Otosclerosis
  ○ May involve round window
- Cholesteatoma
- Round window or oval window fistula
- Cochlea ossificans postmeningitis
- Temporal bone fracture
- Acoustic neuroma
- Exostoses

The decision to operate when these findings are encountered is based on a combination of appropriate concordance of the radiographic findings with the patient's clinical presentation. The proposed diagnosis should match the patient's symptoms and the type of hearing loss on his or her audiogram.

Operative Pitfalls

Operative intervention for hearing loss aims to achieve sustained hearing restoration that address the appropriate type of hearing loss, and also to address all potential diagnoses that may be contributing to the patient's symptomatology. In this way, a skilled neuroradiologist has the ability to alert the surgeon to any concurrent findings, subtle or otherwise, that would expand or alter their surgical plan or surgical approach.

For example, combination of CT and MR imaging increases the sensitivity in assessing if cochlear ossicans is present postmeningitis, which is critical in determining whether cochlear implantation is a feasible option for hearing

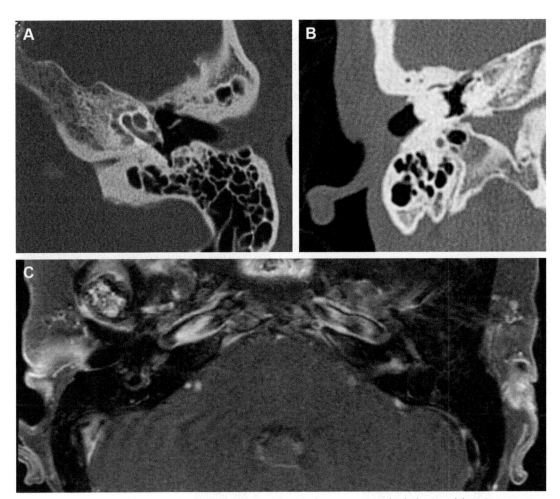

Fig. 8. Acquired causes of hearing loss include (*A*) otosclerosis demonstrating the halo sign, (*B*) EAC exostoses on temporal bone high-resolution CT images, and (*C*) cochlear and IAC enhancement on T1-weighted image with gadolinium in inflammatory processes, such as meningitis.

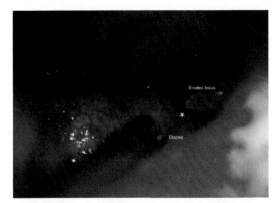

Fig. 9. Ossicular discontinuity. Intraoperative image showing the lenticular process of incus eroded from cholesteatoma resulting in ossicular discontinuity (*asterisk*) with the stapes.

restoration. In the evaluation of EAC atresia, the Jahrsdoerfer criteria, which are based on radiographic findings on preoperative temporal bone CT and the appearance of the external ear, dictate whether atresia repair for hearing is an option.[7]

An unrecognized lateral, dehiscent, or in rare cases of bifid facial nerve could prove disastrous during such an intervention on a pediatric patient who already has abnormal anatomy. In fact, identifying aberrancies in the course of facial nerve is a critical component to preoperative planning and counseling for any patient undergoing middle ear surgery, regardless of the anticipated surgical approach. Similarly, a concurrent finding of superior semicircular canal dehiscence (SSCD) in a patient with conductive hearing loss can steer the surgeon toward SSCD repair rather than stapedectomy surgery.

Take Home Points
- Congenital versus acquired hearing loss has different etiologies.
- Audiogram is critical to the assessment of hearing loss, but radiographic imaging narrows the wide differentials and surgical options.
- Every temporal bone is unique. As such, radiographic imaging provides the surgeon with a road map on what to expect intraoperatively, and avoid pitfalls and risk stratification.

CEREBROSPINAL FLUID LEAK AND TEGMEN DEHISCENCE

Defects of the lateral skull base, also known as tegmen dehiscences, are a diagnostic and management quandary for clinicians. These defects may result in herniation of meninges and cerebral tissue with resultant meningocele or encephalocele, respectively (**Fig. 10**). If the dura mater has also been violated, leakage of CSF from the subarachnoid space to the sinonasal or tympanic cavities can develop. The identification and repair of these communications is paramount because they can result in serious intracranial infections and complications. However, there is incipient literature that certain patients with spontaneous tegmen dehiscences can also be monitored because the rate of severe intracranial infection in these patients is low.[8] Tegmen dehiscence can occur in the congenital, postsurgical, traumatic, postinfectious, neoplastic, and spontaneous settings.

With the widespread use of antibiotics for otologic infections, the primary causes of temporal bone dehiscence have changed over the last few decades as chronic otitis media less frequently result in bony erosion, encephaloceles, and CSF leak. Most of these pathologies now occur in the spontaneous, postsurgical, or post-traumatic setting. A recent retrospective review by Sanna and colleagues[9] found that 45.9% of meningoencephalic herniations were iatrogenic, 24.8% spontaneous, 21.8% secondary to chronic otitis media, and 7.5% post-traumatic. The phenomenon of spontaneous tegmen defect has become more common in the past three decades, particularly in obese, middle-aged women.[10,11] Although no definitive mechanism has been described for this pathology, it is hypothesized that hypertrophic arachnoid granulations combined with intracranial hypertension cause erosion of the dura resulting in bony dehiscence and CSF leak. This is further evidenced by higher rates of spontaneous CSF leak and recurrence in patients with thinning of the lateral skull base noted on CT.[12] The presentation and history of patients depends on the cause of their pathology. However, certain common trends remain as listed next.[9]

Presentation of a Patient with Lateral Skull Base Defect
- Headache
- Clear, thin fluid from ear or nose
- Persistent middle ear effusion with aural fullness and hearing loss
- Persistent clear otorrhea after tympanostomy tube placement
- Meningitis
- Pneumocephalus
- Seizures

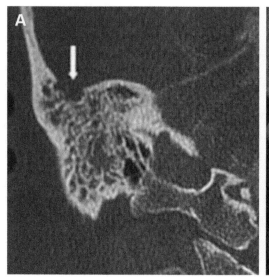 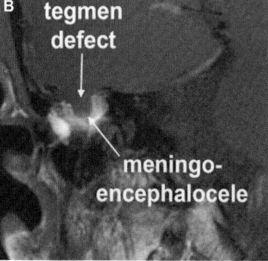

Fig. 10. Tegmen dehiscence (*arrow*) is best appreciated on temporal bone CT images (*A*). However, encephalocele is best appreciated on MR images (*B*).

Pertinent History of Patient with Lateral Skull Base Defect
- General medical history: obesity, medications, hypertension
- Otologic history: hearing loss, previous ear surgeries, previous tympanostomy tubes, ear infections, tinnitus, vertigo, facial nerve deficits
- Neurologic history: seizures, meningitis, and idiopathic intracranial hypertension
- Traumatic history
- Miscellaneous: other past medical and surgical history, especially rhinologic and skull base

Clinical history, imaging, and sampling of any draining fluid are the most important factors in diagnosing a CSF leak. Sampled fluid must be sent for a β2-transferrin assay, a protein specific for CSF and perilymph. In patients for whom fluid cannot be obtained and suspicion is high, imaging can become essential to diagnosis and treatment planning. The primary imaging modality for clinicians is high-resolution CT of the temporal bones. This examination enables evaluation of bony integrity with thin cuts to detect even small areas of dehiscence that may suggest cause of the leak. Up to 45% of patients with spontaneous CSF leaks have been found to have multiple tegmen defects.[12] Patients in whom encephalocele or meningocele are suspected also require MR imaging to differentiate cerebral herniation from other soft tissue pathology. In some patients, high-resolution CT scanning does not indicate the location of the skull base defect. For these cases, other tests for CSF leak diagnosis include radionuclide cisternography, CT cisternography, MR imaging cisternography, and MR myelogram.[13]

Surgical Approaches

Most iatrogenic and traumatic CSF leaks can be treated conservatively. Surgical treatment is reserved for patients with CSF leaks that do not improve with appropriate trial of conservative management, or those with history of meningitis. Decision making for surgical treatment and type of approach is guided by the location of the CSF leak, size of the defect, and patient-specific clinical factors including tolerance of temporal lobe retraction or the potential of conductive hearing loss. The options for approach to the lateral skull base for tegmen repair are transmastoid, middle cranial fossa (MCF), or a combined approach. The site of dehiscence is then repaired with a variety of measures ranging from fat, muscle, and cartilage to hydroxyapatite bone cement or fibrin glue.[11] Choice of repair material affects postoperative appearance on imaging and may make evaluation difficult should the leak persist or the surgery have complications.

Conservative Management of CSF Leaks
- Bed rest
- Lumbar drain
- Intracranial pressure precautions: diuretics, laxatives, cough suppression

Surgical Routes for Repair of CSF Leak[9]
- Transmastoid
  - Smaller defects
  - Defects within the tegmen mastoideum
  - Posterior fossa involvement
  - Advantage: does not require temporal lobe retraction, quicker postoperative recovery
- Middle cranial fossa
  - Larger defects
  - Multiple defects
  - Defect in tegmen epitympanum/petrous apex
  - Significant encephalocele
  - Advantage: does not require manipulation and possible dislodgement of ossicles

Take Home Pearls
- Skull base dehiscence can present with conductive hearing loss, complications of otitis media, vertigo, CSF otorrhea, meningitis, or seizures.
- Patient history is important in diagnosing causes of skull base dehiscence.
- First-line imaging is thin-cut CT of the temporal bones.
- Surgical approach via the transmastoid or MCF depends on the size and location of the defect, and patient's clinical status.

SUPERIOR SEMICIRCULAR CANAL DEHISCENCE

The phenomenon of SSCD was described in 1998 as sound- or pressure-induced vertigo in the setting of dehiscence of the bone separating the superior semicircular canal from the MCF.[14] Patients are usually of similar demographic to those with spontaneous CSF leaks, and some have hypothesized that these might be different presentations of the same pathology.[15] Although many patients have both hearing loss and vertigo, they may also present with only one of the findings.

Clinical Presentation of Superior Semicircular Canal Dehiscence
- Autophony
- Tullio phenomenon: eye movement induced by loud noises

- Hennebert sign: eye movements caused by pressure in the EAC
- Episodic vertigo: sound or pressure induced
- Conductive hearing loss
- Pulsatile tinnitus

Diagnosis of SSCD is usually not dependent on clinical examination because these results are inconsistent. Vestibular testing using cervical vestibular evoked myogenic potentials can demonstrate lower thresholds in patients with SSCD. This test is based on the vestibulospinal reflex, quantifying sternocleidomastoid activation from saccular stimulation. However, the cornerstone of diagnosis of this syndrome is the clinical picture in conjunction with oblique views on high-resolution temporal bone CT demonstrating dehiscence of the bone (Fig. 11).

Surgical Approaches

The MCF approach for repair of SSCD was first described by Minor and colleagues,[14] and it is associated with high rates of symptom resolution.[16] However, less invasive approaches have been developed to avoid the craniotomy and temporal lobe retraction required for the MCF approach. These include the transmastoid and the endoscopic-assisted transmastoid approaches.[17,18] The decision of the approach depends on the location and extent of the dehiscence and the height of the superior arcuate eminence if the anterior limb is involved.[19] Once exposed, the superior semicircular canal is then plugged with a combination of fascia and bone graft, and the skull base is resurfaced with bone cement or graft.

Take Home Pearls
- SSCD is a syndrome characterized by hearing loss and sound- and pressure-induced vertigo

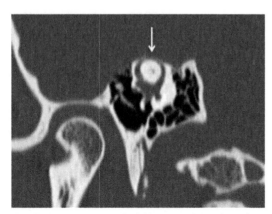

Fig. 11. Superior canal dehiscence (*arrow*) is best appreciated on oblique views on temporal bone CT.

in the setting of bony deficiency over the superior semicircular canal.
- Diagnosis depends primarily on clinical history in conjunction with radiologic findings on high-resolution temporal bone CT.
- Surgical approach is via MCF or transmastoid approach, depending on size and location of the dehiscence.

ACOUSTIC NEUROMA

Vestibular schwannomas are benign neoplasms generally arising from the vestibular divisions of cranial nerve VIII. Although some of these tumors, particularly those associated with neurofibromatosis 2, are aggressive and can grow quickly, most of these tumors are slow growing and some may not have clinically significant growth at all. For this reason, patient symptomatology and imaging findings of interval growth are important in the decision to intervene. Furthermore, intervention takes the form of either surgery or radiation therapy. A general overview of the decisions is discussed next, and a more complete treatment of this pathology is found elsewhere in this issue. (See Apoorva T. Ramaswamy and Justin S. Golub article, "Management of Vestibular Schwannomas for the Radiologist," in this issue.)

Surgical and Therapeutic Approaches

Because vestibular schwannomas are benign and slow-growing lesions, their therapeutic approach centers on functional preservation, particularly of hearing and the facial nerve, although other structures may be implicated. For many patients, the initial diagnosis is followed by an observation period to understand the growth trajectory of the neoplasm, if no factors necessitate immediate intervention. Although patients are being observed, they are usually monitored with serial MR imaging of the internal auditory canal with and without gadolinium contrast. These lesions tend to be isointense to hypointense to cerebral tissue on T1 and T2 series, and they enhance with contrast (Fig. 12). In some cases, they may also have a cystic component.

Decision to Observe in Vestibular Schwannoma
- Elderly or poor surgical candidate
- Patient with small tumor and excellent hearing
- Patient preference
- Tumor on the side of the only hearing ear

Once the decision to intervene has been made, the mode of surgical versus stereotactic radiation therapy must be determined. This decision is made based largely on patient preference,

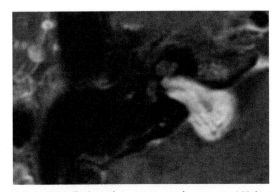

Fig. 12. Vestibular schwannoma enhances on MR imaging T1 with gadolinium.

although certain factors, such as size greater than 3 cm and the presence of obstructive hydrocephalus, necessitate surgical intervention.

Stereotactic Radiation Therapy
- Advantages
  - Decreased length of stay
  - Decreased cost
  - Lower periprocedural morbidity
- Contraindications
  - Active vestibular symptoms
  - Large tumors (>3 cm)
  - Absolute indications for surgical intervention Surgery
- Indications
  - Obstructive hydrocephalus (absolute)
  - Size >3 cm (relative indication)
  - Vestibular symptoms
  - Patient preference
- Contraindications
  - Poor surgical candidate

The surgical approach for vestibular schwannoma depends on size, location, and functions to be preserved, particularly hearing and the facial nerve. The three main approaches are the MCF, retrosigmoid, and translabyrinthine. The MCF and the retrosigmoid allow for hearing preservation, whereas the translabyrinthine approach necessitates obliteration of the cochlea and vestibular structures. Clinically, preoperative hearing status and vestibular testing may predict ability to preserve hearing with surgical intervention. Radiologically, tumor size and location are helpful in deciding on approach.

Radiologic Findings Favoring Hearing Preservation Surgery
- Medial IAC over lateral IAC enhancement
- Cuff of CSF lateral to enhancement within IAC on T2
- Tumor thought to originate from superior vestibular nerve

Take Home Pearls
- Vestibular schwannomas are slow growing lesions in which functional preservation is paramount when deciding on therapy.
- Observation with serial MR imaging screening is an option for elderly patients without indicators for immediate intervention.
- Size greater than 3 cm and obstructive hydrocephalus necessitate prompt surgical intervention.
- Stereotactic radiation therapy may be an option for patients with growing tumor who do not have brainstem compression.
- The decision to attempt hearing preservation surgery depends on clinical findings and radiologic information regarding tumor size and location.

VASCULAR MALFORMATIONS OF THE TEMPORAL BONE

The differential diagnosis of pulsatile tinnitus is an extensive one because multiple anomalies can result in this symptom. The types of pulsatile tinnitus are divided based on whether they are synchronous with arterial or venous pulsations. Table 1 provides an overview of the different causes of these types of pulsatile tinnitus. For the purposes of this review, the focus is glomus tumors and carotid diverticulum.

Glomus Tumors

Glomus tumors, or paragangliomas, are highly vascular and generally benign neoplasms derived from neural crest cells that can occur along multiple neurovascular structures. The subtypes that cause pulsatile tinnitus are those that occur in the temporal bone: glomus tympanicum and glomus jugulare. Some lesions, glomus jugulotympanicum, may involve both the jugular bulb and the tympanic cavity. Presentation varies based on the location and size of the tumor, although pulsatile tinnitus and conductive hearing loss are the primary reasons for presentation. A careful examination of the lower cranial nerves is important in these patients, because up to 10% may have silent neuropathies.[20] Although usually sporadic, 10% of these lesions are familial. The familial subtypes are often related to succinate dehydrogenase mutations that may require further work-up for pheochromocytoma.

Imaging is critical for work-up of these tumors, the primary examination being high-resolution CT of the temporal bone with contrast (Fig. 13). This examination allows visualization of the mass and any local bony erosion that may be caused by the lesion. If jugular foramen involvement is

Table 1
Differential diagnosis of pulsatile tinnitus

Arterial	Venous
1. Dural, skull base, and cervical region AVMs/AVFs	1. Idiopathic intracranial hypertension syndrome
2. Atherosclerotic carotid and subclavian artery disease	2. Jugular bulb abnormalities: high location, dehiscence, and diverticula
3. Glomus tumors of jugular foramen and middle ear	3. Transverse-sigmoid sinus stenosis and aneurysms
4. Tortuous internal carotid artery	4. Abnormal condylar and mastoid emissary veins
5. Dehiscence of the superior semicircular canal	5. Increased ICP associated with Arnold-Chiari syndrome and stenosis of the sylvian aqueduct
6. Fibromuscular dysplasia of the carotid artery	6. Idiopathic or essential tinnitus
7. Increased cardiac output (anemia, thrombocythemia, thyrotoxicosis, and pregnancy)	
8. Carotid artery dissection	
9. Brachiocephalic artery stenosis	
10. External carotid artery stenosis	
11. Vascular anomalies of the middle ear	
12. Aberrant artery in the stria vascularis	
13. Vascular compression of the eighth nerve	
14. Aortic murmurs	
15. Paget disease	
16. Otosclerosis	
17. Hypertension, antihypertensive agents	

Abbreviations: AVF, arteriovenous fistula; AVM, arteriovenous malformation; ICP, intracranial pressure.

From Sismanis A. Pulsatile tinnitus: contemporary assessment and management. Curr Opin Otolaryngol Head Neck Surg 2011;19:348–57.

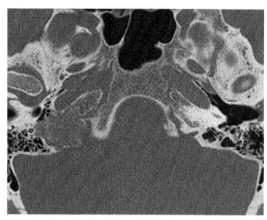

Fig. 13. Right glomus jugulares showing expansive mass within the jugular foramen and characteristic bony erosion. MR imaging would show characteristic "salt and pepper" appearance from the flow voids.

pharyngeal being the most characteristic feeding vessel. There are two well-established classification systems for these tumors based on location that are important for surgical planning. The Glasscock-Jackson and Fisch-Mattox scales are listed in **Box 1**. The Fisch-Mattox scale is preferred because of its clarity with regards to the involvement of the internal carotid artery (ICA), and it is largely based on CT imaging.[20]

Surgical treatment

Management of glomus tympanicum is surgical, and procedures are generally well tolerated. The approach is transcanal or transmastoid, depending on the extent of the tumor. Glomus jugulare are more complicated because of their proclivity to involve lower cranial nerves, particularly the vagus. Although young patients generally tolerate surgical intervention well, older patients often are not able to compensate for dysphagia because of a high vagal injury. In these situations, a serial imaging approach can guide need for intervention and radiotherapy may be a valuable option for patients with growing lesions.[20]

Internal Carotid Artery Diverticula

Although ICA diverticula in the middle ear are usually asymptomatic, they can present similarly to glomus tumors with pulsatile tinnitus and conductive hearing loss. On otoscopy, both also can present as red blanching masses behind the TM. However, anomalies of the ICA are rare, and therefore a high index of suspicion is necessary to prevent disastrous complications. Imaging work-up is similar to that of glomus tumors with high-resolution CT with the addition of MR angiography to further visualize vascular anatomy. It is thought

suspected either because of symptomatology or CT findings, MR imaging can allow for visualization of intracranial structures. Given its high vascularity, the lesion characteristically has a "salt-and-pepper" appearance on MR imaging because of flow voids. MR angiography can further delineate the feeding vessels that might be targets for preoperative embolization, with the ascending

Box 1
Classification of glomus tumors

Fisch-Mattox Classification System

A. Limited to middle ear cleft

B. Limited to tympanomastoid complex, no infralabyrinthine involvement

C. Involves labyrinthine compartment, extends to petrous apex

  1. Limited involvement of vertical portion of carotid canal

  2. Invades vertical portion of carotid canal

  3. Invades horizontal portion of carotid canal

D. Intracranial involvement

  1. Intracranial extension less than 2 cm

  2. Intracranial extension greater than 2 cm

Glasscock-Jackson Classification System

Glomus tympanicum

  I. Limited to the promontory

  II. Completely fills the middle ear space

  III. Fills the middle ear and extends to the mastoid

  IV. Extends into the external auditory canal, may extend anteriorly to the internal carotid artery

Glomus jugulare

  I. Involves jugular bulb, middle ear, and mastoid

  II. Extends underneath IAC, may have intracranial extension

  III. Extends into petrous apex, may have intracranial extension

  IV. Extends into clivus and infratemporal fossa, may have intracranial extension

that these vascular anomalies occur because of disturbances in embryologic vascular development, and they often cooccur with persistent fetal branches of the external carotid artery.

Surgical/Therapeutic Approaches

For patients in whom symptom burden is low, either asymptomatic or with pulsatile tinnitus, the conservative approach of minimal intervention with clinical follow-up is preferred. Intervention is required in patients with debilitating symptoms or with the potential to develop devastating neurovascular complications or destruction of adjacent

structures. In these situations, interventional angiography may provide benefits. Operative resurfacing of carotid dehiscence has been described but is fraught with serious consequences, such as intracranial ischemia. Acute hemorrhage may require packing of the middle ear cavity or ligation of the artery altogether.[21–26]

Take Home Pearls
- Pulsatile tinnitus has a broad differential, but it is broken down into venous or arterial subtypes.
- Glomus tumors are benign highly vascular lesions with variable involvement of the cranial nerves.
- The Fisch-Mattox grading scale for imaging findings of glomus tumors is important for treatment planning, particularly with respect to carotid involvement.
- ICA diverticula can present similarly to glomus tumors.
- ICA diverticula management is conservative, but knowledge of anatomy and coexisting abnormalities is crucial for control in context of emergencies.

CONCLUDING REMARKS

Anatomic understanding of the temporal bone is essential for appropriate diagnosis of otologic and neuro-otologic processes. The role of the ear organs as constituents of the lateral skull base is an important concept in understanding the interplay between otologic and neurosurgical pathologies. Often, lesions of the cerebellopontine angle or internal auditory canal may present with hearing loss, tinnitus, or imbalance, whereas complicated otologic processes may result in meningitis or dural sinus thrombosis. An understanding of the temporal bone and possible diagnoses and the relevant decision points in treatment are critical in the relationship between the radiologist and surgeon.

REFERENCES

1. Jackler RK, Schindler RA. Role of the mastoid in tympanic membrane reconstruction. Laryngoscope 1984;94(4):495–500.

2. McGrew BM, Jackson CJ, Glasscock ME. Impact of mastoidectomy on simple tympanic membrane perforation repair. Laryngoscope 2004;114(3):506–11.

3. Eliades SJ, Limb CJ. The role of mastoidectomy in outcomes following tympanic membrane repair: a review. Laryngoscope 2013;123(7):1787–802.

4. Cho YS, Lee HS, Kim SW, et al. Tuberculous otitis media: a clinical and radiologic analysis of 52 patients. Laryngoscope 2006;116(6):921–7.

5. Walshe P, Walsh RM, Brennan P, et al. The role of computerized tomography in the preoperative assessment of chronic suppurative otitis media. Clin Otolaryngol 2002;27(2):95–7.

6. Potsic WP, Korman SB, Samadi DS, et al. Congenital cholesteatoma: 20 years' experience at The Children's Hospital of Philadelphia. Otolaryngol Head Neck Surg 2002;126(4):409–15.

7. Jahrsdoerfer RA, Yeakley JW, Aguilar EA, et al. Grading system for the selection of patients with congenital aural atresia. Otol Neurotol 1992;13(1):6–12.

8. Rao N, Redleaf M. Spontaneous middle cranial fossa cerebrospinal fluid otorrhea in adults. Laryngoscope 2016;126:464–8.

9. Sanna M, Fois P, Russo A, et al. Management of meningoencephalic herniation of the temporal bone: personal experience and literature review. Laryngoscope 2009;119:1579–85.

10. Stucken EZ, Selesnick SH, Brown KD. The role of obesity in spontaneous temporal bone encephaloceles and CSF leak. Otol Neurotol 2012;33:1412–7.

11. Lobo BC, Baumanis MM, Nelson RF. Surgical repair of spontaneous cerebrospinal fluid (CSF) leaks: a systematic review. Laryngoscope Investig Otolaryngol 2017;2:215–24.

12. Stevens SM, Rizk HG, McIlwain WR, et al. Association between lateral skull base thickness and surgical outcomes in spontaneous CSF otorrhea. Otolaryngol Head Neck Surg 2016;154:707–14.

13. Reddy M, Baugnon K. Imaging of cerebrospinal fluid rhinorrhea and otorrhea. Radiol Clin North Am 2017;55:167–87.

14. Minor LB, Solomon D, Zinreich JS, et al. Sound- and/or pressure-induced vertigo due to bone dehiscence of the superior semicircular canal. Arch Otolaryngol Head Neck Surg 1998;124:249–58.

15. El Hadi T, Sorrentino T, Calmels MN, et al. Spontaneous tegmen defect and semicircular canal dehiscence: same etiopathogenic entity? Otol Neurotol 2012;33:591–5.

16. Nguyen T, Lagman C, Sheppard JP, et al. Middle cranial fossa approach for the repair of superior semicircular canal dehiscence is associated with greater symptom resolution compared to transmastoid approach. Acta Neurochir (Wien) 2018;160(6):1219–24.

17. Carter MS, Lookabaugh S, Lee DJ. Endoscopic-assisted repair of superior canal dehiscence syndrome. Laryngoscope 2014;124:1464–8.

18. Banakis Hartl RM, Cass SP. Effectiveness of transmastoid plugging for semicircular canal dehiscence syndrome. Otolaryngol Head Neck Surg 2018;158:534–40.

19. Lookabaugh S, Kelly HR, Carter MS, et al. Radiologic classification of superior canal dehiscence: implications for surgical repair. Otol Neurotol 2015;36:118–25.

20. Sanna M, editor. Microsurgery of skull base paragangliomas. New York: Thieme; 2013.

21. Brown K, Selesnick SH. Congenital disorders of the middle ear [Chapter 48]. In: Lalwani A, editor. Current diagnosis & treatment- otolaryngology head and neck surgery. New York: McGraw-Hill; 2012.

22. Ishman SL, Friedland DL. Temporal bone fractures: traditional classification and clinical relevance. Laryngoscope 2004;114:1734–41.

23. Dahiya T, Keller JD, Litofsky SN, et al. Temporal bone fractures: otic capsule sparing vs otic capsule violating clinical and radiographic considerations. J Trauma 1999;47:1079–83.

24. Brodie HA, Thompson TC. Management of complications from 820 temporal bone fractures. Am J Otol 1997;18:188–97.

25. Lambert PR, Brackmann DE. Facial paralysis in longitudinal temporal bone fractures: a review of 26 cases. Laryngoscope 1984;94:1022–6.

26. Quaranta A, Campobasso G, Piazza F, et al. Facial nerve paralysis in temporal bone fractures: outcomes after late decompression surgery. Acta Otolaryngol 2001;121:652–5.

Advanced MR Imaging of the Temporal Bone

Sachin Jambawalikar, PhD*, Michael Z. Liu, MS, Gul Moonis, MD

KEYWORDS

- Temporal bone MR imaging • 3D MR imaging • DWI of inner ear • Cholesteatoma

KEY POINTS

- For detailed anatomy of the internal auditory canal and inner ear, heavily T2-weighted fast MR imaging techniques such as 3-dimensional driven equilibrium fast spin echo or 3-dimensional coherent gradient echo play an important role.
- Advanced 3-dimensional flip angle optimized MR imaging of the temporal bone allows for high resolution 3-dimensional fluid-attenuated inversion recovery imaging with reduced artifacts.
- Advanced multishot nonechoplanar imaging and echoplanar imaging diffusion-weighted imaging techniques allow for higher resolution diffusion-weighted imaging acquisition in multiple orientations with minimal distortion.

Temporal bone pathologies are challenging to discern because of their small size and subtle contrast.[1] MR imaging is one of the key modalities in evaluating otologic diseases.[2] Current advancement in MR imaging techniques provide multiparametric information for evaluation of these pathologies. The aim of this article was to review state-of-the-art 3-dimensional (3D) morphologic and diffusion sequences for otologic MR imaging.

INTRODUCTION

MR imaging has been a key modality in evaluation of otologic complaints[2–4] over the past decade. Over this time, there has been vast advances in MR imaging technology, including multichannel coil arrays, advanced shimming techniques, gradient linearity corrections, and improvements in sequence development. The standard of care sequences used for MR temporal bone imaging include heavily T2 weighted 3D images, high-resolution 3D fluid-attenuated inversion recovery (FLAIR) images and diffusion-weighted imaging (DWI). In this article, we discuss different vendor MR imaging terminology and sequences behind these 3 main techniques used for otologic imaging. Table 1 provides vendor specific names for these sequences for the 3 major MR vendors.

MR IMAGING ADVANCED 3-DIMENSIONAL IMAGING

MR imaging produces unparalleled image contrast for soft tissues imaging. In an attempt to improve the spatial resolution to detect minute pathologies in the temporal bone, a lot of work has been done over the years to develop high resolution 3D sequences. High-resolution fast spin echo (FSE) and gradient echo sequences are widely used as an alternative or adjunct to T1 postcontrast images in temporal bone imaging.[5]

Heavily T2-Weighted 3-Dimensional Sequences

To demonstrate the detailed anatomy of the internal auditory canal and inner ear, high-resolution MR imaging sequences using heavily T2-weighted 3D

Disclosure Statement: No disclosures.
Department of Radiology, Columbia University Medical Center, 622 West 168th Street, Presbyterian Building, FL01, Room/Suite 0331, New York, NY 10032, USA
* Corresponding author.
E-mail address: sj2532@cumc.columbia.edu

Neuroimag Clin N Am 29 (2019) 197–202
https://doi.org/10.1016/j.nic.2018.09.009
1052-5149/19/© 2018 Elsevier Inc. All rights reserved.

Table 1
Terminology for Inner ear imaging sequences from 3 major vendors

Sequence Name	GE	Siemens	Philips
3D GRE	3D FIESTA + C	3D CISS	3D b-SSFP
3D heavily T2-weighted FSE	FRFSE	RESTORE	DRIVE
3D variable flip angle FLAIR	Cube FLAIR	SPACE FLAIR	FLAIR VISTA
DWI EPI	MUSE	RESOLVE	Multishot EPI
DWI 2D FSE	PROPELLER	BLADE and HASTE	MULTI-VANE
Small FOV DWI EPI	FOCUS	ZOOMit	Zoom Diffusion

Abbreviations: 2D, 2-dimensional; 3D, 3-dimensional; DWI, diffusion-weighted imaging; EPI, echoplanar imaging; FLAIR, fluid-attenuated inversion recovery; FOV, field of view; FRFSE, fast recovery fast spin echo; FSE, fast spin echo; GRE, gradient echo; MUSE, multiplexed sensitivity-encoding; PROPELLER, periodically rotated overlapping parallel lines with enhanced reconstruction.

fast imaging techniques play an important role in the evaluation of various diseases of the temporal bone. Two basic techniques are widely used to provide high spatial resolution MR imaging of the temporal bone with a cisternographic effect: 3D gradient echo–based techniques and 3D FSE-based techniques.

Three-dimensional coherent gradient echo-based sequences

Steady-state free precession (SSFP) sequences (FIESTA or trueFISP or balanced SSFP) are a group of gradient echo sequences in which a steady state develops between pulse repetitions for both the longitudinal and transverse relaxation values. These sequences are acquired with the shortest possible repetition time and echo time to minimize susceptibility effects and optimize scan efficiency. SSFP provides high signal in tissues with high T2/T1 ratios, such as cerebrospinal fluid and fat, and enables submillimeter spatial resolution, allowing isotropic 3D acquisitions, which can be used for multiplanar reconstructions. A pulse sequence diagram for 3D balanced SSFP is shown in **Fig. 1**. Even with a short TR and echo time, the balanced SSFP sequence will produce dark bands (banding artifacts), as shown in **Fig. 2**, owing to magnetic field inhomogeneities and distortions introduced by the patient.[6] A modification of the SSFP sequence (FIESTA-C/CISS)[7,8] with 2 acquisitions with and without radiofrequency phase alternation is generally acquired to mitigate these artifacts. The scanner combines the paired data with maximum intensity value for each voxel, thereby producing an artifact free image. This makes FIESTA-C/CISS a mainstay in the evaluation of the cerebellopontine angles and inner ear imaging. It allows for the accurate detection of small masses such as schwannomas and detailed evaluation of

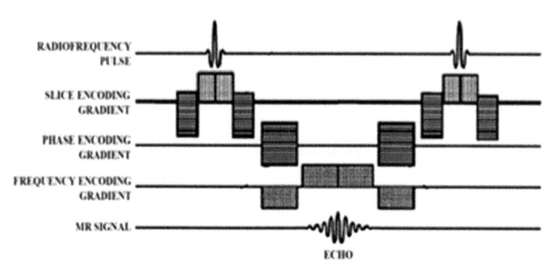

Fig. 1. Pulse timing diagram of 3-dimensional balanced steady-state free precession MR imaging sequence.

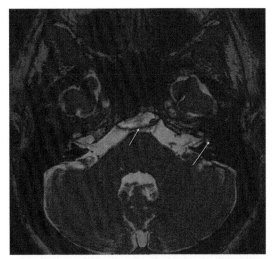

Fig. 2. Axial 3-dimensional balanced steady-state free precession heavily T2-weighted image with banding artifact in the inner ear and prepontine cistern (*white arrows*).

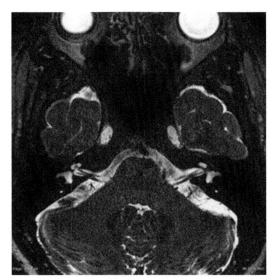

Fig. 3. Axial 3-dimensional driven equilibrium turbo spin echo heavily T2-weighted image though the inner ear.

the small structures such as the internal auditory canals and the labyrinth of the inner ear.

Three-dimensional fast spin echo–based sequences

Driven equilibrium (DRIVE, Philips Healthcare, Andover, MA), fast recovery fast spin echo (GE Healthcare, Chicago, IL) or (RESTORE, Siemens Healthcare, Erlangen, Germany) are FSE or turbo spin echo–based heavily T2-weighted sequences that are routinely used for temporal bone imaging. These sequences apply a set of additional −90° recovery pulses at the end of the echo train to accelerate recovery of the remaining transverse magnetization back to the longitudinal axis.[5,9] The 3D DRIVE-based sequences (**Fig. 3**) generally have less susceptibility artifacts compared with 3D balanced SSFP sequences.[10]

Three-Dimensional Fluid-Attenuated Inversion Recovery Sequences in the Inner Ear

In addition, 3D imaging can be obtained using special FSE techniques, such as sampling perfection with application optimized contrasts using variable flip angle (VFA) evolutions (SPACE; Siemens Healthcare), volumetric isotropic turbo spin echo acquisition (VISTA; Philips Healthcare) or 3D FSE Cube (GE Healthcare). These are classified as high-resolution isotropic 3D sequences. VFA refocusing radiofrequency pulses provide increased signal in gray and white matter tissues compared with fixed refocusing pulses. Additionally, these VFA pulses suppress blurring in the substantially longer echo train length acquisition required for

high-resolution, submillimeter isotropic imaging in the temporal bone. These are mostly used in inner ear imaging for FLAIR contrast rather than T2 contrast, because the VFA will produce a higher brain tissue signal compared with the cisternographic contrast produced in heavily T2-weighted 3D sequences discussed in the preceding segment. VFA-based 3D-FLAIR sequences produce high-resolution 3D images with a suppressed fluid signal. The 3D-FLAIR sequence allows separate visualization of endolymphatic and perilymphatic components and has become a new diagnostic tool for the visualization of endolymphatic hydrops in Menière disease. Both gadolinium-enhanced 3D FLAIR[11,12] and nonenhanced 3D FLAIR[12,13] imaging have been shown to be useful in detecting inner ear pathology. The 3D FLAIR VISTA images are able to reveal labyrinthine hemorrhage as a cause of sudden sensorineural hearing loss.[13] The cochlear signal on 3D FLAIR images has been suggested to be an additional parameter to use when monitoring the degree of functional impairment in patients with vestibular schwannomas (**Fig. 4**).[14]

Diffusion-Weighted Imaging for Cholesteatoma Detection

DWI reflects the microanatomy of tissues based on the molecular diffusion of protons corresponding to the Brownian motion. In DWI, the signal is obtained by applying a pair of opposing magnetic field gradients along a defined diffusion direction. If a particular tissue has high diffusion, the opposing gradients will cause signal attenuation

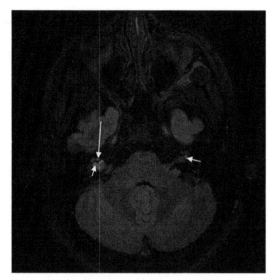

Fig. 4. Axial 3-dimensional volumetric isotropic turbo spin echo acquisition fluid-attenuated inversion recovery sequence in a patient with bilateral vestibular schwannomas (*white arrows*) demonstrates increased signal in the bilateral distal internal auditory canals and right cochlear basilar turn.

and produce low signal in a diffusion-weighted image. The apparent diffusion coefficient estimates the mobility of protons moving within tissue. The apparent diffusion coefficient is limited in dense hypercellular tissues such as tumor and increased in edema, inflammation, and fibrosis with low cellularity. DWI has become an essential complementary sequence to standard MR imaging sequences. A variety of different DWI techniques are used, which are divided into echoplanar imaging (EPI)-based and non–EPI-based techniques.

Echoplanar imaging sequences
Single-shot (SS) EPI-DWI is a widely available standard DWI technique and is used as a fast diagnostic method and additional valuable tool in workup of suspected cholesteatoma.[15] It is relatively insensitive to motion, but prone to susceptibility artifacts, chemical shift, and geometric distortion, and has a limited spatial resolution and relatively thick sections. To decrease susceptibility and distortion artifacts, multishot or segmented EPI approaches are becoming popular. In addition, segmented/multishot EPI can acquire images at higher spatial resolution than SS methods. REadout Segmentation Of Long Variable Echo trains (RESOLVE) DWI[16,17] is a new segmented EPI DWI technique that delivers sharp, high-quality images at high spatial resolution and reduced slice thickness. Besides higher spatial resolution, RESOLVE DWI is capable of producing

distortion-free coronal images in the evaluation of cholesteatoma.[18] It uses the same diffusion preparation as SS EPI. By dividing the k-space trajectory into multiple segments in the frequency encoding direction, the echo time can be decreased to increase the quality of the acquired images. Furthermore, RESOLVE DWI is largely free of distortion, susceptibility, and T2* blurring artifacts. Multishot techniques, however, are susceptible to motion-induced phase errors. RESOLVE uses navigator echoes to correct these errors at the expense of additional scan time. A novel multishot DWI technique, termed multiplexed sensitivity encoding, provides robust high-resolution diffusion-weighted MR imaging without the use of navigators for correction of motion induced phase errors.[19] Reduced field of view (FOV) diffusion techniques with EPI readout using 2-dimensional excitation pulses allow for small FOV diffusion with s shorter echo time and s higher spatial resolution. FOCUS DWI[20] (GE Healthcare) and ZOOMit[21] (Siemens Healthcare) are 2 reduced FOV DWI techniques available for small FOV in organs such as the prostate, pancreas, and inner ear to produce high-resolution, reduced distortion DWI images.

Nonechoplanar imaging sequences
Standard EPI DWI may be significantly limited by artifacts from the skull base. Turbo spin echo–based DWI is a spin echo–based SS or multishot technique with a longer echo time and a higher signal-to-noise ratio than SS EPI-DWI. Non–EPI sequences[22] are capable of being acquired at greater spatial resolution and additionally do not exhibit the susceptibility artifacts that are observed with standard EPI-DWI. Furthermore, thinner slices can be obtained than with EPI sequences. The SS version of turbo spin echo-DWI is a diffusion-weighted half-Fourier acquisition single-shot turbo spin echo imaging sequence with excellent motion insensitivity and less sensitivity to susceptibility artifacts and geometric distortion than the EPI sequence shown in **Fig. 5**. A non-EPI multishot DWI sequence called periodically rotated overlapping parallel lines with enhanced reconstruction (GE Healthcare) has been reported as useful in avoiding geometric distortion and accurate in assessing location extent and size as well as foci of cholesteatoma.[18,23] Similar DWI sequences BLADE (Siemens Healthcare) and MultiVane (Philips Healthcare) are also provided by other vendors. The k-space data are acquired in the form of rotating sections (blades). The resulting oversampling of the central k-space leads to an improved signal-to-noise ratio (SNR) and to the reduction

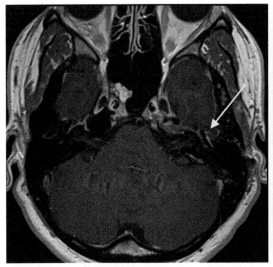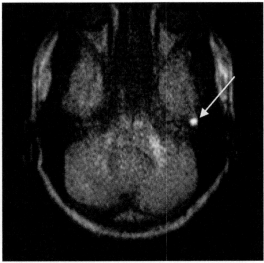

Fig. 5. Axial T1 postcontrast and axial half-Fourier acquisition single-shot turbo spin echo imaging diffusion-weighted imaging sequence demonstrate a peripherally enhancing lesion in the left anterior epitympanum with restricted diffusion compatible with cholesteatoma.

of motion and susceptibility artifacts. This allows for distortion free multishot DWI acquisitions in the coronal plane[24] as shown in **Fig. 6**. Slice thickness for the DWI (and its corresponding anatomic T1w or T2w) should not exceed 3 mm. Cholesteatoma appears hyperintense on DWI obtained with b-factors of 800 or 1000 s/mm^2; this is similar to a histologically identical lesion, the epidermoid cyst. Non-EPI DWI have been shown to accurately predict residual and/or recurrent cholesteatomas after primary cholesteatoma surgery.[25] DWI may also replace delayed gadolinium-enhanced T1w sequences. Images from non-EPI sequences or newer EPI techniques such as RESOLVE can even be fused with anatomic images (T1w and T2w) in coronal and/or axial orientation to better localize suspected lesions.

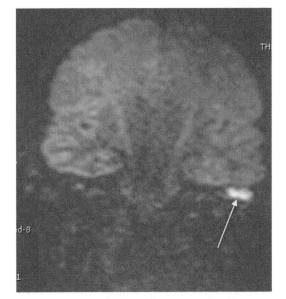

Fig. 6. Coronal multishot diffusion-weighted imaging sequence demonstrates a cholesteatoma (*white arrow*) in the left mastoid air cells.

REFERENCES

1. Schulze M, Reimann K, Seeger A, et al. Improvement in imaging common temporal bone pathologies at 3 T MRI: small structures benefit from a small field of view. Clin Radiol 2017;72(3):267. e1–12.
2. Lingam RK, Connor SEJ, Casselman JW, et al. MRI in otology: applications in cholesteatoma and Ménière's disease. Clin Radiol 2018;73(1):35–44.
3. Forgues M, Mehta R, Anderson D, et al. Non-contrast magnetic resonance imaging for monitoring patients with acoustic neuroma. J Laryngol Otol 2018;1–6. https://doi.org/10.1017/S0022215118001342.
4. Phelps PD, Lloyd GAS. Diagnostic imaging of the ear. Springer-Verlag London; 2012.
5. Schmalbrock P. Comparison of three-dimensional fast spin echo and gradient echo sequences for high-resolution temporal bone imaging. J Magn Reson Imaging 2000;12(6):814–25.
6. Casselman JW, Kuhweide R, Deimling M, et al. Constructive interference in steady state-3DFT MR imaging of the inner ear and cerebellopontine angle. AJNR Am J Neuroradiol 1993;14(1):47–57.

7. Widmann G, Henninger B, Kremser C, et al. MRI sequences in head & neck radiology – state of the art. Rofo 2017;189(05):413–22.

8. Dai YL, King AD. State of the art MRI in head and neck cancer. Clin Radiol 2018;73(1):45–59.

9. Naganawa S, Koshikawa T, Fukatsu H, et al. MR cisternography of the cerebellopontine angle: comparison of three-dimensional fast asymmetrical spin-echo and three-dimensional constructive interference in the steady-state sequences. AJNR Am J Neuroradiol 2001;22(6):1179–85.

10. Byun JS, Kim HJ, Yim YJ, et al. MR imaging of the internal auditory canal and inner ear at 3T: comparison between 3D driven equilibrium and 3D balanced fast field echo sequences. Korean J Radiol 2008;9(3):212–8.

11. Hida K, Takano K, Yoshimitsu K, et al. Inner ear enhancement on gadolinium-enhanced 3D FLAIR images in a patient with Vogt–Koyanagi–Harada disease. BJR Case Rep 2017;3(1):20160090.

12. Berrettini S, Seccia V, Fortunato S, et al. Analysis of the 3-dimensional fluid-attenuated inversion-recovery (3D-FLAIR) sequence in idiopathic sudden sensorineural hearing loss. JAMA Otolaryngol Head Neck Surg 2013;139(5):456–64.

13. Kim DS, Park DW, Kim TY, et al. Characteristic MR findings suggesting presumed labyrinthine hemorrhage. Acta Otolaryngol 2017;137(12):1226–32.

14. Reimer P, Parizel PM, Stichnoth F-A. Clinical MR imaging: a practical approach. Springer-Verlag Berlin Heidelberg; 2012.

15. Fitzek C, Mewes T, Fitzek S, et al. Diffusion-weighted MRI of cholesteatomas of the petrous bone. J Magn Reson Imaging 2002;15(6):636–41.

16. Porter DA, Heidemann RM. High resolution diffusion-weighted imaging using readout-segmented echo-planar imaging, parallel imaging and a two-dimensional navigator-based reacquisition. Magn Reson Med 2009;62(2):468–75.

17. Wan H, Sha Y, Zhang F, et al. Diffusion-weighted imaging using readout-segmented echo-planar imaging, parallel imaging, and two-dimensional navigator-based reacquisition in detecting acute optic neuritis. J Magn Reson Imaging 2015;43(3):655–60.

18. Karandikar A, Loke SC, Goh J, et al. Evaluation of cholesteatoma: our experience with DW propeller imaging. Acta Radiol 2015;56(9):1108–12.

19. Chen N-K, Guidon A, Chang H-C, et al. A robust multi-shot scan strategy for high-resolution diffusion weighted MRI enabled by multiplexed sensitivity-encoding (MUSE). Neuroimage 2013;72:41–7.

20. Banerjee S, Nishimura DG, Shankaranarayanan A, et al. Reduced field-of-view DWI with robust fat suppression and unrestricted slice coverage using tilted 2DRF excitation. Magn Reson Med 2016;76(6):1668–76.

21. Liney GP, Holloway L, Al Harthi TM, et al. Quantitative evaluation of diffusion-weighted imaging techniques for the purposes of radiotherapy planning in the prostate. Br J Radiol 2015;88(1049):20150034.

22. Migirov L, Wolf M, Greenberg G, et al. Non-EPI DW MRI in planning the surgical approach to primary and recurrent cholesteatoma. Otol Neurotol 2014;35(1):121–5.

23. Suzuki H, Sone M, Yoshida T, et al. Numerical assessment of cholesteatoma by signal intensity on non-EP-DWI and ADC maps. Otol Neurotol 2014;35(6):1007–10.

24. Schwartz KM, Lane JI, Bolster BD Jr, et al. The utility of diffusion-weighted imaging for cholesteatoma evaluation. AJNR Am J Neuroradiol 2011;32(3):430–6.

25. Dremmen MHG, Hofman PAM, Hof JR, et al. The diagnostic accuracy of non-echo-planar diffusion-weighted imaging in the detection of residual and/or recurrent cholesteatoma of the temporal bone. AJNR Am J Neuroradiol 2012;33(3):439–44.

Moving?

Make sure your subscription moves with you!

To notify us of your new address, find your **Clinics Account Number** (located on your mailing label above your name), and contact customer service at:

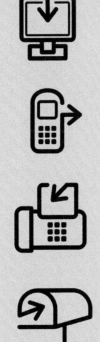

Email: journalscustomerservice-usa@elsevier.com

800-654-2452 (subscribers in the U.S. & Canada)
314-447-8871 (subscribers outside of the U.S. & Canada)

Fax number: 314-447-8029

Elsevier Health Sciences Division
Subscription Customer Service
3251 Riverport Lane
Maryland Heights, MO 63043

*To ensure uninterrupted delivery of your subscription, please notify us at least 4 weeks in advance of move.

Printed and bound by CPI Group (UK) Ltd, Croydon, CR0 4YY

03/10/2024

01040306-0004